WOMAN'S DAY
BOOK OF
FAMILY MEDICAL
QUESTIONS

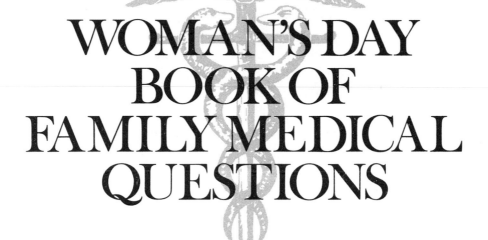

WOMAN'S DAY
BOOK OF
FAMILY MEDICAL
QUESTIONS

JOHN G. DEATON, M.D.
ELIZABETH JEAN PASCOE

Medical Editor: Philip R. Alper, M.D.

A Woman's Day/Random House Book
New York

Library of Congress Cataloging in Publication Data

Deaton, John G 1939–
Woman's Day book of family medical questions.

Bibliography: p.
Includes index.
1. Medicine, Popular—Miscellanea. I. Pascoe,
Elizabeth Jean, joint author. II. Alper, Philip R.
III. Title.
RC81. D29   616'.024   79–4804
ISBN 0–394–41468–3

Manufactured in the United States of America

24689753

FIRST EDITION

To Lilian B. Fine

Acknowledgments

W. Gerald Rainer, M.D., William E. Smith, M.D., and Karen Teel, M.D., helped with the early parts of the manuscript. Jack W. Moncrief, M.D., Harold Skaggs, M.D., and Dennis Welch, M.D., supplied information about nephrology, neurology and hematology, respectively. James E. Burris, M.D., reviewed the section on the eyes; Stanley L. Harrison, M.D., on pediatrics; and Thomas G. Glass, Jr., M.D., on snakebite. Diana Camacho, R.D., and Kathryn Lloyd, R.N., W.H.C.S., of the Model Cities Clinic in Austin, helped with the nutritional and women's health care sections of the book. Charlotte Mayerson, our editor at Random House, and Dina Von Zweck, director of trade publishing of CBS Publications, made invaluable contributions to the editing, direction and content of the book.

Contents

Introduction

The editors of *Woman's Day* and of Random House conceived this book to answer the medical questions most families encounter. It covers those of major consequence as well as the less serious health problems that arise in daily life.

The book will help you to make intelligent decisions about what doctor to consult and, after you've been to the physician's office, to understand and evaluate what he or she has told you. It first describes the part of the body involved, its function and what can go wrong with it, and then explains what kind of examination and treatment you can expect, the possible complications, the side effects of medication and the chances of recovery.

What is the illness? What is the treatment? Whom should I consult? The book goes to the heart of these questions in language that is clear, direct and to the point. It takes into account the latest medical information available and yet it is conservative, down-to-earth and well grounded in the medical practice and experience of the authors and the medical consultants.

Turn to the chapter on the subject that concerns you—sick babies and children, the brain and nerves, emergencies, skin care or whatever else—read the entries that explain what you need to know, consult the index and cross references for related information. Convenient, reliable and comprehensive, this book will become an important part of your family health care.

THE EDITORS

WOMAN'S DAY
BOOK OF
FAMILY MEDICAL
QUESTIONS

1

GETTING
(or Not Getting)
PREGNANT

How does pregnancy occur?   It occurs when a sperm from the man fertilizes a woman's egg. The latter is released at ovulation, enters the fallopian tube and passes slowly toward the womb. It will die if it isn't fertilized within twenty-four hours in the outer third of the tube. The fertilized egg continues its journey to the womb and implants there six days after fertilization. It grows into an embryo, then a fetus, then a baby.

At what age can a woman become pregnant?   It's possible to become pregnant as soon as the menstrual cycles begin, or at an average age of twelve to thirteen. A sexually active individual may become pregnant before having a menstrual period—the very first egg is fertilized. Pregnancies under the age of twelve are unusual, but have occurred.

To what age does fertility last?   Until the menopause, the cessation of menstrual cycles. Pregnancy after the age of fifty is rare, but an instance of a woman giving birth at the age of fifty-seven is on record, and a medical doctor has reported delivering the baby of a sixty-three-year-old woman.

When does fertility begin in a man?   It commences with the onset of the ability to ejaculate, which coincides with puberty. The customary age for this is twelve to fifteen, but ejaculation may begin as early as age eight or nine.

3

To what age does male fertility last? Men in their eighties have fathered children. Unlike women, men do not have cycles of fertility, though more work remains to be done on whether there is in fact any variability in male fertility.

Does ejaculation have to take place in the vagina for a woman to become pregnant? No, ejaculation on the lips of the vagina may cause pregnancy. Sperm are remarkably motile and can swim easily and rapidly across moist surfaces. Ejaculation onto an object, such as a finger, that is later placed on or in the woman's genitals may also cause pregnancy.

When in the monthly cycle can you actually get pregnant? It varies from woman to woman and month to month, and pregnancies have occurred after intercourse near the first or toward the end of the monthly cycle. Peak fertility for most women occurs fourteen days before the next menstrual period when ovulation takes place, that is, when one ovary releases an egg. The egg is capable of being fertilized until it's twenty-four hours old. Since sperm can live for two or three days in the fallopian tubes, intercourse occurring three days before or up to one day after ovulation can cause a pregnancy.

How can you tell when you're at your peak of fertility? By keeping a temperature chart. Take your oral temperature every morning after waking and before getting out of bed. An ovulation thermometer will enable you to read even a small change in temperature: it registers only between 95 and 100 degrees, and is calibrated at each tenth of a degree. Shake the thermometer down the night before, and don't sit up, eat or do anything else before putting it under your tongue. After three minutes remove the thermometer and record the temperature. On the day that you ovulate, you'll note a rise in temperature of 0.4 degree to 1 degree F., and the higher reading will persist throughout the remainder of the cycle. The first day of higher temperature coincides with your peak of fertility. Body temperature does fluctuate a bit from day to day, and in some months the ovulatory rise may be hard to pinpoint. For best accuracy, keep a chart of your temperature for three months if you need to establish your time of ovulation.

Are there any easier ways of predicting when ovulation occurs? At the time of ovulation, a fourth of women have pain in one side of the lower abdomen. It varies from dull to sharp, and may last several hours. The pain, called *Mittelschmerz* (the German word for "middle pain"), is due to irritation caused by slight bleeding from the ovary that released the egg. The woman who has mittelschmerz may recognize it for what it is. Curiously, the pain doesn't necessarily alternate from one side to the next in successive months. This is because the ovaries don't necessarily take turns in releasing eggs. Ovulation may occur from the same ovary several months in a row.

The calendar method is useful if your periods occur regularly. Keep a record of the first day of bleeding each month for three months. Then average the interval between periods. Using the average number of days between periods (such as twenty-eight days), you can predict when your next menstrual period will begin. Fourteen days before that date is your approximate date of ovulation. Still another way of predicting ovulation is to use the cervical-mucus test that will be discussed later.

What if your periods don't occur regularly? The more irregular you are, the less likely it is that you're ovulating with every period. Anovulatory cycles occur most frequently in teenagers and in women beyond the age of thirty-five or forty. For these persons, predicting the time of ovulation may not be possible.

BIRTH-CONTROL METHODS

What birth-control method is most reliable? The Pill. Taken correctly, it is well over 99 percent effective in preventing pregnancy. The only methods that are more reliable are the sterilization operations: tubal ligation for a woman or vasectomy for a man, both of which are virtually 100 percent effective in preventing pregnancy, although in the case of vasectomy there is a waiting period before the risk of pregnancy is over.

What are some other effective means of birth control? The intrauterine device (IUD), the diaphragm with spermicidal jelly, the condom, spermicidal foam and the new vaginal inserts. The IUD gives 97 to 99 percent protection against pregnancy. The diaphragm and jelly, the condom and spermicidal foam each give 97 percent protection when used correctly and consistently. The actual effectiveness when large numbers of couples are surveyed is somewhat lower, but the main reasons for failure are forgetting to use the method or not using it properly. As to the vaginal inserts, they are too new for conclusive figures to be available on their effectiveness.

How good are the other methods of birth control? Worldwide, the rhythm method may be the most commonly used means of birth control. At best, it gives a success rate of 87 percent in protecting against pregnancy. That is, 13 out of 100 women who use the method correctly and consistently will become pregnant during a year's time. Coitus interruptus (the withdrawal of the penis before ejaculation) can provide about 91 percent protection from pregnancy. In large surveys, couples report its effectiveness to be only 75 to 80 percent.

Which methods are least effective?   Taking a douche is not very effective. The douche doesn't remove all the sperm, and the stream of water may wash some of them into the womb. About 40 out of 100 women who use this method alone will become pregnant during a year's time. Breast-feeding (and the consequent suppression of menstrual periods) also tends to be ineffective as a means of birth control. Forty percent of women who rely on it will become pregnant during a year's time.

Among the methods that don't work but are often thought by the uninformed to be effective are the woman's failure to have an orgasm and the use of a vaginal-hygiene product, such as Norforms, before intercourse. Failure to climax in no way prevents a woman from becoming pregnant, and products such as Norforms were not intended for use in birth control.

THE PILL

When did the Pill become available for general use?   In 1960.

How does the Pill work?   It contains synthetic substitutes for estrogen and progesterone, the hormones produced by the ovaries during the menstrual cycle. When a woman takes the Pill, the synthetic hormones enter her bloodstream, affecting the body's glandular balance, and cause her ovaries to stop making hormones or releasing eggs. This cessation of ovulation is generally thought to be the way the Pill works, though other mechanisms may also be in effect. The progesterone component of the Pill alters the lining of the uterus and cervix in a way that helps to prevent pregnancy, and the Pill may disturb sperm and egg movement within the fallopian tube.

How dangerous is the Pill?   An increase in the tendency to have blood clots was the first serious side effect found to be caused by the Pill. The risk of death from a blood clot is about seven to eight times greater in Pill users than in nonusers. High blood pressure is three times more common among women who use the Pill. All else being equal, the woman who takes an oral contraceptive (another name for the Pill) is more likely to have a heart attack than is a woman who doesn't use the Pill. Among smokers, the person who takes the Pill is five times more likely to have a heart attack than would be the case if she were not taking it. The heart-attack risk is even higher for women over thirty-five or forty who smoke more than a pack a day. The current recommendation is that a woman over forty shouldn't take the Pill; a person between thirty and thirty-nine may take it if she doesn't smoke or have other risk factors for heart disease, or if she is taking the Pill, she stops smoking and seeks treatment for such conditions as high blood pressure and elevated cholesterol.

6

Still another side effect of the Pill is the possibility that it will cause a benign liver tumor. This complication is rare, and doesn't usually occur unless the individual has taken the Pill for at least two to five years. The risk of gall bladder disease and jaundice is also higher among Pill users. We have no hard evidence that the Pill causes cancer, but the Food and Drug Administration warns doctors to keep an eye out for breast lumps and uterine bleeding in women taking oral contraceptives. "Sequential" oral contraceptives have been taken off the market because of evidence that they may cause endometrial cancer.

Though these side effects are alarming, most are relatively rare. And, since pregnancy itself poses a threat to health, a woman may feel justified in accepting some risk from the Pill.

Which women should not take the Pill? Women over the age of forty, women who smoke or have high blood pressure or an elevation of scrum cholesterol, and women with a history of blood clots, stroke or heart disease. The woman with cancer of the breast or reproductive organs should not take the Pill. Nor should the individual with liver disease, gall bladder disease or sickle cell anemia. The woman who suffers from depression, migraine, diabetes, varicose veins or fibroid tumors of the uterus should take the Pill only under special circumstances and under close medical supervision.

Although the link between possible birth defects and the Pill is not yet established, the FDA warns that a woman should stop taking it three months before she tries to get pregnant and not start it again until after she has delivered her baby. She should also stop the Pill at least four weeks before undergoing surgery because of the risk of blood clots.

Is it safe for an epileptic to take the Pill? It depends on the type and severity of the epilepsy. Taking the Pill may cause additional seizures around the time of the menstrual period, but some epileptic women who use it report no increase in their number of seizures.

What are the warning signs that the Pill isn't safe for you? The danger signals are:
 · Severe or blinding headaches, nosebleeds or ringing in the ears, which may signal high blood pressure or an impending stroke.
 · Blurred vision, flashing lights, blindness or dizziness, again indicating high blood pressure or an impending stroke.
 · Severe pain or swelling in the calf or thigh, in the absence of injury, may signal a blood clot in the leg.
 · Chest pain or shortness of breath, pointing to a possible blood clot in the lungs or a heart attack. The pain may strike in the rib areas or in the front or back of the chest.

7

· Pain in the abdomen, swelling beneath the right rib cage, or jaundice, which may be signs of gall bladder disease or a benign liver tumor.

Should you experience any of these symptoms, stop the Pill and see your doctor immediately.

What are the most common side effects of the Pill?   About 40 percent of women who use the Pill have nausea, weight gain or headaches. Fatigue and breast soreness may occur. Spotting between the periods is probably the most troublesome minor side effect of the Pill. This can usually be controlled by raising the content of estrogen in the Pill, but the spotting may naturally stop after two or three cycles when the body has adjusted to the Pill.

Which Pill is best?   Current evidence indicates that the lower the estrogen content of the Pill, the safer it is to use. The original birth-control pills contained three times the amount of estrogen that was necessary to prevent ovulation. A Pill containing fifty micrograms or less of estrogen is just as effective. Some authorities favor a Pill with thirty or thirty-five micrograms of estrogen (it also contains progesterone). In China only two kinds of pills are available; both contain thirty-five micrograms of estrogen, have been in use there since 1968 and seem to suit the Chinese.

Is the sequential Pill better than the combination Pill?   No. The sequential Pill contains estrogen for only the first fourteen to sixteen days of the cycle, then estrogen and progesterone for the last five to seven days of hormone stimulation. The combination Pill contains both hormones throughout the cycle. The pregnancy risk is at least 1 percent greater with the sequential than with the combination Pill.

Acting on orders of the FDA, drug manufacturers stopped the sale of sequential contraceptives in 1975. The reason was the probable relationship between taking sequential pills and developing endometrial carcinoma.

How do you obtain the Pill?   It must be prescribed by a doctor, preferably a specialist in obstetrics and gynecology. The physician will (or should) examine you, discuss with you the various forms of birth control and prescribe an oral contraceptive. That's only the beginning. The woman taking the Pill should report any problems to her physician, and she should be seen by the physician and examined completely at least twice during the first year on the Pill and then once a year thereafter.

What questions should you ask the doctor about the Pill?   Don't hesitate to ask for a Pill with fifty micrograms or less of estrogen. If you're bothered by spotting between periods, you may have to take a Pill with a higher dose

8

of estrogen, but you won't know until you try the low-dose form. The progesterone content of the Pill is also important. Progesterone may cause oily skin or the growth of hair. Thus, if you have a problem with acne or body or facial hair, you need a Pill with a low dose or a different kind of progesterone. The comparative cost of the various oral contraceptives is yet another thing to inquire about. Most doctors have on hand a goodly supply of samples given to them by drug salesmen. Ask if you can have several free packets of the Pill you'll be taking. That way, you haven't spent anything for pills if the first brand causes problems. The physician who refuses to discuss the type you need, or who tells you that all pills are alike, is the wrong doctor to prescribe the Pill.

How do you take the Pill?   Follow the directions according to the type of Pill. Some come in twenty-one-day packs, others in twenty-eight-day packs. With the first type, you start on the first Sunday after your period or the fifth day after your period began and take them daily for twenty-one days; then, after a week you begin a new pack. With the twenty-eight-day pack, you start on the first Sunday after your period and take them for twenty-eight days, and then start a new pack immediately.

It's best to use another method of birth control, such as the diaphragm and jelly, during your first month on the Pill. You may not be fully protected until your second month of being on the Pill.

What do you do when you miss a Pill?   Associate taking the Pill with a regular activity, such as your morning toilet, and maybe you won't forget. If you miss one, take it as soon as you remember, and go ahead with the current day's dose on schedule. Your chances of becoming pregnant are remote. But forgetting two pills is another matter. Take them as soon as you remember and continue the pills the rest of the cycle; you must also use another means of birth control the rest of that cycle. Forgetting to take three or more pills either greatly increases your chances of becoming pregnant or you may start your period. Begin using another method of birth control, and check with the doctor about how to begin a new cycle of pills. The advice may be to start a new pack immediately or to wait a week. At any rate, you'll have to use a second form of birth control for at least two weeks after you begin your new package of pills.

Does taking the Pill change your nutritional needs?   The estrogen in the Pill may impair your absorption of certain vitamins, especially pyridoxine. The current recommendation is that a woman taking the Pill may need ten times the usual dietary allowance of pyridoxine (vitamin B_6). This can be supplied by supplements prescribed by a physician or by increasing the dietary intake of milk, meat, liver, fish, corn and other grains.

9

What is the mini-Pill?　It is a low-dose birth-control pill containing only progesterone—not estrogen and progesterone, as the regular Pill does. The mini-Pill is less reliable than the regular Pill. Two or three out of a hundred women who rely on it for a year will become pregnant.

At one time it was thought that the woman who didn't qualify to take the regular Pill could use the mini-Pill. This has been found not to be the case, since a small amount of the progesterone in the pill is converted by the body to estrogen. Moreover, the mini-Pill causes a troublesome irregularity of the menstrual cycles.

Is a long-term Pill in the offing?　A once-a-month Pill has been tested, but it hasn't proven as effective as the regular Pill. Spotting is also a problem with the monthly type.

Hormone injections may eventually become available as an alternative to the Pill. Provera, the one studied most extensively, is a progesterone drug that has been available to doctors for years to treat menstrual irregularities. In its long-acting form (Depo-Provera), the drug is given as an injection every three months and provides 100 percent protection against pregnancy during this time. It has been turned down by the FDA for use as a contraceptive because beagle dogs given high doses of it showed an increased incidence of breast cancer. Depo-Provera also causes irregular menstrual bleeding or an absence of the menses. Still another problem is that the person receiving it may fail to regain her fertility for up to a year after the injections are stopped.

What other long-term agent is being tested?　In Brazil and Chile a rod containing norgestrel (a synthetic progestogen) has been tested. It is implanted under the skin of the arm or buttocks. Because the hormone is released slowly, the contraceptive effect may last for up to ten years. Fertility returns when the rod is removed through a small incision. About 30 percent of women who've tried this method noted irregular menses or prolonged periods of bleeding; some also developed ovarian cysts.

Theoretically, a woman could be immunized against sperm by injection of a birth-control vaccine. The vaccine would give her body the capacity to destroy sperm before fertilization occurs. Research to develop such a vaccine is under way. To date, promising results have been obtained in sheep and other animals, but human tests haven't been done.

A long-term contraceptive pill for men is now being tested in China. Even if it proves to be effective, it will take a long time for the drug to be approved in the United States.

What is the morning-after Pill?　It is not one pill, but five days of treatment with diethylstilbestrol (DES), a synthetic estrogen. Taken after un-

10

protected intercourse, the DES will cause the uterus to expel a fertilized egg. Its main use is in the treatment of a victim of rape. The DES should be started as soon after intercourse as possible, and no later than seventy-two hours afterward. The pregnancy rate after DES therapy is only 0.3 percent, but the high doses of estrogen may cause nausea, vomiting and menstrual problems. Also, the drug can seriously harm the developing embryo if the pills fail and a pregnancy ensues.

Some physicians prefer to give ethinyl estradiol, another form of estrogen, as a morning-after Pill. Although it seems to be better tolerated than DES, it causes very similar effects. A newcomer to the field is prostaglandin. Like estrogen and progesterone, this hormone can be reproduced in the laboratory. It is used in a tablet that is inserted into the vagina the morning after. It works, but causes such severe pain and menstrual irregularities that only two out of fifty women in one study continued to use it for more than three months. Scientists are trying to develop a form of prostaglandin that will be effective and well tolerated when taken by mouth the morning after.

What are the advantages and disadvantages of the morning-after Pill? The advantage is that it can be used to prevent pregnancy even though conception may have already occurred. The disadvantage is that it exposes a woman to very high doses of estrogen and causes the side effects mentioned above. A woman would be well advised to use the morning-after Pill no more often than once a year.

Is there anything else that can be taken after intercourse to prevent pregnancy? Menstrual extraction can be used to terminate a suspected pregnancy before it is diagnosed. The procedure may be done when a period is one day or one week late or up to three weeks overdue. Beyond the three-week limit, menstrual extraction becomes a vacuum-aspiration abortion, since the techniques are virtually the same.

After inserting a thin tubing into the cervix, the physician uses a syringe or a suction machine to aspirate the uterine contents. The extraction may be painless, though some women experience cramps or severe pain. Bleeding similar to that in a menstrual period occurs afterwards. A follow-up exam and pregnancy test are done two weeks later to make sure that a pregnancy, if one existed, was terminated by the procedure.

The fee for a menstrual extraction ranges from fifty to a hundred dollars, which is less than for an abortion.

How successful is menstrual extraction? This depends on the technique used. Aspiration performed with a very small tubing resulted in continuation of the pregnancy in 5 percent of women in one series. The use of a slightly larger tubing resulted in a pregnancy continuation rate of less than 1 percent. (Of course, many women who have menstrual extraction aren't pregnant, and thus have no risk of continued pregnancy.) Some doctors will agree to perform an abortion at no cost if it is found later that the menstrual extraction did not stop a pregnancy. That's something to discuss with him or her in advance.

THE IUD

What is an IUD?   It is a device that is inserted into the uterus through the cervical opening. "IUD" stands for *intrau*terine *d*evice. Through mechanisms that are not completely understood, the IUD prevents pregnancy in 95 to 99 percent of women who use it.

What does an IUD look like?   It's a small piece of plastic formed into the shape of a "T," a "Y," a "7," or a series of loops or coils. The Dalkon Shield (now withdrawn from the market) resembles a shield, but has spines projecting from its sides. All IUDs have a tail of nylon thread.

What are the advantages of the IUD?   Since the IUD is worn inside the womb, there's no need to use the Pill or other contraceptive measures— theoretically; the wearer is advised to use an additional means of birth control during the first few months after the IUD is in place. Low expense is another advantage: once the unit's in place, that's it, except for follow-up visits to the doctor. Many women find this an ideal means of birth control, especially if they have trouble remembering when using other methods.

What are the disadvantages of the IUD?   It fails to protect against pregnancy in as many as 5 percent of women who use it for a year. Among the causes of failure is the expulsion of the device, which is most likely to occur during the first few months after insertion. The risk of expulsion is greater when the wearer has never been pregnant, and some doctors believe that the IUD is best suited to the woman who's had at least one child. In other women, tubular infections may occur, sometimes causing sterility. Pelvic pain and menstrual irregularities are frequent complaints. The woman jogger may experience discomfort from an IUD, and pregnancy that occurs with an IUD in place can pose a serious risk. The IUD exposes the woman to a potentially fatal infection should a miscarriage occur: the risk of death from a spontaneous abortion is fifty times greater in a woman continuing a pregnancy that occurred despite an IUD than in a pregnant person who has not used an IUD. Many of the deaths from this complication have occurred in women using the Dalkon Shield, which was taken off the market in 1974. The Dalkon Shield has a tail consisting of several hundred fibers that apparently serve as a wick to allow germs access to the womb. Spontaneous breakage is another problem with the Shield. Thousands of women are still wearing a Dalkon Shield, and the current recommendation is that it be removed even though the person has no symptoms and is not pregnant. Other IUDs have also been associated with fatal infections, and any brand of intrauterine device should be removed when pregnancy is diagnosed. Removing the IUD will induce an abortion a fourth of the time. When a careful insertion technique is employed, perforation of the uterus by the IUD occurs once in every 10,000 insertions, though the rate of perforations with the Dalkon Shield was much higher. Pelvic inflammatory disease (PID) occurs more commonly in users of the IUD. There is also a higher risk of tubular pregnancy.

Are the new IUDs better than the previous ones?　Yes. The first IUDs were nonmedicated. They worked by keeping the fertilized egg from becoming implanted in the womb, and they had an average success rate of about 95 percent. The first medicated IUD to win FDA approval had copper as its active ingredient, which exerts a sperm-killing action inside the womb. In 1975 the FDA approved an IUD that is made of silicon rubber impregnated with progesterone. Released slowly, the progesterone acts on the lining of the womb to prevent a fertilized egg from taking root. That this device must be replaced every year is a disadvantage in comparison to nonmedicated IUDs, which may be worn for five to ten years or more. Medicated IUDs do cause side effects, though fewer than nonmedicated ones, and their success rate is 99 percent.

Who can safely wear an IUD?　Almost any healthy woman who wishes to avoid pregnancy. Rarely, the shape of the womb will not conform to the insertion of the IUD. Uterine polyps, a history of excessive menstrual bleeding and trouble with recurring pelvic infections are other contraindications. So is pregnancy or a suspicion of pregnancy. The woman with known or suspected cancer of the cervix or uterus should not use an IUD.

Does a previous tubal pregnancy disqualify a woman from using an IUD? Yes. The woman who has survived a tubal pregnancy will have had that tube removed, and she may have a partial obstruction in her remaining tube. That's where the problem may arise with the use of the IUD. Unlike barrier methods, it doesn't prevent sperm from entering the womb. Some of the sperm may swim past the IUD and travel all the way up to the tube to cause conception. The IUD would prevent the fertilized egg from implanting in the womb, but it might remain trapped in a damaged tube to cause tubal pregnancy. For this reason the woman who has had a tubal pregnancy should choose a method of contraception other than the IUD.

How is the IUD inserted?　It's usually done during or right after the menstrual period, when the opening in the cervix (the narrow neck of the uterus) is at its largest. The doctor measures the uterus with a probe and

13

inserts the tube-like injector loaded with an IUD of the appropriate size and shape. The IUD is made of a resilient substance, so that even though it can be drawn into the injector tube, it will spring out to its previous shape when released inside the uterus.

What about the IUD tail?　It protrudes through the cervix into the vagina, and is similar to a tampon string (though not as thick). The tail serves several purposes. It lets you feel to see if the unit is still in place, and it enables the doctor to remove the IUD by pulling on the string. Because the tail of each type of IUD is of a certain color and consistency, one can identify the device by looking at the string.

Will the string cause discomfort during intercourse?　The tail is cut so that only a couple of inches of it protrude into the vagina. The woman cannot feel it, but her partner may. As the string softens and becomes coated with secretions, it is less noticeable to the man. If it persists in causing him discomfort, it can be trimmed off so that it barely extends beyond the cervix.

Will I note any discomfort after the IUD is inserted?　You may. Some women, particularly those who've never had a baby, develop cramps after the IUD is in place. The cramps are caused by contractions of the uterus as it attempts to empty itself. The pain may be most severe in the low back. On rare occasions, excruciating pain develops after the insertion of an IUD.

What can be done for the pain?　The doctor may have to remove the device immediately if the pain is very severe. More likely, the cramps will subside after a day or two, and can be relieved by taking aspirin or acetaminophen.

One cause of persistent pain is an IUD that doesn't fit well or has stretched the walls of the womb. Changing to an IUD of a different size and shape may relieve the discomfort.

Will my periods become heavier after the IUD is inserted?　Yes. Heavy periods and spotting are the most common side effects of the IUD. These tend to disappear after the first two or three months, but not always. Excessive bleeding is the most frequent reason for removing the IUD, and even the woman who adjusts to the device can expect to lose up to twice the amount of blood that she did before she began wearing it.

Does the IUD have any other effects?　It increases the likelihood that the wearer will develop a pelvic infection, though the incidence of infections is only 2 or 3 percent. Fever, lower abdominal pain and an abnormal discharge are signs of infection. Treatment, which should be started early, consists of removing the IUD and administering antibiotics.

14

The discharge of an infection should not be confused with the watery, odorless discharge some IUD wearers may note. The latter is related to irritation of the cervix by the IUD tail. Shortening of the tail may reduce the amount of discharge.

What precautions should the IUD wearer take?   Check regularly to make sure the device is still in place. Once a week, bear down while seated on the toilet and reach into the vagina until you feel the dimple-like opening of the cervix. If you can feel the tail of the IUD, it's still in place. If you can't, notify the doctor, and use another means of birth control until the physician has examined you. Another thing to check for is change in the length of the string. An increase or decrease in length may mean the IUD has changed position, and this, too, is reason to notify the doctor. After the device has been in place for four to six months and you've had no trouble with it, you needn't continue checking it every week. You can check just once a month, right after the menstrual period.

Probably the most important thing for the IUD wearer to remember is to notify the doctor should any signs of pregnancy occur. A missed menstrual period, breast soreness, nausea and other symptoms suggest pregnancy. The IUD should be removed at once.

What can be done if the IUD comes out?   You and the physician may elect to insert another one. Reinsertions are usually successful and a second expulsion is unlikely.

How do you know if the missing IUD has entered the abdomen?   Because they contain barium, all IUDs show up on X-ray. A film of the pelvic region will show if the device has perforated the uterus and entered the abdomen.

Do you need to use foam with the IUD?   Most authorities recommend the use of spermicidal foam in conjunction with the IUD during the first six months of its use. Some women prefer to use foam during mid-cycle no matter how long the IUD has been in place, and as an alternative, the man can use a condom during mid-cycle. But the additional protection provided by the foam or condom is not great; the IUD itself is sufficient to provide a high degree of protection against pregnancy.

How often is a follow-up exam needed?   Several checkups are advisable during the first six months after an IUD is in place. After that, a yearly examination is usually sufficient.

How long will the IUD last?   Medicated IUDs have the shortest life. The Progestasert must be removed during its twelfth month in the uterus. The

15

Copper 7 (Gravigard) has to be removed after three years. In both instances a new IUD can be inserted when the old one is removed.

Nonmedicated IUDs tend to last at least five years. In a study of the Lippes Loop, it was determined that a third of women who had the device inserted were still wearing it ten years later. An advantage of keeping the IUD for several years is that the degree of protection goes up the longer the device is in place. The wearer who elects to become pregnant can simply have the IUD removed.

Does the IUD cause cancer?   We have no evidence that it does.

THE DIAPHRAGM AND JELLY

What is the diaphragm?   It is a dome-shaped cup of latex rubber. At the base of the dome is a flexible metal ring which can be bent for insertion into the vagina, and which will then spring open to encircle the cervix and prevent the entry of sperm. The diaphragm acts as a barrier between the vagina and the womb.

What is the jelly?   A spermicidal agent that comes in a tube and can be squeezed out in much the same way as hair oil or toothpaste can— "spermicidal" refers to the ability to kill sperm on contact. Spermicidal cream is also available, but it is not as easy to manipulate or as effective as the jelly.

How does the method work?   Before inserting the diaphragm, the jelly is applied to the rim and the inside, or the cup, of the diaphragm; the jelly is thus held next to the mouth of the womb. Two effects are in operation: the diaphragm is a barrier to sperm, and the jelly will kill any sperm that manage to make it around the barrier.

What are the benefits of the diaphragm-and-jelly method?   Safety and ease of use are the main benefits. Serious side effects do not occur. Unlike the Pill and the IUD, the diaphragm does not have to be used except during intercourse, and can be inserted up to six hours beforehand. Once it's in place, it can't be felt during intercourse. The cost is low. Most of the expense is in the visit to the doctor for the prescription and in the purchase of the unit, which should cost less than ten dollars, even allowing for drugstore markup. After that, the only expense is the spermicidal jelly. It comes in large or small tubes at a cost that averages about twenty-five cents per application.

What are the disadvantages of the diaphragm?   It is slightly less effective than the IUD and the Pill. It requires a certain amount of paraphernalia

—the diaphragm and jelly—that must be carried along if the woman is away from home and expects to have sexual relations. This means that the forgetful person shouldn't rely on this method. Some women object to putting the unit into the vagina, but this hesitancy tends to disappear after the first few times, and the couple may even make insertion of the diaphragm a part of their love play. Rarely, a woman or a man is allergic to the jelly or to the latex rubber of which the diaphragm is made.

Who can use the diaphragm?   Almost any woman who is willing to tolerate the slight inconvenience of this method. The only contraindication is a pelvic configuration that won't accommodate the diaphragm. Relaxation of the pelvic muscles or an unusual position of the uterus may prevent the unit from fitting properly.

How effective is the diaphragm?   The woman who uses her diaphragm and jelly properly can get almost complete protection against pregnancy. The effectiveness is at least 97 percent. Large studies show a failure rate of up to 15 percent, but these figures reflect improper usage of the diaphragm or failure to use it.

What are the causes of failure?   Not using it or using it incorrectly. Correct insertion means that the front edge of the cup rests behind the pubic bone and the back edge extends beyond the cervix. Neglecting to put spermicidal jelly into the cup and around its rim is another cause of failure. It is a good idea to keep an extra tube of jelly on hand.

Not having periodic checkups to ensure that the diaphragm is the right size may be a cause of failure. It is also important to regularly check the rubber of the diaphragm for holes or tears.

Does your diaphragm size change?   It may. Since a woman will experience some enlargement of the vagina during the first few months of active sex life, a diaphragm fitted before the beginning of sexual relations may become too small in several months. The woman should have another fitting about three months later and again after the birth of a child. Weight loss or weight gain of more than ten or fifteen pounds may change the dimensions of the vagina. With a loss of weight you may need a larger diaphragm, while with a gain of weight you may need a smaller one.

How do I use the diaphragm?   Have it fitted, prepare it correctly, insert it the right way, leave it in for a sufficient time after intercourse, and take proper care of it:

1. *A doctor's prescription* is required for the diaphragm, because it must be fitted to your own measurements. It is important that the unit fit snugly in the top of the vagina while covering the cervix.

2. *Prepare the diaphragm* by dipping it in warm water and squeezing about

17

three inches (a teaspoonful) of spermicidal jelly into the cup of the unit. Spread the jelly around the bottom of the cup and along the inside rim. Some physicians also recommend applying the sperm-killing agent to the outside of the diaphragm.

3. *Correct insertion* should be taught you by the doctor who prescribes the diaphragm. Practice putting it in while you're still in the examining room, or if you don't have it yet, use one of the fitting rings to make sure that your insertion technique is right. The usual position for insertion is with one foot elevated and resting on the commode or bathtub rim. Spread the main lips with one hand, and fold the unit with the fingers of your other hand. Insert it so that it locks in place with the front edge behind the pubic bone and the back edge beyond the cervix. Then feel through the cup for the cervix, which is round and about the size of a small nose, and has a small dimple in its center. The unit should entirely cover the cervix.

4. *Leave the diaphragm in* for at least six to eight hours after intercourse. This length of time is necessary to make sure that all the sperm are killed. If you have intercourse several times within a short period, insert another teaspoonful of spermicidal jelly into the vagina before each act of intercourse. Do not remove the diaphragm until six to eight hours after the last lovemaking; it will then be safe to remove the diaphragm and to douche. Don't douche with the unit in place, as the stream of water might dislodge it.

5. *Remove the diaphragm* by hooking a finger under its rim. Wash it with soap and water, dry it and dust it with cornstarch. It should not be left in direct sunlight and should be kept in its container. Hold it up to the light now and then to check for holes. It's necessary to get a new diaphragm about every two years.

What if I forget to remove the diaphragm?   No harm done. Some women leave it in for a day or two just out of forgetfulness and notice no problems. Leaving it in longer might cause vaginal irritation or discharge, so the best idea is to remove and clean the unit at least once a day.

What keeps the diaphragm from coming out during intercourse?   It fits snugly in the vagina out of the way of most of the thrusting motions of the penis. Nonetheless, it is possible for the unit to come out during intercourse, especially if it wasn't inserted properly. Dislodgement of the diaphragm is more likely to occur during intercourse if the woman is in the superior position. If the front rim of the diaphragm slips out during intercourse, simply reposition it and continue with lovemaking. If dislodgement becomes a problem, check with your physician.

Can the diaphragm hold back the menstrual flow?   Yes. Some women use it to allow tidier lovemaking during the menstrual period. Still others have used it in a nonsexual emergency when a period started and they had no tampons or pads available.

Does the diaphragm cause cancer?   We have no evidence that it does.

What's the difference between the diaphragm and the cervical cap?
Each acts as a barrier to sperm, but the cervical cap is made to fit tightly over the cervix in the same way that a thimble fits over a finger. It stays in place by suction. The cap may be worn throughout the month (except during the menstrual period), or, like the diaphragm, used intermittently with spermicidal jelly. Since it is made of lucite, rubber or plastic, the cervical cap is not as vulnerable to injury as the diaphragm. Some authorities claim that it is easier to fit than a diaphragm because the cervix is less variable in size than the vagina.

Is the cervical cap still available?   It may be obtained through some physicians, but it is no longer made in America. It is manufactured by Lamberts (Dalston) Limited, of London, and is used more commonly in Europe than here. Some experts believe that the cap is too unreliable for widespread use, and others don't like it because of the cervical irritation that may result from wearing it throughout the month.

What other methods of birth control are being tested?   A ring that is two inches wide and a third of an inch thick has been designed for insertion into the vagina after the menstrual period. Collapsible like a diaphragm, it resumes its shape inside the vagina and can be worn comfortably for three weeks. The progesterone it contains is released slowly during this time to prevent ovulation. A menstrual period begins a few days after the ring is removed, and the device is reinserted on the fifth day after the onset of bleeding. The side effects are apparently less than those of the Pill, though the ring itself may cause vaginal discharge or irritation. The vaginal ring works, but more studies are needed to evaluate its efficacy and its side effects.

The use of a medicated sponge has shown some promise. Containing a spermicidal agent and also acting as a barrier, the sponge is inserted after the menstrual period and left in the vagina until the next period, or it may be removed, washed and reinserted as necessary. The modern contraceptive sponge is being tested in medicated and nonmedicated forms, but it is much too early to judge its effectiveness.

19

FOAM

What is foam?   A sperm-killing aerosol that is released into the vagina before intercourse. It can be purchased without a prescription. The container resembles a can of shaving cream, and pressure on the nozzle releases the foam into a plastic applicator. This contraceptive also comes in the form of tablets, suppositories and cream.

What are the advantages of foam?   You don't have to see a doctor to get it. Other than a rare occurrence of allergic reactions, it causes no side effects. Foam is relatively inexpensive.

What are the disadvantages of foam?   Some brands may irritate the man's penis, but others may not. Foam may have an unpleasant taste, hindering oral-genital sex. Many women find it messy, both during sex and in the time that it remains in the vagina.

How effective is foam?   When used alone, foam is less effective than other barrier methods of birth control. It does give a success rate of 97 percent among conscientious users, but the ways to fail are numerous and the actual success rate is 78 percent among large numbers of women who rely on this as their only means of birth control.

How do you use foam?   Buy one of the major brands of spermicidal foam. Get the can of foam, not the tablets, suppositories or cream, all of which do not disperse as well in the vagina and are less effective. Shake the can well before use, at least twenty times, to mix the foam and add bubbles. Follow the directions and insert one or two applicators of foam into the vagina within half an hour before intercourse. Position the applicator so that the foam is instilled near the cervix. Wait at least eight hours after intercourse before douching. (It's all right to insert a tampon to keep the foam from leaking out if you have to go somewhere.) Be sure to keep an extra container of foam; the one you're using may run out at the wrong moment.

How can I make foam more effective?   By using it exactly as directed before every act of intercourse, and by asking your partner to assist you in its use. Even better, he can do his part by wearing a condom for additional protection. If you're still worried about getting pregnant, try using the diaphragm-and-jelly method.

Does foam protect you from venereal disease?   Not really, though some doctors believe it offers a slight protection against contracting gonorrhea.

RHYTHM

What is rhythm?   It is a method of birth control accomplished by refraining from intercourse during the mid-cycle days when a woman is most likely to get pregnant.

What are the advantages of rhythm?   It costs nothing, requires no medical examination and is acceptable to most religious and ethnic groups.

What are the disadvantages of rhythm?   It calls for restraint on the part of both partners during the middle of the monthly cycle when the woman's sexual drive is apt to be at its peak. Also, a woman must be able to calculate her date of ovulation. This may be impossible if her periods occur irregularly, unless she employs the cervical mucus method discussed below. Sickness and emotional upset may disrupt the cycles and lead to unwanted pregnancy.

How effective is rhythm?   The average effectiveness is 80 percent, meaning that twenty out of a hundred women who rely solely on this method will get pregnant during a year's time.

How do you use rhythm?   Calculate your time of ovulation using the calendar method or the basal-body-temperature method. (See p. 4.) Refrain from intercourse during the seven "unsafe" days of the month. The unsafe time begins three days before the predicted date of ovulation, includes the day of ovulation and lasts until three days afterward. If you do have intercourse during the time of peak fertility, you should use another means of birth control.

An alternative method that is growing in popularity is the use of the Billings, or cervical-mucus, test popularized by Drs. John and Lynn Billings. Following the menstrual period vaginal secretions are slight; as a woman approaches ovulation a progressive increase in secretion occurs and may be noted as wetness at the vaginal lips. The mucus, which may be obtained by wiping the vulva with white toilet tissue, is thin and stretchable. Just before and after the time of ovulation it has the consistency of raw egg white and can be drawn apart in a thin thread for a distance of four inches. Following ovulation the quantity of mucus decreases and it takes on a thick, sticky consistency. Intercourse is avoided from three days before until three days after the height of the cervical-mucus secretion. A woman who learns to note and record the amount and type of her cervical mucus can use the rhythm method even if her menstrual periods occur irregularly. This method is now being taught in many women's health centers.

THE CONDOM

What is the condom? It is a sheath, made of either latex rubber (hence the slang term "rubber") or the linings ("skin") of sheep's intestines, that is worn over the penis during intercourse. By collecting the ejaculate, it prevents sperm from reaching the womb.

All skin condoms are premoistened, and they provide a more natural feel to intercourse than do latex condoms, although they are more likely to slip off during intercourse. Latex condoms come in either dry or premoistened form; the latter type is available with a liquid lubricant or with a powdery, silicone-type of lubricant. Like skin condoms, premoistened latex condoms must be used shortly after the package is opened.

What are the advantages of the condom? It is safe, easy to use and inexpensive. It can be purchased without a prescription and is small enough to be carried anywhere. It is the only method of birth control that offers good protection against venereal disease.

What are its disadvantages? It may reduce the man's or the woman's sexual sensitivity. Because it must be rolled up over the penis before intercourse, it requires an interruption of foreplay, and also, the penis must be withdrawn soon after ejaculation. The rare instance of allergy to latex rubber can be overcome by the use of a skin condom.

How effective is the condom? More so than generally thought. In England among married couples the condom offered a 97 to 98 percent success rate in protecting against pregnancy. In large studies in the United States the success rate was reported to be about 90 percent. As with other methods, the effectiveness of the condom depends on the skill and diligence of the users.

How good is the condom combined with other methods? The condom used in conjunction with spermicidal foam or the diaphragm and jelly provides better than 99 percent protection against pregnancy.

Are condoms manufactured with care? Yes. The manufacturing and testing of the product have been automated, and the FDA requires that each condom be "safe, effective and properly labeled." In 1968 FDA tolerance levels were set to allow seizure of shipments containing more than 0.25 percent faulty units.

Better marketing than in previous years has accompanied the improvement in quality. Once an item that was bought at a filling station or from a druggist who reached under the counter to do the selecting himself, the condom has now gained a measure of respectability. Over forty states have laws permitting drugstores to display condoms openly. One result is that the number of women purchasing condoms for their partners has gone up 500 percent.

How should the condom be used?   It should be put on just before the start of intercourse, and innovative couples can do it in a sensual manner. The condom should be rolled all the way to the hilt of the erect penis. To serve as a receptacle for semen, a space should be left between the tip of the condom and the penis (some condoms are made with such a receptacle). Premoistened condoms are less likely to break than the dry kind, for which a small amount of spermicidal jelly can be used as a lubricant. K-Y jelly is an excellent lubricant. Vaseline or other forms of petrolatum jelly should not be used, as they cause rubber to disintegrate. Make sure that the rubber ring remains securely around the base of the penis during intercourse. Remove the penis soon after ejaculation, and hold the rubber in place so that no semen can escape. Use a new condom for each act of intercourse.

What if the condom breaks?   Keep spermicidal foam or jelly available, and insert two applicators of it into the vagina immediately. Wait eight hours before douching. By using foam with the condom, you'll increase the effectiveness of this method and be protected in the event the rubber breaks.

Do condoms get too old to use?   Yes. At most, they have a storage life of two years—less if exposed to heat. Use fresh ones if possible, and remember that the condoms you buy today may have been on the drugstore shelf for some time. Check with the druggist to find out how long they've been in stock. The aging of condoms is one reason why you should purchase them only from dispensing machines in busy locations or from druggists who have a fairly active trade.

COITUS INTERRUPTUS

What is coitus interruptus?   It means birth control achieved by withdrawing the penis just before ejaculation. It is said by some authorities to be the leading birth-control method in the world, though others claim that the rhythm method is number one. In this country, coitus interruptus is most apt to be used by young persons.

What are the advantages of coitus interruptus?   It costs nothing, requires no paraphernalia or preparation (except mental), has no side effects, and can be used when intercourse occurs at an unanticipated moment.

What are the disadvantages?   It interrupts lovemaking just at the moment of greatest pleasure for the man and often for the woman. Since the responsibility for withdrawal rests on the man, it places the control of contraception with him, rather than with the woman.

How effective is coitus interruptus?   It has an average success rate of 75 to 80 percent in protecting against pregnancy. About one out of four women relying on this method can expect to become pregnant during a year's time.

What are the causes of failure?   The man must withdraw when his natural urge is to do the opposite: a rational act may not be possible at such an irrational moment. Or, the woman may become sufficiently excited to prevent withdrawal.

Even with flawless performance of coitus interruptus, pregnancy may still occur. The man's pre-ejaculatory fluid begins to escape before he has an orgasm, and it may contain enough sperm to cause a pregnancy. The most common reason for failure, though, is resumption of intercourse after the man has ejaculated. His penis still contains enough sperm to impregnate his partner. For these reasons, coitus interruptus is not recommended except as a backup method when no other means of birth control is available.

How can you make coitus interruptus more effective?   By making sure that withdrawal occurs well ahead of ejaculation, that ejaculation occurs as far away as possible from the woman's genitals, and that additional intercourse is not attempted for eight hours—a long enough time to make possible the purchase of condoms or foam.

STERILIZATION

What is sterilization?   It is the operation to make a man incapable of fertilizing an egg or a woman incapable of becoming pregnant. Vasectomy is performed on the man; tubal ligation on the woman.

How effective is sterilization?   It is virtually 100 percent effective if the surgery is adequate and the patient follows instructions.

How is tubal ligation done?   Usually, by closing off the passageway (the fallopian tube) from the ovary to the womb. The traditional method is an abdominal operation to make surgical stitches about an inch apart in the middle section of each tube; the part of the tube between the stitches is then removed. Each tube is thus tied twice and partially amputated. The surgery must be done in a hospital, and it usually takes several days for the woman to be able to get back to her regular activities. The operation is frequently done a few days after delivery of the baby.

Will tubal ligation keep me from having menstrual periods?   No.

Will it affect my sex drive? There is no anatomical or physiological reason why it should. Because they no longer have to worry about birth control, most women report increased sexual desire after undergoing sterilization.

Is the operation reversible? In a certain percentage of women, yes. The standard operation to reopen tied tubes is reported to have been successful in allowing pregnancy in 20 to 40 percent of women, but that statistic has been questioned recently. Now, a microsurgical technique has been developed which may allow the operator a much better chance of restoring fertility—up to 70 percent or better is the claim. The microsurgical technique is not available in all parts of the United States, and it *is* major surgery requiring general anesthesia and hospitalization. The number of pregnancies occurring after this procedure remains to be established.

Doctors are developing methods of tubal ligation that may be easier to reverse. One is the placement of Silastic bands around each tube; another is to close off the tubes with metal clips. Removal of the bands or the clips, should reversibility become desirable, may restore fertility. It will be several years before we know if these methods are as good as they sound. It is almost certainly not a good idea to undergo tubal ligation if there is *any* possibility that you may change your mind and want to have children.

Is there an easier way of closing off the fallopian tubes? Yes. By looking through a laparoscope (somewhat like using a telescope to peer inside the body), a specialist can perform a procedure having the same effect as tubal ligation through a small incision in the navel (and sometimes an additional cut lower down). Carbon dioxide gas is pumped into the abdomen to make the viewing easier, and an electrocautery is used on the tubes. Instead of being tied, the tubes are coagulated in one or more places by a touch of the electric current. Since the abdomen isn't opened, the surgery can be done in an outpatient center. When the woman is released several hours later, she generally will need someone to drive her home. She has to stay in bed the rest of the day and part of the next day, after which she can resume her normal activities.

What are the side effects of laparoscopic sterilization? Soreness in the navel and slight vaginal bleeding may occur (the latter is due to manipulation of the cervix during the surgery). Though an attempt is made to remove the carbon dioxide from the abdomen at the end of the operation, not all of it can be removed; even though the patient is lying in bed, the gas may irritate the sensitive diaphragm muscle high in the abdomen. This can produce pain in the chest and shoulders, which may last from two days to a week.

Is the procedure dangerous?   Not really, though the complication rate is inversely related to the skill of the operator. This is why it's best to have the laparoscopic procedure done by a specialist who averages doing at least one such procedure a week. Don't be afraid to ask the doctor how much experience he or she has had; if you have any doubts, ask your physician or internist to recommend another specialist. Still another way to find out who's good and who isn't is to talk either to a nurse or physician in training at the hospital where the surgery is to be done or to someone at a community or women's health service who will have information about the track record of various physicians.

Possible complications include a burn of the bowel or bladder when these organs are accidentally touched by the electrocautery. Sometimes the tube bleeds from the site of the cauterization. The rate for major complication (that is, surgery is required to correct a bowel, bladder or bleeding problem) is less than four out of every 1,000 women having the operation. The death rate from laparoscopic sterilization is 2.5 deaths per 100,000 women having the procedure. One can contrast this with the 1973 statistic that the mortality rate for women bearing children was 16 maternal deaths per 100,000 live births.

How soon does the procedure have a contraceptive effect?   Immediately. You can stop worrying about pregnancy even if you have intercourse later the same day.

What are the causes for failure of a laparoscopic procedure?   Pregnancy occurs in fewer than one out of 10,000 women having the operation. It's possible that the novice operator of the electrocautery may coagulate the round ligament of the uterus rather than the tube, or that the tube may somehow reopen on its own in spite of adequate coagulation.

What about hysterectomy?   Removal of the womb, hysterectomy, makes a woman sterile. Since it is major surgery, it is not usually done unless the woman has valid and serious medical reasons for removing the uterus, such as severe endometriosis or the other problems discussed in Chapter 4. Hysterectomy ends the menstrual periods.

What does vasectomy entail?   The tubes carrying sperm from the testicles to the penis are tied and a section of each is removed. Vasectomy can be done in the doctor's office under local anesthesia, and the man can walk out afterward.

What are the side effects of vasectomy?   Soreness and swelling in the scrotum persist for several days, but these symptoms tend to be mild.

26

Rarely, a clot or infection will occur. Even more rarely, one or both testicles may become inflamed. Sometimes the sperm, which are still produced but now have no place to go, build up to form a painful nodule that may have to be removed by additional surgery. In the vast majority of men the sperm are simply broken down and resorbed by the body. The mortality rate from vasectomy is zero.

Does the operation prevent the man from ejaculating?   No. Sperm make up only 5 to 10 percent of the volume of a man's ejaculate. Most of the semen comes from the prostate gland and seminal vesicles, which aren't affected by a vasectomy.

Will vasectomy affect sex drive?   Usually not. Psychological factors figure strongly in a man's ability to achieve an erection, and it's possible for him to feel (or be made to feel) that the loss of fertility has taken away his maleness or potency. The kind of man most likely to feel this way does not usually submit to a vasectomy. In a survey of more than a thousand men who had vasectomy, it was found that almost 99 percent had no regrets. Three-fourths claimed an increase in sexual pleasure, and only one and a half percent had less sex drive.

When is it safe for the man to resume sexual relations?   For a week after surgery the man should not have an ejaculation; his body needs this time to heal. Even then, he's not yet sterile. Sperm are present in his genital tracts above the site of the vasectomy, and may live there for several weeks. The couple must use another means of protection until a physician has examined the semen and certified that it is free of sperm. A dozen or more ejaculations may be necessary before this is the case and intercourse is safe.

What are the causes for failure of a vasectomy?   Failure occurs in one to four out of every thousand men who have the operation, and the usual cause is for one or both of the sperm ducts to reopen spontaneously.

Is vasectomy reversible?   With the use of the old technique, reversal was possible in only one out of four men. The new, microsurgical technique apparently has made it possible to reverse the operation in over 70 percent of men, but even then, fertility may not return. Half of the men who've had a vasectomy develop antibodies against their own sperm, and these antibodies may make the sterilization permanent. So if there is a chance that you may want children, do not consider sterilization.

What about using a sperm bank?   Sperm banks are in operation in many cities, and a man contemplating vasectomy can submit semen specimens for freezing and storage. Should he later decide to have children, the sperm can

27

be thawed and used to artificially inseminate his wife. Freezing apparently doesn't harm the sperm, and many normal children have been conceived after fertilization from frozen sperm. Still, there's no guarantee that insemination will work, especially if the sperm have been stored for more than three years. Thus, a man or woman seeking sterilization should presume that it will be permanent.

ABORTION

What is an abortion?   It is the ending of a pregnancy through a means other than the birth of a baby. A miscarriage is a "natural" abortion. In medical parlance the word "abortion" has always been used to refer not only to an induced abortion but also to a miscarriage.

How dangerous is an abortion?   The risk is small during the first twelve weeks of pregnancy—2.6 deaths per 100,000 abortions. After the first three months of pregnancy, abortion is more difficult and the risk to the mother increases. Used at this point in the pregnancy, the saline method, where a sterile solution of salt and water is injected into the fetal sac, caused one death per every 5,500 abortions. When hysterotomy (surgical incision of the uterus)—an operation that is similar to a cesarean section —was necessary to remove the fetus, the maternal death rate was 2.7 deaths per 1,000 abortions. To keep her risk at a minimum, the woman who wishes to have an abortion should make the decision as early in her pregnancy as possible.

How do I obtain an abortion?   Visit a gynecologist who offers the procedure, or ask your family physician to refer you to a specialist or clinic where you can have the abortion. Clinics that may help include those run by various family-planning groups, Planned Parenthood or a women's health care center that specializes in abortions. Investigate thoroughly to find the best place that is available to you.

How much does it cost?   In some parts of the country you can get an abortion for $125. You shouldn't have to pay more than $200 if it is done during the first three months of pregnancy. Watch out for higher prices— and less dependable medical services—at some of the commercial, profit-motivated abortion clinics. Try to avoid these places. Also inquire about aftercare. How much will it cost, and who will be available to take care of you at night or on weekends?

Realize, too, that a first-trimester abortion is medically easier and less expensive than an abortion after twelve weeks of pregnancy. An early abortion can be done in an office or clinic, but a second-trimester abortion is usually done in the hospital and may cost up to $500 to $750. This

28

underscores the logic for reaching a decision about abortion as early as possible.

What are some ways to evaluate an abortion clinic? Ask to tour the facility. Make sure the clinic has good new equipment, plenty of space, nurses to take care of you, and an adequate supply of drugs, intravenous solutions and emergency equipment. Ask what arrangements have been made to transport a patient to a hospital should that become necessary. (The transfer should take no more than ten minutes.) Ask to see the suction apparatus that will be used to perform the abortion. Some doctors still perform first-trimester abortions with a metal scraper, or curette. The complication rate with this method is greater, so find a clinic where the suction method is routine.

What questions should you ask beforehand? You may want to ask about the size of the suction cannula (vacurette) that the physician intends to use to end your pregnancy. It's important that not too large a cannula is used because the less dilation there is, the less pain and bleeding there'll be. Then, too, the greater the amount of stretching of the cervical opening, the more likely it is that you will sustain a permanent injury to the cervix which could prevent your carrying a future, wanted pregnancy to completion. But too small an instrument may be insufficient to remove all the tissue of the pregnancy. The cannula should be no larger than one millimeter in diameter for each week of pregnancy, and it may be a little smaller than that. A six-millimeter cannula is sufficient to evacuate up to an eight-week pregnancy, and a ten- or eleven-millimeter cannula for a twelve-week pregnancy.

What is involved in preparing for an abortion? The first step is to establish fully that you are pregnant. The doctor will examine you and order a pregnancy test. Other lab work will include a blood and urine test, blood typing and Rh factor determination. If you are Rh negative, you should receive an injection of Rhogam after the abortion. This is a type of gamma globulin used to prevent you from becoming sensitized to an Rh-positive child. If you were to become sensitized, it might harm a future wanted pregnancy. (You do not need the Rhogam injection if you know that your sexual partner is also Rh negative.)

How is the abortion done? It is treated like any other surgical procedure. You mustn't eat within eight to twelve hours beforehand. You will be positioned on a table that is similar to a delivery table. For an early abortion, the doctor administers a local anesthetic, dilates the cervix (if it isn't already dilated) and inserts a plastic cannula into the womb. The cannula is attached to a suction machine, the machine is turned on, and the uterine contents are evacuated in only about five minutes. Most women are able to leave the clinic one or two hours later.

Abortion after the twelfth week of pregnancy is usually done in a hospital or surgical outpatient clinic. With the amnioinfusion technique, saline or the chemical prostaglandin is infused into the fetal sac and causes labor to begin within forty-eight hours. After a few hours of labor, the fetus is expelled. Amnioinfusion can't be done until the fetal sac is large enough to accept the injection—which means at least sixteen weeks of pregnancy. Thus a woman who is too far along to have a suction abortion but who isn't yet sixteen weeks pregnant is asked to wait so that amnioinfusion can be attempted. If this procedure fails, hysterotomy can be done. As mentioned before, this is a major operation to open the abdomen and remove the fetus from the uterus.

How painful is an abortion?   The uterine muscle may begin contracting during the abortion, and this can cause cramps; usually the pain is over in half an hour. The dilation of the cervix that is necessary to insert the vacuum aspirator can be painful. You may want to consider requesting dilation with the seaweed lamineria. With this method, a small stem of sterilized lamineria is inserted into the cervix the day before the abortion, and it absorbs water from the tissues to expand and produce relatively painless dilation. The incidence of infection is slightly higher using lamineria, so it's a choice between this risk and the greater pain caused by enlarging the cervical opening with metal probes. Abortion after the first third of pregnancy tends to be more painful. Amnioinfusion involves an injection into the uterus and causes labor pains, and hysterotomy is major surgery requiring a week to ten days of recovery.

How much bleeding will the abortion cause?   You'll have bleeding as heavy as a menstrual period afterwards, and you may pass clots. The bleeding tends to lessen in several days and stops after about a week. Most clinics will give you an ergot drug that will reduce the amount of bleeding during the first day after the abortion. A sudden increase in bleeding or persistently heavy bleeding should be reported to the doctor immediately.

What are the complications of an abortion?   The worst ones are hemorrhage, a perforated uterus and infection. Hemorrhage that occurs immediately may be due to a perforated uterus or to a tear in the cervix. Hemorrhage that begins more than a day after the procedure usually means incomplete evacuation of the uterus, and may require another suctioning or scraping of the uterine cavity. A perforated uterus is a serious complication that may cause lower abdominal pain and other problems. It must be managed in the hospital, and surgery may be needed to repair the perforation. Infection is signaled by fever, a foul-smelling vaginal discharge, and generalized discomfort and pain in the pelvic region. Overall, the complication rate for first-trimester abortion is less than 1 percent.

Experience to date with amnioinfusion of prostaglandin shows a fairly high complication rate, which is why this technique is still under study and the substance used is limited in availability.

How do I know if I'm having a complication?   Take your temperature several times a day for the week after the abortion and report any fever to the doctor. If the amount of bleeding seems too heavy or increases, or is accompanied by a foul-smelling discharge, call the doctor. Swelling of the abdomen, persistent abdominal pain and anything else unusual should be reported.

What follow-up care is needed?   You should be examined two weeks after the abortion to make sure the uterus and cervix are back to normal. This is a good time to discuss birth-control measures with the physician.

Will abortion affect my future chances of having a normal baby?   It may, but this is unlikely. An early abortion usually has no effect on fertility, but one done after the first trimester of pregnancy may damage the cervix and increase the risk of miscarriage during a subsequent pregnancy. Repeated abortion may weaken the cervix and hinder its ability to remain closed during the last part of pregnancy.

How late can an abortion be done?   Medically speaking, it can be done until the time when the fetus becomes viable, or capable of surviving on its own. The time of viability is usually taken to be after about twenty-four to twenty-six weeks of pregnancy. As a practical matter, most doctors won't do an abortion beyond the twentieth week of pregnancy. The Supreme Court's ruling was that during the first third of pregnancy, the abortion is solely the concern of the woman and her doctor. The state may regulate the abortion procedure after the first trimester, and may prohibit abortion if the pregnancy is of more than twenty-four to twenty-six weeks' duration. The usual exception to this rule is when, in the judgment of the doctor, the abortion is necessary to preserve the life or health of the mother.

Can a minor get an abortion without her parents' consent?   Theoretically, yes, since an early abortion is a private matter between the doctor and the patient. In fact the doctor may insist on calling in the parents. If he or she does so without the girl's permission, that's a betrayal of her confidence. Some physicians prefer to ask a third party, such as a medical colleague, social worker or psychologist, to enter into the decision-making process. Most abortion clinics, including those run by Planned Parenthood, don't require parental consent unless—and here's the rub—the state has gotten around the matter by requiring consent for a test or clinical procedure involved in the abortion. Any clinic that handles abortions can tell you what your state's law is on this matter.

Does a woman need her husband's or partner's consent to get an abortion?
In many cases, physicians will not perform an abortion without the consent of the spouse or partner. This may have to do with the physician's personal philosophy or his concern over the risk of malpractice suits.

What is menstrual extraction?   Also known as "menstrual regulation" or "minisuction," menstrual extraction is like a suction abortion, except that it is done when the period is no more than three weeks late. The suction may be accomplished with a syringe or a suction machine, and because the cannula is so small, no dilation of the cervix is necessary.

Some feminist groups have advocated menstrual extraction as a way of avoiding several days of bleeding and of ending an early pregnancy. However, the potential hazards of menstrual extraction are too great for its routine use. Among the possible complications are excessive bleeding, infection and, about 1 percent of the time, continuation of a pregnancy. Still, menstrual extraction can be a useful procedure for a woman who is a week or two late, believes she is pregnant and wants to end immediately her worry about having a child.

INFERTILITY

What is infertility?   A couple's inability to achieve a pregnancy after a reasonable length of time of having intercourse during the fertile period of the woman's menstrual cycle. Most physicians believe that the period of trying should be at least a year before infertility is considered a problem.

If we're both normal, what are our chances of achieving pregnancy?   If you're both twenty-five and healthy, the chances are better than 60 percent in only six months of trying; the chances are 75 percent by the end of nine months, and 80 percent by the end of the year. Another 10 percent of couples will have a pregnancy in the ensuing six months, making a total of 90 percent of couples achieving pregnancy in a year and a half of trying.

What causes infertility?   One must consider first what constitutes *fertility.* The man must produce adequate quantities of normal sperm and introduce these into the vagina during sexual relations. The sperm must penetrate the cervical mucus, swim through the uterus and reach the fallopian tubes, where fertilization occurs. The woman must produce an egg and have patent, or unobstructed, tubes so that the egg can be fertilized and delivered to the uterus, where it implants and grows into a baby. Her body must be capable of carrying the pregnancy to term.

About 40 percent of the time the man is responsible for infertility. He may not produce enough sperm or his sperm may be abnormal. A bad case of the mumps and certain endocrine disorders are among the causes of infertility. Another problem may be a sperm duct obstruction that prevents him from depositing sperm in large enough quantities into the vagina. Diabetes and chronic inflammation of the epididymis are among the causes of this condition.

The woman may not produce an egg each month, or she may have a tubal obstruction that prevents the egg from being fertilized and reaching the womb. Because of endometriosis, a fibroid tumor, hormonal imbalance or a disease of the cervix, the woman may not be able to carry the pregnancy to term even after it begins successfully.

Another consideration is that fertility reaches its peak at age twenty-four or twenty-five in either sex. Beyond the age of thirty, and especially beyond the age of forty, the fertility rate declines rapidly. This is particularly true for the woman, and it means that couples in their thirties or older may have more difficulty achieving a pregnancy.

Can infertility be cured?   Frequently, yes. In one large clinic, the success rate was 65 pregnancies per 100 couples over a period of four years. Most of the pregnancies occurred during the first year of investigation and treatment.

What should we do if we suspect we're infertile?   Visit a specialist whose main field of interest is helping couples to overcome reproductive failure. In most instances the specialist will be an obstetrician and gynecologist. Both partners should go, though the woman often is screened first. The doctor will do a complete physical examination, order tests of certain body functions, and ask her to keep a temperature chart to determine if she is ovulating (releasing an egg each month). It generally takes three months of keeping the temperature chart before valid information is obtained. Depending on what the temperature charts show, she may need further studies, such as an X-ray of the uterus and tubes, a postcoital examination to study the cervical mucus or a laparoscopic examination.

The husband is examined to see if his general health and genital organs are normal. One important historical point is whether he has fathered children in the past. If he has, it's unlikely, though possible, that he is now infertile. By the same token, if the wife has had children by a previous husband but now cannot get pregnant, her present husband may be the source of the infertility. The main part of the man's workup is an examination of the semen. Since frequent ejaculation may reduce the sperm count and volume of semen, he should refrain from having an ejaculation for two

33

or three days before collecting the specimen. He may collect the specimen by masturbation or by coitus interruptus. Some men prefer to collect it in a condom, which is okay so long as the condom contains nothing that will harm the sperm and if the specimen is delivered to the lab within a couple of hours of its collection.

The volume of a normal ejaculate is about a teaspoonful (though some men produce two teaspoonfuls). It contains about 80 to 120 million sperm per milliliter, or a total of 400 to 500 million sperm per ejaculation. A man may be infertile if he produces less than 20 to 40 million sperm per ejaculation. At least 60 percent of his sperm should show normal motility, and 60 percent should appear normal in size and shape.

How long do these studies take? The time varies, depending on what is found during the investigation. Often, several months are allowed between each stage of the workup. It's not unusual for the couple to achieve pregnancy during the studies before the actual cause of the "infertility" is uncovered.

What are the specific methods of treatment? The most frequent cause of infertility in a woman is an obstruction of the fallopian tubes. An X-ray can tell if this is the case. The X-ray dye injection may open up the tubes or they can be blown open with carbon dioxide gas. Sometimes tubal surgery is necessary. The woman who is unable to ovulate may respond to treatment with the drug clomiphene. It is the best drug yet developed to stimulate ovulation, and it will allow conception in about two-thirds of such women. Injection of human chorionic gonadotropin may be effective in causing ovulation if clomiphene therapy fails. Sometimes a minor surgical procedure on the cervix is necessary, or hormone therapy may be needed to make the cervical mucus more receptive to sperm.

When the man's problem is an anatomical defect, such as a varicocele (a collection of varicose veins above the testicle), surgery may be curative. In some instances, hormone therapy may raise the sperm count. Reduction of stress, smoking and alcohol consumption may also help. Recent findings indicate that certain types of tranquilizers and blood-pressure-lowering agents often interfere with fertility. A thorough review of drug therapy and a switch to alternate forms of treatment are in order.

Do fertility drugs cause multiple births? The rate of multiple births (mostly twins) is about 6 percent higher than average after treatment with clomiphene.

Is a "test-tube baby" a possibility? Yes. In the summer of 1978 the first test-tube baby, a girl, was born in England to a woman who had been infertile because of a problem with her tubes. The case gained much public-

34

ity, in which the test-tube aspect was overplayed. What actually happened was that one of the mother's eggs was removed from an ovary and placed in a culture dish where it was fertilized by the husband's sperm; the fertilized egg was then implanted in her uterus. Though conception occurred outside the womb, the baby developed inside her mother's body.

In what situation is artificial insemination done?　When it's determined that the man is infertile, he and his wife may decide to use sperm from an anonymous male donor. The doctor will determine the date that the woman is most likely to become pregnant and will then make arrangements to obtain semen from someone who matches the husband's physical characteristics and who is unlikely to be a carrier of a congenital disease. A small amount of the semen is injected into the cervix, and the rest is placed in the vagina beneath the cervix. More than one insemination may be necessary, but the success rate is high. About 70 percent of fertile women who are inseminated artificially will become pregnant within four or five months. Some doctors believe that it is psychologically beneficial for the man and his wife to have intercourse the same day as the artificial insemination so that it's not clear that one of the husband's own sperm didn't cause the pregnancy.

What can be done on our own before going to the specialist?　Someone has calculated that intercourse four times a week (without contraception) is most likely to induce a pregnancy. The tendency among couples anxious to have a child is to make love more frequently than that. Because frequent ejaculation may temporarily lower the man's sperm count, the emphasis should be placed on quality rather than quantity. By keeping a temperature chart or following the calendar method, the wife can tell when she is most likely to become pregnant. The use of the cervical-mucus test described earlier may also help. Intercourse the day of ovulation is most likely to lead to conception. The couple may have relations in any position, but ejaculation in the male superior position is most apt to allow the semen to remain in the vagina. The woman can help by remaining on her back for twenty minutes after the man's orgasm. A pillow placed under her hips will further expose the mouth of the womb to the sperm. Douching should be delayed for at least eight hours after lovemaking.

Why is it that when some infertile couples adopt a child, they almost immediately achieve a pregnancy of their own?　No one knows for sure, but the general feeling is that once a couple adopts a child, both tend to relax. Their lovemaking becomes less pressured by the desire for pregnancy, and this in itself seems to favor conception. Some persons have theorized that maternity stimulates a woman's body to produce hormones conducive to conception.

35

2

HAVING A BABY

How can you tell if you're pregnant? You may, of course, know you had an unprotected sexual experience and be alert to the possibility of pregnancy. A missed or late menstrual period in a woman who was previously regular is the most reliable sign of pregnancy, but early symptoms include nausea, frequent urination, fatigue, soreness in the breasts and a heavy feeling in the pelvis.

What's the earliest a pregnancy test will be positive? About two weeks after a missed period. This corresponds to four weeks after conception, and the test is positive in 80 percent of pregnant women. By a month after the missed period, the test is positive in 95 percent of pregnant women. The test depends on the presence in the urine or in the blood of a substance, chorionic gonadotropin, that is produced by the developing fetus. If a urine test is done, the first morning sample of urine should be submitted, and it should be kept on ice or frozen if there's any delay in getting it to the lab.

Are the tests ever wrong? Yes. False-positive tests, though rare, may be caused by taking birth-control pills, marijuana, tranquilizers and certain other drugs. A very rare type of tumor of the womb and a few other pelvic conditions may cause a false-positive pregnancy test. A doctor will be able to tell if any of these is present. The usual reason for a false negative test

36

is that the pregnancy isn't far enough along. The test should be repeated in two weeks to see if it has become positive.

How can you tell when the baby is due? To get an estimate of the due date, recall the day that you began your last menstrual period. Add seven days to this date, then subtract three months, and if necessary, correct for the year. For example, if the first day of your last period was June 1, adding seven days will give June 8. Subtracting three months will give an expected delivery date of March 8 of the next year.

Your chances of having the baby on the predicted date are only one in ten, but two-thirds of pregnant women go into labor within five days before or after the predicted date.

How long does pregnancy last? Under normal circumstances, 280 days. This is forty weeks, ten lunar months or just over nine calendar months.

What are the earliest body changes of pregnancy? The earliest notable changes occur in the breasts, which enlarge and become tender. The uterus grows rapidly, and by the sixth week (about the time of the second missed period) it has softened and turned a dusky blue color. This appearance of the cervix (the mouth of the uterus), known as Hegar's sign, is a reliable early indication of pregnancy.

When should you have the first doctor's appointment? For a first pregnancy an examination two or three weeks after the first missed period is advisable; the diagnosis of pregnancy can be confirmed and potential problems may be uncovered. For subsequent pregnancies the first appointment needn't be made until after you've missed two periods.

So that you can be screened for problems before they arise, many obstetricians believe that the optimum time for the first prenatal visit is before you become pregnant. Another reason for doing this is to make you begin looking for the right physician to take care of you and deliver the baby. But before selecting a physician, you have to make some other choices involved in having the baby.

CHOOSING HOW TO HAVE THE BABY

What are the choices one has to make in having a baby? There are three: the method of childbirth, where to have the baby, and the physician who will follow your condition during pregnancy. The choices should be made in the order given because one dictates the other that follows. If you're going to have the baby by natural childbirth, you have to decide this before you select the hospital and doctor; if you choose the doctor first, you may end up letting the physician make the other choices for you.

What are the methods of childbirth?   The main ones are prepared child-birth, natural childbirth and home delivery.

Prepared childbirth is the traditional method of delivery employed by doctors for the last several generations. The woman is followed through her pregnancy and given painkilling drugs during labor. She's offered a choice of agents during delivery and may be put to sleep or have a spinal or local injection of anesthetic. After delivery the baby is taken to the nursery and is brought to the mother only at prescribed times.

Natural childbirth involves prenatal education and breathing exercises to reduce labor pains by emphasizing natural processes and preventing fear. Drugs for pain are either not necessary or used minimally. The pubic hair is not shaved, and the child's father remains in the delivery room to help with the control of contractions and to witness the birth. Lying-in, a service offered by some hospitals, allows the baby to stay with you all the time or most of the time while you're in the hospital.

In home delivery, natural childbirth is usually accomplished with the aid of a midwife, though some physicians also do home deliveries. A doctor must regularly check your condition during pregnancy just as if you were going to have the baby in the hospital, and arrangements have to be made for transport to the hospital in the event of a complication before, during or after the delivery.

How do I choose a method?   The choice is up to you, and will be influenced by what you know about the various methods. Some of the reasons that prepared childbirth has lost its popularity are the higher risk of damage to the fetus by the use of anesthetic drugs, the treatment of birth as a "disease" rather than as a natural process, and the dehumanizing procedures (such as tying her hands) that the mother may be subjected to during labor and delivery.

The favorable aspect of natural childbirth is that the emphasis is shifted from the doctor to the mother. She is in charge of her labor and delivery; she learns how to control pain naturally and to coordinate her contractions with the stage of labor. The father is an active partner in the delivery and is present throughout the birth process. Some women who elect to have natural childbirth may find that they do want anesthetics during delivery; they should discuss this possibility freely with the physician.

Home delivery is, of course, the most natural method of all. It's also the least expensive—and, currently, the least common. It is best suited to the woman who has had one or more children previously and had no complica-tions during labor and delivery. Three musts for the woman contemplating this method of childbirth: a good hospital is nearby; reliable transportation is readily available; and a contingency plan will take effect should complica-tions arise.

What are the factors to consider in selecting a hospital? Some hospitals are better than others, and you may want to visit several before deciding where you'd like to have the baby. A shiny new one in the best part of town isn't necessarily the best. Evaluate the hospital's roominess or lack of it and the availability of doctors and nurses. Hospitals that have physician- and nurse-training programs are generally better than those that don't. The modernness of the equipment is important, as are an adequate blood bank, a good laboratory and comprehensive capability for handling obstetrical emergencies.

Ask if the hospital conducts training classes for the mother and father. If you want natural birth, find out if the hospital will let your husband stay with you in the labor room and accompany you into the delivery room. If you want lying-in does the hospital have it? If you choose to breast-feed the baby, will you be allowed to do it on demand or only at the hospital's official feeding times? The head nurse in charge of the obstetrics service, as well as the obstetrician you are considering or the doctor's nurse, should be able to answer these questions for you.

How do I find the right doctor to deliver my baby? Begin by making a list of the physicians available to you. Your gynecologist, who usually also practices obstetrics, might go on the list. Your internist or family physician might make a recommendation, and so might a friend who's recently had a baby. One possibility is to call the obstetrics ward of the hospital you are interested in and ask a nurse to recommend a physician whose views on childbirth are compatible with your own. You'll probably need an office visit to reach a decision about the doctor. Do not hesitate to see as many physicians as necessary to select the right one for you.

What questions should I ask the doctor? Stress that you want to have a trusting relationship with the doctor, and that you want to discuss certain matters that should be aired before they come up. Remember that although you're the patient, you're also a consumer of medical services. The decisions you make will affect your health and the baby's, and you deserve to know what to expect before contracting for the physician's services. The following questions can be broached in a polite and friendly fashion:

· *What hospitals are you affiliated with?* Since the doctor and the hospital go together, you need to know where the doctor has admitting privileges. In large cities the physician usually has privileges at more than one hospital.

· *How do you feel about natural childbirth?* If you've chosen to have the baby by a method other than prepared childbirth, find out how the doctor feels about it. Is he or she skilled in its use? Does the doctor object to the father being present during labor and delivery? Can the physician refer you to a good source for childbirth training classes?

39

· *How do you feel about weight control during pregnancy?* Physicians are trained to watch for excessive weight gain during pregnancy, but some physicians take the matter too far. They become alarmed at even slight increases above average weight, and may advise weight reduction during pregnancy for the overweight woman. Studies have shown that even an overweight woman should continue to gain weight during pregnancy. To do otherwise is to risk harming her baby. It's important to choose a physician who's aware of the nutritional needs of both the mother and the fetus.

· *Do you give diuretics routinely to all or most of your patients?* In the 1960s the vogue was to give diuretics freely to pregnant women. Now it is known that the great majority of pregnant women don't need these drugs, which may harm the mother or her unborn child.

· *Under what circumstances would you do a cesarean section?* Many people believe that the operation is being done too frequently. Your doctor can't always predict whether cesarean section will become necessary, but it doesn't hurt to explore his or her attitude about this form of delivery. Ask how often in the doctor's practice the operation becomes necessary. A cesarean section rate of over 10 percent of deliveries is probably excessive.

· *Will the doctor be available to deliver your child?* Increasing numbers of doctors practice in associations, so that the one who sees you initially may not be the same one who sees you the next time, and yet another physician may be present at the time of delivery. If this worries you, and you prefer to see one physician throughout your pregnancy and have this person deliver the baby, nail this down as a part of the initial agreement with the doctor.

· *Does the doctor mind your asking questions that relate to your care during pregnancy?* Schedule a first appointment that allows enough time to ask what you want to know. Certain physicians may be put off by your asking questions about the care you'll receive during pregnancy. The physician who answers questions with "Just leave that to me," is saying, in effect, that he or she will make all the decisions. If you have a choice, find another physician.

Is it best to have a specialist (obstetrician) deliver the baby?　A nurse midwife is perfectly capable of managing a normal birth, and so is a general physician. The real need for a specialist arises when a complication develops. The crucial point is that the complication may occur so quickly that it requires immediate attention to save the baby's or the mother's life. Thus, your risk and that of the baby are lowest when you are cared for and delivered by a specialist. It's best to go to a specialist from the start if you have diabetes, high blood pressure or another medical problem, or if you anticipate an Rh incompatibility or other problem during the pregnancy. But if it's your second or third child and you've had no difficulty before, you probably won't need the services of a specialist.

40

What are the credentials of a specialist?   A fully qualified obstetrician has served a four-year postgraduate training program in obstetrics and gynecology, and has been certified by the American Board of Obstetrics and Gynecology, the examining authority that conducts the certification tests. He or she may also be a Fellow of the American College of Obstetrics and Gynecology. Signs of additional qualifications include teaching appointments, authorship of scientific papers and membership on medical advisory committees.

CARE DURING PREGNANCY

What does the first doctor's visit involve?   The doctor will take a history and do a physical exam, including taking measurements to see if there's room in your pelvis for the baby to pass through. Routine tests include a Pap smear, blood count, blood typing and Rh factor determination, urinalysis and tests for syphilis and German measles antibodies. After the exam you can ask questions and get advice on such matters as nutrition, bowel habits and exercise.

How often should you see the doctor?   At least once a month until the seventh month of pregnancy. After that you should go every two weeks until the last month, when you should be seen weekly.

What should you eat during pregnancy?   If you are in good health and follow a well-balanced diet, you don't need to change your regular eating habits. A well-balanced diet consists of foods from each of these four food groups:
   · *Meats,* such as beef, veal, poultry, liver, fish, or high protein foods such as eggs, beans or dried peas
   · *Fruits and vegetables,* including citrus fruits, and green and yellow vegetables
   · *Breads and cereals,* such as bread made from whole grain or enriched flour, hot and cold cereals, brown rice, groats or other grains
   · *Milk and milk products,* such as cheese, yogurt, ice cream and butter (or its nondairy substitute margarine)
   Special emphasis should be placed on getting enough protein. The Food and Nutrition Board recommends a daily intake of sixty-five grams of protein during pregnancy. You need a daily minimum of three cups of milk, two or three servings of vegetables (including one dark green or deep yellow vegetable), two servings of meat or meat substitute (eggs, beans, fish or dried peas), four servings of whole-grain or enriched bread or cereals, one serving of citrus fruit, one serving of other fruit and a tablespoon of butter or margarine.

Consider, as well, what you should not eat. Candy, potato chips, soft drinks and similar products supply "empty" calories that aren't accompanied by much in the way of vitamins or minerals. You would do well to select the basic foods given above in preference to "junk" foods.

What about the teenager who is pregnant?   The pregnant teenager has a growing body within a growing body. Nutritional and calorie-intake requirements are higher than for a grown woman. A dietary consultation is indicated. In fact, consultation with a nutritionist is a good idea for any pregnant woman.

Do you need prenatal supplements?   You may not need supplements if you're healthy and you eat properly, but many doctors and nutritionists favor giving them routinely. It's possible, for example, to eat enough meat, liver and meat substitutes to get the eighteen milligrams of dietary iron needed each day during pregnancy. On the other hand, one iron tablet a day will supply this need. Good supplements contain a balanced amount of vitamins and minerals, including such essentials as calcium, folic acid and vitamin C.

What about salt intake?   So long as your blood pressure remains normal during pregnancy and you don't develop an undue amount of swelling, you can continue using the same amount of salt you did before pregnancy. Your physician, who is concerned with your health as well as the baby's, will tell you if you need to reduce your salt intake, but this should be done only if an abnormal condition warrants it. The current consensus is that salt restriction should not be prescribed routinely for pregnant women.

How much weight should you gain?   If your weight was normal before pregnancy, most physicians recommend a gain of about twenty-four to twenty-six pounds. If you were underweight before pregnancy, you might need to gain more than this amount; if you were overweight you might need to gain less. Rigid calorie restriction is certainly not indicated. Even the overweight mother or the woman who gains too much weight at the start of pregnancy should continue to gain weight right up until the time of delivery; to do otherwise is to risk harming the baby. Failure to gain enough weight can cause the baby to have a delay in development or a lower-than-average birth weight, which is associated with a higher fetal mortality rate. On the other hand, many an overweight woman can look back to a pregnancy as the beginning of her obesity. She gained an inordinate amount of weight, and never quite lost it after the baby was born. If you eat to appetite and choose nutritious food while restricting "junk" food, this isn't likely to happen.

How is the weight gain distributed?   A gain of twenty-five pounds would be distributed like this:

Weight of baby=seven and a half pounds
Weight of bag of water=two pounds
Weight of placenta=one pound
Weight gain of uterus=two and a half pounds
Weight gain of breasts=two pounds (one pound per breast)
Increase in weight of mother's blood=three and a half pounds
Increase in mother's fat stores=six and a half pounds

Since most of the baby's growth occurs in the last part of pregnancy, that is when most of the weight should be gained. As an average, the recommended gain is about two pounds during the first three months, eleven pounds during the second three months and twelve pounds during the last three months.

What medicines are safe during pregnancy?   You shouldn't take *any* drug of *any* kind at *any* time during pregnancy without first checking with your doctor. Even nonprescription drugs, such as aspirin, are not considered entirely safe during pregnancy. Sometimes medicines must be given during pregnancy, but these should be prescribed only when the danger of the illness outweighs the risk to the baby.

Especially important to avoid during pregnancy is the drug diethylstilbestrol (DES). At one time it was commonly given to pregnant women because it was thought to help prevent miscarriages. Babies born to mothers who took DES during pregnancy have shown an increased incidence of vaginal cancer and malformations of the reproductive organs. Since hormones similar to DES are present in birth-control pills, you shouldn't take the Pill if you have the slightest suspicion that you are pregnant.

Is smoking all right during pregnancy?   A woman who smokes a pack or more of cigarettes a day during her pregnancy will, on the average, have a baby weighing about twelve ounces less than the average weight of babies born to nonsmokers. Smoking does not affect the incidence of miscarriages or the fetal survival rate, but most obstetricians recommend that the expectant mother stop smoking.

Can I drink during pregnancy?   Alcohol in small amounts won't harm the baby, so you can safely have a cocktail a day. The consumption of large amounts of liquor is another matter. Babies born to alcoholic mothers may be underdeveloped (perhaps because of the poor nutrition so common to alcoholics), and the baby may show alcohol withdrawal effects shortly after it is born.

How much rest do I need during pregnancy? You need a good night's sleep and at least two rest periods during the day. Sleep eight hours or longer if you want to. A good way to tell if you're getting enough sleep is whether it takes the alarm clock to wake you every morning. If you're getting the rest you need, you ought to be waking up on your own. Plan to rest half an hour each morning and about an hour in the afternoon. Don't sleep during these daytime rest periods, as that might interfere with your sleeping at night. Just relax in a comfortable chair with your legs propped up. Turn off the TV, unplug the phone and don't read. Let your mind drift, and relax. Extra amounts of rest are indicated if you're carrying twins.

What activities can I tolerate during pregnancy? You can continue your usual activities, with one exception. Don't do things that cause you to be overly tired. Avoid long trips, staying up late and hard physical labor. You can safely continue on most jobs and you can swim, play tennis, dance, golf, bowl and do just about anything else you normally enjoy, so long as you're used to it and it doesn't exhaust you. Severe or prolonged fatigue may increase your risk of getting toxemia of pregnancy or of delivering your child prematurely.

What about walking? This is an excellent form of exercise during pregnancy. Begin with one brisk walk a day, and as your strength permits, increase it to two walks a day. Walking is good for the psyche as well as the body.

Is it all right to jog? Pregnant women have run the marathon distance. One person did it not too long before her baby was born and the baby was normal. Some joggers report that being in shape makes labor and delivery easier. So if jogging is a regular activity for you, it is probably safe to continue it after you're pregnant, so long as your doctor doesn't have any medical objections. You may have to cut down on your distance and speed, especially during the second half of pregnancy, and you should keep your obstetrician posted on any unusual symptoms you may develop. Fatigue must be avoided, and calorie intake may have to be adjusted depending on the amount of jogging you do. Most doctors feel that pregnancy is not the time to *begin* a jogging program, nor that pregnancy is conducive to competitive running.

Will sexual relations harm the baby? No. You're free to enjoy sex right up until the time of delivery if you wish, provided yours is a normal pregnancy and the doctor hasn't advised otherwise. Of course, the development of bleeding or discomfort following sexual relations should be reported to the doctor.

It may be best to avoid sex during the last month of pregnancy if you've had trouble with premature deliveries or episodes of premature labor pains. Contractions of the uterus may occur during orgasm, and these could bring about premature labor in a susceptible person.

What are the best positions for intercourse during pregnancy?   During the first third of pregnancy, intercourse is comfortable in any position. The woman-on-top position is suitable for the middle months of pregnancy. The wife can support her weight and keep her abdomen from pressing against her husband's body. The rear-entry position is best for the last months of pregnancy. The wife rests on her side while the husband enters her from the rear. The sitting position is another way of having coitus late in pregnancy. The husband sits in a chair or on the edge of the bed, and his wife takes a position on top of him. The usual sitting position is with the couple face to face, but late in pregnancy the wife may find it more comfortable to sit facing her husband's feet.

What form of sex is not safe during pregnancy?   Cunnilingus is not safe during the last three months of pregnancy. Presumably because of the increased blood flow to the vagina and womb, it's easier for air to be absorbed into the bloodstream, where it could cause harm. Several fatalities from this practice have been reported.

What about douching during pregnancy?   You should not douche. Deaths from air entering the bloodstream have occurred with the use of a hand bulb, and it is not a good idea to insert the nozzle or anything else more than two and a half or three inches into the vagina during pregnancy.

What about bathing?   This is all right in the shower or the tub, since bath water does not enter the vagina.

POSSIBLE PROBLEMS

Is swelling of the hands and feet a serious problem?   Not unless it's accompanied by a rapid, excessive weight gain or puffiness of the face or eyes. A certain amount of swelling is normal during pregnancy. It occurs in about two-thirds of pregnant women and is most noticeable in the hands, feet and ankles. Most of this swelling should disappear during the night, when the feet and hands are kept level with the heart by the flat surface of the bed.

What causes the swelling?   By virtue of being pregnant, the expectant mother retains fluid. Her blood volume expands to one and a half times its original amount, and her total increase in body water by the end of pregnancy will be about six and a half quarts. All this water places some strain on the heart and circulation. The insignificant swelling of the feet and ankles that may normally occur in dependent parts of the body becomes exaggerated during pregnancy, and this causes the swelling.

What can be done for the swelling?   Keeping the feet elevated when resting is one way of helping. Walking several blocks a couple of times a day is another way of reducing the amount of swelling. A moderate reduction in the use of table salt or salty foods may be necessary if the swelling persists, but this should be done only under careful supervision.

When is the swelling dangerous?   When it is accompanied by rapid and sizable gain in weight. A gain of a pound a week from about the fourth month on is permissible, but a gain of two pounds a week suggests excessive fluid retention. A gain of four pounds or more in a week is very suggestive of excessive fluid retention. This is one of the danger signs suggesting toxemia, and it calls for prompt treatment by the doctor.

What is morning sickness?   The nausea and vomiting that about half of pregnant women are bothered by during the first few months of pregnancy. After throwing up first thing in the morning, the expectant mother may feel fine; or she may have an upset stomach throughout the day.

What causes morning sickness?   Doctors aren't sure, but the hormone-rich environment of early pregnancy is thought to be the cause. The nausea tends to leave by about the third or fourth month of pregnancy, which corresponds to the time when the blood level of chorionic gonadotropin falls to a much lower level than was present earlier in pregnancy.

What can be done for morning sickness?   Eat a light breakfast of juice and toast. Avoid greasy foods, and space your eating into four small meals rather than three large ones. Try to get outside and breathe fresh air several times a day. If vomiting becomes a problem, the doctor can prescribe something for it. Among the common treatments are anti-vertigo drugs, but these should be used sparingly, and only after more natural methods have been tried. On rare occasions, a woman will develop nausea and vomiting that is severe enough to require treatment in the hospital.

What causes constipation during pregnancy?   From the stomach to the rectum, the digestive tract works more sluggishly during pregnancy. The weight of the womb on the lower intestine, reduced activity and a generalized relaxation of smooth muscle are other factors that contribute to constipation.

What can be done for the constipation?   The expectant mother should develop a regular bowel habit. Moderate amounts of exercise will aid in elimination, and so will eating high-fiber foods and drinking lots of fluids. Prune juice, apple juice, apples, peaches, pears, bananas, figs and apricots are foods that have a laxative effect. A mild laxative or a mild stool softener may become necessary, but these should be used with caution. Again, the best policy during pregnancy is to avoid, wherever possible, the use of any drugs.

What other symptoms are normal during pregnancy?   Backache is a frequent complaint. It may be relieved by wearing low-heeled shoes, getting adequate amounts of rest and wearing a well-fitting maternity girdle. Hemorrhoids occur more commonly than in nonpregnant women. Prevention of constipation and the use of anal suppositories may provide relief. Varicose veins may become a problem in susceptible persons. Elevation of the legs for thirty minutes at least four times a day will help, and elastic support stockings can be worn to prevent the veins from distending. Heartburn is a common complaint. The use of Gelusil, Riopan, Maalox or a similar antacid preparation should provide relief.

Is vaginal discharge anything to worry about?   Vaginal and cervical secretions increase during pregnancy and may cause a discharge. The amount is usually small to moderate. The new "mini pads" are useful for making you feel more comfortable. Discharge that persists or smells bad should be brought to the attention of the doctor.

What about spotting during pregnancy?   Any amount of bleeding should be reported to the physician, especially if it is accompanied by pain. Perhaps a fourth of pregnant women experience some spotting in the first months, but it is also one of the early signs of a miscarriage. The doctor may order mild sedatives and bed rest, and the bleeding will usually stop. The chances of the pregnancy continuing normally are good. Sexual intercourse should be avoided while spotting is present and for at least two weeks after the bleeding stops.

Bleeding during the later part of pregnancy tends to be more serious, for the uterus is large and its blood supply is great. The bleeding should be considered an emergency and no time should be wasted in getting to the hospital.

How do you know when a pregnancy is in trouble?   The danger signs are:
· Vaginal bleeding, meaning threatened miscarriage or premature labor
· A gush of fluid from the vagina, signifying rupture of the bag of water

· Severe abdominal pain, indicating miscarriage, premature labor or another complication

· Chills and high fever, indicating an infection

· Rapid weight gain, marked swelling, severe headache or visual disturbances, which point to toxemia of pregnancy

· Vomiting that goes on for several hours or more, signifying any of several possible complications

· Cessation of fetal movements for more than a day, when these were previously active, indicating possible death of the fetus

How often does miscarriage occur?   About 15 percent of pregnancies end in miscarriage.

What causes the miscarriage?   More than half of fetuses miscarried during the first half of pregnancy are found on examination to have developmental defects. The miscarriage was nature's way of eliminating what would have become a handicapped baby or one unable to survive on its own.

Surgery on the mother, such as an appendectomy, may cause her to miscarry. The mother who has kidney disease, high blood pressure, toxemia of pregnancy, diabetes or any serious illness runs an increased risk of having a miscarriage. Poor nutrition, thyroid disease and blood incompatibilities between the mother and the fetus are additional causes of miscarriage.

A condition known as "incompetent cervix" may lead to miscarriage in the second half of pregnancy. Losing its plug of mucus, the cervix opens and lets the fetus slip through. Abruptio placentae and placenta previa are other causes of miscarriage late in pregnancy. "Abruptio" refers to premature separation of the placenta, which loses its hold on the womb, and the woman notes vaginal bleeding and, perhaps, abdominal pain. In placenta previa, the placenta overlies the point where the uterus opens into the cervix. As a result, bleeding and loss of the baby may occur as the cervix begins to dilate during the last three months of pregnancy.

What can be done to prevent miscarriage?   Many doctors doubt that any treatment really helps, and the woman who is going to miscarry an early pregnancy will do so no matter what. Nevertheless, bed rest and mild sedation are prescribed when spotting occurs early in pregnancy. Good nutrition, healthy living and prompt medical therapy of any illness will increase a woman's chances of carrying a pregnancy to completion.

Miscarriage from an incompetent cervix can be prevented by applying a suture that acts as a drawstring to close the mouth of the womb. The suture must be removed at the onset of labor; or delivery can be by cesarean section. Prompt diagnosis and cesarean section may save the baby when abruptio placentae or placenta previa occurs.

What happens when a baby dies in the womb? Sooner or later it will abort spontaneously. In fact, most miscarriages occur after the fetus has already been dead for several weeks. The medical term "missed abortion" is applied when the products of conception are retained for two months or more after the death of the fetus. The woman, after some vaginal bleeding earlier in the pregnancy, may lose weight and note that her breasts are returning to their previous size. Very occasionally the fetus may be retained in the womb indefinitely. The danger in letting this happen is that it exposes the woman to the development of a serious and possibly fatal bleeding problem that is somehow triggered by the dead fetus. For this reason, the management of missed abortion is to induce labor with an oxytocin drip ("pit drip") or by injecting a saline solution into the womb.

ILLNESS DURING PREGNANCY

If I get sick, will it hurt the baby? Minor illnesses, such as a cold or sore throat, won't harm the baby, nor will bladder infection, skin infection, ear infection or similar problems. If drug therapy is required, penicillin or another antibiotic that doesn't harm the baby may be used.

Flu (influenza) might hurt the baby if the mother had a severe case of it during the first two or three months of pregnancy. Viral hepatitis, mumps, regular ("big red") measles, chicken pox and German measles are other infections capable of harming the baby during the first part of pregnancy. One virus, the cytomegalovirus, may cause only mild flulike symptoms in the expectant mother, yet severely infect her unborn child. It's best to avoid contact with children or adults who have any illness characterized by fever and rash or jaundice. Or if you're exposed to any of these conditions, notify your physician. An injection of gamma globulin to keep you from getting the disease may be indicated.

Are X-rays during pregnancy safe? Not really, though we don't yet know enough to say that a given amount of radiation will cause a certain defect in the developing fetus. We do know that the *ideal* amount of exposure is zero, especially in the first half of pregnancy. You don't need a chest X-ray, and you shouldn't have dental or other X-rays. The routine use of X-rays to measure pelvic size or to see how the baby is developing is no longer justified. An apparently safe procedure, ultrasound (see p. 53), can be used to check the baby's position or growth if necessary. If you get sick before you're sure you're pregnant, tell the doctor. X-ray studies can be postponed until you're sure you're not pregnant or until after the baby is born.

What are the dangers of German measles during pregnancy? The expectant mother who has German measles (rubella) during the first third of pregnancy may give birth to a child with defective vision or hearing, a heart murmur or mental retardation. About half of fetuses exposed to rubella during the first month of pregnancy will contract the infection. The incidence of congenital defects is lower when the infection occurs in the second or third month of pregnancy, but some risk persists should the mother have rubella even during the middle months of pregnancy.

A test for rubella antibodies is indicated in the initial evaluation of pregnancy. About 85 percent of adults will have the antibodies, and the mother can be reassured that she doesn't have to worry about German measles. If she doesn't have protective antibodies and contracts the disease, she may elect to have an abortion.

Since rubella vaccine is now available, all children between the ages of one and puberty should be inoculated. A pregnant woman cannot be immunized against German measles, since the live vaccine could infect the child she is carrying. However, she should be vaccinated right after her baby is born. Women who have the vaccination must take care not to get pregnant for three months afterward.

What about venereal disease during pregnancy?   Caught early, gonorrhea and syphilis can be treated and cured during pregnancy. The penicillin that is used to treat the mother will pass through the placenta and cure the baby, too. Since the causative virus does not respond to antibiotic therapy, the venereal disease known as herpes cannot easily be cured. The usual mode of spread to the fetus is by direct contact during delivery. For this reason an active herpes infection of the mother's genitals is an indication for delivery of her child by cesarean section.

Will diabetes affect my pregnancy?   Yes, control of diabetes is more difficult during pregnancy, and diabetic mothers have a higher risk of developing toxemia, having a serious infection or losing the baby through stillbirth. Even so, most diabetic women can carry and deliver a normal infant. Close care during the pregnancy is necessary, and the mother is often admitted to the hospital about four weeks ahead of her expected delivery date. Since babies born to diabetic mothers tend to be large, premature induction of labor or cesarean section may be indicated. Sometimes diabetes has its onset during pregnancy.

Will high blood pressure affect my pregnancy?   Yes, high blood pressure prior to pregnancy raises one's risk of developing toxemia of pregnancy. If drug therapy has controlled the blood pressure before pregnancy, it should continue to do so afterward. Thiazide diuretics, such as Esidrix or HydroDiuril, are standard drugs for controlling hypertension, but their usage during pregnancy must be weighed against the possibility of drug-induced jaundice or platelet deficiency in the fetus. A similar risk/benefit trade-off exists for the use of reserpine, Apresoline (hydralazine) and other antihypertensive drugs during pregnancy. Most of the newer antihypertensive drugs have not been tested for use during pregnancy.

What is toxemia of pregnancy?　　A condition that is unique to pregnancy, toxemia is characterized by sudden onset of high blood pressure, excessive weight gain and the appearance of protein in the urine. It is a disease of the first pregnancy and rarely occurs in subsequent ones. An exception is a situation where it complicates the pregnancy of a woman who had high blood pressure or diabetes prior to the pregnancy. Though diabetes or hypertension raises a woman's risk of developing toxemia, in most instances the cause of this complication is unknown.

How frequently does toxemia occur?　　Toxemia—or preeclampsia, a more modern term for the condition—occurs in 6 or 7 percent of pregnancies.

When do the symptoms of toxemia appear?　　Usually in the three or four months preceding delivery.

What are the risks stemming from toxemia?　　The most serious risk to the mother is the development of convulsions and coma, known as eclampsia. Though the incidence of eclampsia is quite small, one in ten women who develops it will die. The risk to the fetus is much greater: a reported 25,000 stillbirths a year occur as a result of toxemia of pregnancy.

What can be done for toxemia?　　Hospitalization is usually indicated. Complete bed rest will help to lower the blood pressure, and a low-salt diet may reduce the amount of swelling, which is usually most pronounced in the face and extremities. The source of difficulty in toxemia seems to reside in the kidneys, which tend to retain salt, hence the need for restricting its use. There is some controversy over this treatment, however. Drug therapy may be indicated to control the blood pressure or to prevent the onset of convulsions. The only specific treatment is to end the pregnancy. Doctors try not to resort to this until the last month of pregnancy, when the baby is big enough to have a good chance of surviving. Special techniques are available to check on the baby's maturity. Premature delivery in preeclampsia is usually done via cesarean section.

KNOWING ABOUT THE BABY

How does the Rh factor affect pregnancy?　　The condition doctors call "hemolytic disease of the newborn" was known to Hippocrates, but its cause was not unraveled till modern times. It is due to an Rh factor incompatibility between the pregnant woman and the fetus she is carrying.

51

The Rh factor is one of the blood types that are present on the surface of red blood cells. About 85 percent of people are Rh-positive, meaning they have the Rh factor on their red cells. The remaining 15 percent of the population are Rh-negative. These persons don't carry the Rh factor, but they are capable of forming serum antibodies against it if they are exposed to it through a blood transfusion or a pregnancy. Some mixing of the mother's blood with the fetal blood does occur late in pregnancy or at the time of delivery, and if an Rh-negative mother has an Rh-positive child, she may form antibodies against the Rh factor. In a subsequent pregnancy, these antibodies may attack an Rh-positive child to cause anemia, jaundice and the other features of hemolytic disease. Many such children are stillborn.

It's only when the mother is Rh-negative and the father is Rh-positive that problems may occur, and blood typing at the start of pregnancy will show if this is the case. If the pregnancy is at risk, further testing can be done to see if the mother's titer of antibodies rises. When necessary, a small amount of the amniotic fluid from around the fetus can be withdrawn for testing. Should this procedure—known as amniocentesis—show that the fetus is under attack by Rh antibodies, doctors may elect to give it transfusions while it is still in the womb. The more common method of treatment, however, is to induce labor early and give exchange transfusions to the newborn.

What can be done to prevent an Rh problem?　The incidence of hemolytic disease of the newborn has dropped since 1967, when a way of preventing the sensitization became available. Rhogam, a type of gamma globulin, is given to an Rh-negative mother within seventy-two hours after she has delivered an Rh-positive baby. The gamma globulin destroys any Rh-positive red cells that may have entered her bloodstream, and thus prevents her from forming antibodies against them. Rhogam should also be given to an Rh-negative woman who undergoes an abortion or miscarriage after the eighth week of pregnancy.

What causes a birth defect?　About 4 percent of babies have a birth defect, and among the things that predispose to it are:
· *Family history of an inherited disease,* such as hemophilia or Tay-Sachs disease (a blood test can show if you carry Tay-Sachs disease—see Chapter 5)
· *Previous pregnancy resulting in a child with a birth defect,* such as Down's syndrome (mongolism) or muscular dystrophy
· *Pregnancy complicated during the first few months by German measles or a generalized viral infection*
· *Exposure to harmful drugs, chemicals or X-rays* during pregnancy
· *Pregnancy occurring in a woman over forty years of age*

Can you tell if a baby will be defective?　　This may be possible through the use of amniocentesis, ultrasound or fetoscopy. Amniocentesis is the insertion of a needle into the womb and the removal of a small amount of the liquid surrounding the fetus. Studies can be done on this fluid to see if the child has a chromosomal or biochemical abnormality that is associated with a known birth defect. Since amniocentesis is ideally done between the fourteenth and sixteenth weeks of pregnancy, the parents may elect to have an abortion if the findings are positive for a defect. Amniocentesis also makes it possible to tell the sex of the fetus. This information may prove useful, as in the case of hemophilia, a condition that may appear in a boy but not in a girl when the mother carries the trait. Thus, the parents might elect to have an abortion when a fetus at risk of developing hemophilia is shown by amniocentesis to be a boy.

Ultrasound scanning of the womb is done in conjunction with amniocentesis so that the appropriate place for withdrawing fluid can be selected. The scan itself is also a screening test. Conditions such as hydrocephalus, microcephaly or anencephaly may be detected by ultrasound.

Fetoscopy is a new but promising technique for detecting fetal abnormalities. Through an instrument that resembles a tiny telescope, the doctor is able to visualize individual parts of the fetus, and even draw a blood sample if one is needed.

Do these tests ever cause miscarriage?　　Ultrasound doesn't, but the incidence of miscarriage following amniocentesis is about one out of every three or four hundred such studies. Obviously, amniocentesis is not a routine test. It shouldn't be done unless the risk of having a defective child outweighs the risk of causing a normal fetus to be miscarried. The same may be said for fetoscopy. It, too, may induce a miscarriage, though how often this occurs is not yet known.

Does amniocentesis ever fail to diagnose a defect?　　Yes. In a small percentage of cases, the amniocentesis indicates a normal pregnancy but a defective child is born. Conversely, the amniocentesis may indicate that a defect is present, yet on examination the aborted fetus is found to be normal.

Who should decide whether amniocentesis should be done?　　The parents should make the decision in collaboration with the obstetrician and a medical geneticist.

TUBAL PREGNANCY

What is a tubal pregnancy?　It's a form of ectopic pregnancy occurring in the tube instead of the uterus. Normally, fertilization takes place in the tube; the fertilized egg, or zygote, passes slowly to the uterus, where it implants and grows into a baby. In tubal pregnancy the zygote never reaches the uterus. Instead, it stops along the way and grows inside the thin walls of the tube.

What causes tubal pregnancy?　The most common cause is infection or scarring of the tubes by gonorrhea or some other infection. A complete obstruction of both tubes would make the woman infertile, so the obstruction is only partial—enough to allow the sperm to pass through on its way to fertilize the egg, but not enough to allow the egg to escape to the uterus. Other causes of tubal obstruction are endometriosis and scarring from pelvic surgery. A woman who's had trouble getting pregnant seems to have a higher risk of tubal pregnancy, and some experts believe than an endocrine or ovarian condition is responsible for many instances of tubal pregnancy.

How common is tubal pregnancy?　It occurs in about a third of a percent of pregnancies, or one in 300 women who become pregnant.

What are the symptoms of tubal pregnancy?　At first there are no symptoms. The woman may feel she is pregnant, or her periods may continue suggesting that she isn't. The fetus is usually three or four weeks more developed than would be expected from the number of missed periods. Spotting several days each month is not uncommon, and mild pain in the lower abdomen may be noted.

Between the sixth and twelfth weeks of pregnancy, the placenta ruptures through the thin wall of the tube causing hemorrhage into the abdominal cavity. This catastrophe is accompanied by excruciating lower abdominal pain and pain that may be referred to the shoulders. Dizziness, fainting and the other signs of shock (circulatory collapse) occur. Rarely, the bleeding is less calamitous and creates a condition resembling appendicitis or peritonitis.

What is the treatment of tubal pregnancy?　Because this is a life-threatening emergency, the first step is to get the woman to the hospital as quickly as possible. Once the diagnosis is made, the hemorrhaging tube must be removed by surgery.

Can you get pregnant again after having a tubal pregnancy?　Yes, about half of women who've been treated for tubal pregnancy get pregnant again.

The chances for carrying the subsequent pregnancy to term are better than three out of four.

THE GROWING FETUS

When does most of the baby's growth occur?   During the last three months of pregnancy. The baby weighs about a pound at the end of the sixth month, two and a half pounds at the end of the seventh month, five pounds at the end of the eighth month, and seven pounds or more at the end of the ninth month.

When, during pregnancy, does the baby start kicking?   The mother usually notices fetal movement about halfway through pregnancy, during the fifth month. The motion is very faint at first and becomes more noticeable later on. The movements start much earlier than the fifth month; it's only then that the fetus becomes large enough for the mother to detect the movement. A thin woman tends to be more aware of kicking than does an obese person, because fat insulates the fetal movements. The baby tends to be more active during a second or third pregnancy because the uterus gets larger and the baby has more room to move around.

What's the significance of the kicking?   It tells that the baby is alive and developing. The fetus doesn't just sleep and wait during pregnancy, it exercises! It grasps the cord, changes positions, makes sucking motions or hits the wall of the womb with a foot or a knee or an elbow. It tends to be most active during the sixth and seventh months of pregnancy, and less so afterwards because of its relatively large size and tight fit in the womb.

What if the kicking stops?   Periods of activity alternate with periods of rest, so it's normal for the kicking to stop for one or two days during the fifth or sixth month of pregnancy. If movement stops for more than two days during the last three months of pregnancy, notify the doctor. In the rare instance that a baby dies in the womb, the mother's sensation that the kicking has stopped is usually the earliest sign.

When can the doctor first hear the baby's heartbeat?   About the twentieth to twenty-second week of pregnancy. The sound is something like the distant ticking of a watch, and the heart rate is around 140 beats a minute.

What if the fetal heartbeat can't be heard later on during pregnancy? It's not unusual for the baby to shift position, making it harder at some times than at others to detect a fetal heartbeat. So long as the fetus continues its kicking and the expectant mother feels well, there's no need to worry. Most likely, the heartbeat will be heard at the next examination. When the doctor or mother is worried that something is amiss, an ultrasound test will tell for sure. The sound waves are reflected by the pulsing flow of blood, and the test will show whether or not the fetal heart is beating.

Can you tell if it's a boy or a girl?   Not by the amount of kicking, by the fetal heart rate or by the number of boys or girls you've had previously. The chances of it being a boy (or a girl) are fifty-fifty, and the only sure way to diagnose the baby's sex before labor and delivery is with amniocentesis. This procedure is not indicated for sex determination unless the fetus is at risk of an hereditary disease that strikes one sex but not the other.

The actual determination of sex is made by growing fetal cells in tissue culture, then counting their chromosome content. A boy has one "X" chromosome and one "Y," while a girl has two "X" chromosomes.

TWINS

How frequently do twins occur?   Twins occur once in every 80 or 90 live births. Triplets occur once in every 10,000 births; quadruplets once in every 500,000 births. The odds against having quintuplets are 50 million to one.

What causes twins?   A woman may release two eggs at ovulation, and if both are fertilized they will become fraternal, or nonidentical, twins. These twins may be of the same sex or one may be a boy and one a girl, and they will resemble each other more or less like normal siblings. The other cause of twins is a situation where one egg is fertilized by one sperm, then divides into two separate masses that grow in the womb as identical twins. These twins are always of the same sex and are identical in appearance.

Are some people more prone to have twins?   Yes, factors that increase the risk of twinning are:
  · *A family history of twin births,* especially if the mother or father is a twin
  · *Pregnancy occurring when the mother is thirty-five or older,* though a young woman may have twins as her first pregnancy
  · *Therapy with fertility drugs,* such as clomiphene
  · *Miscellaneous factors,* such as race and number of previous pregnancies. The chance of having twins increases with each pregnancy, and you're three times as likely to have twins if you're black than if you're white or Oriental. It has been determined that the frequency of twinning is related to the frequency of coitus. A high incidence of twin births occurred in the post–World War II years when servicemen first returned home, and twin births are more common when a couple is married or living together than when pregnancy occurs after a single act of intercourse.

How can you tell if you're carrying twins? The signs of multiple pregnancy are rapid weight gain not due to swelling or obesity, unusually large uterus for the number of months of pregnancy, and the sensation by the expectant mother that she has more than one baby kicking in her womb. The doctor may be able to make the diagnosis by hearing more than one fetal heartbeat.

The most accurate way to diagnose twins, triplets or the like is with an ultrasound study. Sound waves of an intensity too high to hear are beamed into the abdomen and reflected back by the underlying structures to give a visual image of what's in the uterus. Ultrasound is widely used and apparently safe, but because some questions have been raised about its long-term effects, it should not be employed unless there are definite indications for the study.

Are twins harder to deliver? Because twins are generally born about three weeks prematurely, each weighs about two pounds less than the average singleton. Thus, labor and delivery may not be more difficult. The woman carrying twins does have a greater risk of toxemia of pregnancy, and is more likely to have excessive blood loss at the time of delivery. The second twin is usually born five to fifteen minutes after the first one, but the second birth may be delayed for several days. In one instance, twin births occurred fifty-six days apart. The first twin weighed only three and a half pounds, but the birth weight of his brother, born two months later, was almost six pounds. By that time the first twin also weighed six pounds.

What causes Siamese twins? They are always identical twins, and it is thought that the egg that divided into two masses to form them did not divide completely. Thus, they were left joined at the head, abdomen or pelvic area.

LABOR

Can you get abdominal pains before the onset of labor? Yes, the pains of false labor, known as Braxton Hicks contractions, are most noticeable during the last month of pregnancy. During the week before delivery they may occur every ten or twenty minutes. One purpose of these contractions is to help flatten out the cervix and prepare it for the dilatation that will be necessary during the child's birth.

How can you tell between actual labor and false labor? The pains of false labor occur irregularly and at long intervals. They are most prominent in the lower abdomen. The pains may last two minutes or more, but they tend to be short. They don't increase in severity, and they aren't made worse by walking. Actual labor pains begin at the top of the womb, move down through its muscular walls, and radiate into the back. The pains occur at regular intervals, last half a minute to a minute, and tend to become more frequent and more severe as labor progresses. The pains of actual labor are usually intensified by walking.

One fairly sure sign of actual labor is the so-called bloody show. The "show" is a small amount of blood-tinged mucus which is discharged from the vagina after labor begins. It represents the release of the mucus plug that has been in the mouth of the womb during pregnancy.

When should you go to the hospital?   At the onset of actual labor. Since you may not know when this begins, call your doctor and describe the pains you're having and how often they are occurring. Pains that are regular and that occur every five or six minutes (or more often) usually indicate actual labor.

What if the sac of water breaks?   The chances that this will happen are only one in ten, and you should not be disturbed if it does occur. You'll note the sudden escape of a cup or more of warm fluid. Call the physician to explain what's happened, and he or she will probably want to examine you or admit you to the hospital. In most instances, labor begins within twenty-four hours of the rupture of the sac of water.

Will the ruptured water sac make delivery more difficult?   Not usually. For one thing, not all the fluid will come out, and for another, the fluid itself is not what lubricates the birth passage. The main problem with a ruptured sac is that infection may occur if the baby isn't delivered within a day or so. This is why it's best to go into the hospital once the sac ruptures. In some instances, protective antibiotic therapy may be given if delivery is delayed for more than a day after the sac breaks.

What do you do if a part of the cord or a part of the baby comes out before you reach the hospital?   Lie down so that the force of gravity will not be directed downward. Call an ambulance to transport you to the hospital, or, if you're already en route, proceed there as quickly and safely as possible. *Do not try to push the protruding part back inside.* Especially to be avoided is any attempt to hold the baby's head in or to keep the mother's legs closed until arrival at the hospital. It's better to have the baby in a taxi than to risk damaging its brain at this critical point in the birth process.

How long does labor last?   The average length of labor for the first baby is about fourteen hours. The length of labor for subsequent babies averages eight hours or less. Your labor may be shorter or longer than average.

Factors that favor a short labor are second or subsequent baby, small baby, head-first position and a previous history of short labor. Factors that suggest a longer labor are first baby, large baby and breech birth. All else being equal, the woman with large bones and a roomy pelvis will have a shorter labor than the small-boned woman with a small pelvis.

What are the three stages of labor?   The first stage begins at the onset of labor and lasts until the cervix is flattened and completely dilated; this stage lasts for about twelve and a half hours when it's the first baby. The second stage of labor begins when the cervix is fully dilated and ends when the baby is born. It lasts about an hour and a half. The third stage begins with the birth of the baby and ends when the placenta is delivered. It lasts only five minutes.

How wide does the cervix have to dilate before the baby can get out?   It has to reach a diameter of ten centimeters, a little more than four inches. The last five centimeters of dilation go much more quickly than the first five.

When can pushing down begin?   Once the cervix is fully dilated, pushing down will help to expel the baby. The woman who has practiced natural childbirth will know how to coordinate her breathing and muscular effort with the uterine contractions.

NATURAL CHILDBIRTH

What is natural childbirth?   It is the opposite of prepared childbirth. Instead of relying on drugs, anesthesia and obstetrical maneuvers such as the use of forceps, the woman learns about the physiology of birth, practices breathing techniques and does abdominal exercises, all of which prepares her to have the baby in the encouraging presence of her family and friends. She is not tied down, shaved, forced to lie in one position or put to sleep during the delivery. The main difference between prepared and natural childbirth is a shift in emphasis. The mother is in control; the doctor or midwife is an assistant.

How did natural childbirth develop?   It came about through the efforts of women who had gone through the traditional, prepared method of child-birth and found it less than satisfactory. They looked to Europe for a better way, and found it in the "childbirth without fear" method of Dr. Grantly Dick-Read of England, and the "childbirth without pain" method of Dr. Ferdinand Lamaze of Paris. Though the medical establishment in the United States resisted natural childbirth (and continues to resist it in many ways), the popularity of the method along with the women's movement of the 1960s and 1970s helped to force its acceptance.

In defense of American doctors, it must be said that prepared childbirth was itself developed in response to a women's movement. In the early part of this century, feminists berated the medical profession for its seeming indifference to the pain of childbirth. When it was discovered that German doctors were able to treat labor and delivery in a way that allowed painless childbirth, the technique was brought to America. It was known as "twilight sleep," and involved the use of morphine and scopolamine during labor; the mother was given ether or chloroform during the actual birth. A few American doctors tried the technique and rejected it as unsafe. However, in 1914 Dr. Eliza Taylor Ransom, a Boston physician, opened the Twilight Sleep Maternity Hospital. Prominent women, such as Mrs. John Jacob Astor, helped to publicize the new method. Soon other American doctors had taken it up. With the modification that safer drugs and more technology have been added, twilight sleep has remained the traditional method of prepared childbirth.

In time, women began to complain that childbirth was being treated like a disease. The woman in labor was admitted to the hospital and kept isolated from her husband and friends. Doctors and nurses were often cavalier in their attitude ("You got it in there, honey, so you're going to have to get it out") and gave painkilling drugs with inadequate thought to the respiratory depressant effects the injections might have on the fetus. The birth itself was like an operation: drugged and tied to the delivery table, the woman woke up with stitches in her bottom and no memory of what had happened. Perhaps most frustrating of all, the baby was whisked away as soon as it was born, and except for a few visits, held physically separated from the mother until she left the hospital. Small wonder that so many women wanted a change!

What does natural childbirth entail?   Most of all, it is a learning process. The woman and her partner attend the training sessions regularly during the last two months of pregnancy, and they learn to work as a team in coordinating their breathing efforts and relaxing between pains. Since fear may contribute to pain, they are taught the physiology of childbirth. They learn about the stages of labor and when it is and isn't best to bear down. They learn the technique of blowing air in and out to keep from pushing, and take exercises to make the muscles stronger for the time when pushing is needed. The woman is taught ways to concentrate on her breathing rather than on the labor pains, and how to move into different positions to make labor more comfortable. She learns that birth is something she accomplishes by her active involvement, and she can take comfort from knowing that her partner will be there to assist her throughout labor and delivery.

What is the Lamaze method?   It is essentially the one outlined above, and it draws on the work of Dr. Ferdinand Lamaze as well as of many others. As early as the 1930s, Grantly Dick-Read stressed that birth could be a moment of supreme triumph for the woman if her fear of it were removed. Ferdinand Lamaze of the Paris metalworkers' clinic came along some years later to offer the psychoprophylaxis method of childbirth. He and his colleague, Dr. Pierre Vellay, based the method on Russian experience that was, in turn, based on Dr. Pavlov's work.

Dr. Lamaze did not claim that every woman who used his method would have painless birth, but he did find that 90 percent of them were able to go through labor and delivery without drugs or anesthetics. His method was given a great boost in popularity in 1959, when Marjorie Karmel, an American living in Paris, published the book *Thank You, Dr. Lamaze.* Since then the terms "natural childbirth" and "the Lamaze Method" have been used interchangeably.

How available is training for natural childbirth? The training classes are available in most cities, though not every hospital will allow birth by this method. A sign of progress is that obstetricians in many areas encourage, or even require, their patients to attend natural childbirth sessions. Still, there are some doctors who pay lip service to natural childbirth while continuing to employ forceps, episiotomy and drug injections even on paticnts who have been assured that the delivery would be "natural." The only way to prevent being deceived is to take careful steps to select the right physician to deliver your baby. It is also important to remember that some circumstances may require departure from the natural childbirth routine.

Many women consider lying-in to be just as important as natural childbirth, because the baby, after all, is what birth is about. Hospitals have tended to be more unyielding than doctors in their insistence that the child bc kcpt in the nursery except at feeding time. However, lying-in is permitted in an increasing number of hospitals; usually, the mother has the option of letting the baby return to the nursery for several hours a day.

How do you know if natural childbirth will work for you? You don't, but you've lost nothing in trying it. At worst, the training wastes time. At best, it can give you a healthier baby, a more secure feeling during labor, and the contentment of being in control during delivery. It can make birth the moment of supreme joy it was meant to be.

HOME DELIVERY

Why the movement toward home delivery? Until this century all deliveries occurred in the home. The return to this method was prompted by the feeling of many women that hospitals removed the joy of birth, subjected the mother and her baby to dehumanizing and even dangerous procedures, and charged exorbitant fees for these "services."

What are the advantages of home delivery? You can have the baby in a natural setting surrounded by family and friends. The cost is less. You don't have to worry about being strapped to a table, shaved or put to sleep. After delivery, you can keep your baby with you.

How is the delivery accomplished? Natural childbirth is employed, and delivery is usually by a midwife, or a nurse-midwife, a registered nurse with special training in obstetrics. Some physicians will perform home deliveries.

How safe is it? In a study of two thousand women, half of whom delivered in a hospital and the other half at home, home birth was as safe or safer than hospital delivery. Home births required less anesthesia and vaginal tears were fewer, in spite of the fact that hospital births routinely involved episiotomies to prevent such tears.

What kind of prenatal care is involved? The woman should have the same kind of prenatal care she would get if she were going to deliver in a hospital. This may create a problem, as most doctors will not give prenatal care to someone planning an out-of-hospital delivery. Getting good prenatal care thus constitutes the main problem of those who want home delivery.

Why are so many obstetricians against home delivery? Physicians have been trained in hospital delivery as a part of centralized medical care. With good reason, they speak of the hospital's sterile environment and ability to cope with infection, hemorrhage or other complications. The disagreement hinges on whether all women need hospital delivery just in the event of a complication. Money is another consideration. The obstetrician derives a good part of his or her livelihood from hospital deliveries, and stands to lose it if women begin having their babies at home.

Who qualifies for home delivery? Even the advocates of this method admit that not all deliveries can take place in the home. A woman with a health problem or the likelihood of a complicated delivery, such as a breech birth, should have the baby in the hospital. Hospital delivery is definitely indicated when the baby is born prematurely. Despite careful prenatal screening, 5 percent of women who attempt home delivery run into a problem and must be taken to the hospital. Here are some guidelines that can help you decide if you're qualified for home delivery:

· You've had at least one baby in a hospital setting and the delivery was normal. (It's best not to attempt the first delivery at home.)

· You've been followed during pregnancy by an obstetrician, and you have no signs indicating a problem with your health, the delivery or the baby's chances of surviving.

· You're sure by dates and size that the baby is full-term, not premature.

· You and your partner have taken natural childbirth training.

· You have the services of a physician or a competent, licensed midwife to perform the delivery.

· You have the means for quick conveyance to a nearby hospital in the event of a complication.

PREPARED CHILDBIRTH

What is prepared childbirth?　It is a hospital delivery done by a doctor on a woman who's usually had little or no childbirth training. At the onset of labor the expectant mother is admitted to the labor room, "prepped" by being shaved and given an enema and perineal scrub, then given analgesics for her pain. She is not allowed to have food or liquid by mouth. Delivery (usually without the father present) is accomplished with the help of anesthesia, low forceps and an episiotomy.

What can be done to ease labor pains?　Natural childbirth training will probably keep you from needing a painkilling drug during labor. By changing positions and controlling your respiration, you learn to concentrate on the labor itself rather than on the pain. When an injection is requested, Demerol and a tranquilizer, such as Phenergan or Vistaril, are usually given.

Timing of the injection is important. It shouldn't be given until labor is well under way, as too early an injection may stop the progress of labor. By the same token, it should be injected no later than about two hours before the baby is born. The painkiller has as one of its actions a depressant effect on respiration, and if it is given shortly before birth it can interfere with the newborn's efforts to breathe.

Can a long labor be speeded up?　Yes, in the same way that labor is induced—provided that the woman's pelvis is large enough to permit normal delivery. In the event that the reason for the delay in delivery is a small or contracted pelvis, giving a drug to stimulate uterine contractions might cause the uterus to rupture.

When should labor be induced?　The doctor may induce labor when the mother has toxemia of pregnancy, is diabetic or has any condition that could affect her health or the baby's if pregnancy is allowed to continue.

Elective induction is done on occasion when the woman and her doctor believe the baby is due or past due and yet labor hasn't occurred. This form of induction is not indicated unless the fetus is fully developed and the woman is ready for labor. Evidence of this is apparent in the cervix: "ripe," it is soft, flattened and partly dilated.

How is induction done? Rupturing the bag of water may bring on labor within an hour or two. If labor doesn't start in this time, an intravenous drip of oxytocin ("pit drip") is begun. Oxytocin is a hormone that has as its main action the ability to cause the uterus to contract. If it is going to work in starting labor, it usually does so within a few hours—eight at most.

Is it dangerous to induce labor? The risk to the mother and her child is greater than with natural onset of labor, which is why induction for the doctor's convenience is never indicated. Even when a valid reason for inducing labor exists, certain precautions must be observed. Someone must watch the mother closely while she's receiving the oxytocin, and someone must monitor the fetal heartbeat to make sure the drug doesn't harm the baby. The dreaded complication of labor induction—a ruptured uterus— is a rare event, but to lessen its likelihood a woman over thirty-five, or one who's had five or more children, should not have labor induced.

What are forceps? This is an instrument the doctor may use to guide the baby's head through the last part of the birth tract. It actually consists of two curved blades that are applied separately around the baby's head, then locked together near the handle. With a steady downward pull, the physician can help to extract the baby's head.

What's the purpose of a forceps delivery? The application of "low forceps" is generally thought to shorten the second stage of labor and reduce the risk of injury to the baby's brain. Misapplication of forceps could have the reverse effect and damage the brain.

Are forceps necessary to deliver the baby? Not in most cases.

What are the "stitches" taken just before the baby is born? The cut is known medically as an *episiotomy.* It may be done in the midline between the vagina and the anus, or at about the seven or eight o'clock position downward from the vagina. "Stitches" refers to the appearance and feel of the cut after it is sewn up.

What's the purpose of the episiotomy? To make it easier for the baby's head to get out. Otherwise the head may become a battering ram that tears the vulva, bladder or rectum (these tears could also require stitches). In effect, the episiotomy substitutes a straight cut for the jagged lacerations that may occur during natural childbirth. An additional benefit claimed by doctors and some women is that the episiotomy helps to prevent the relaxation of pelvic muscles that would occur were the woman to have several children the natural way.

When is the cut made?   Soon after the baby's head begins to bulge against the vulva. If low forceps are used, the episiotomy is done right after the forceps are in place.

Do the stitches have to be removed?   No, the suture material is absorbable.

Can you get by without an episiotomy?   Yes, and more and more women are requesting that episiotomy not be performed routinely.

What anesthesia should I choose?   This depends on your personal preference, the speed with which labor progresses, and how well you tolerate the delivery. It also depends to some extent on the doctor, since he or she may be more skilled at one method than another. All these methods have disadvantages, as listed below. Here are the choices:
  • *Analgesia,* the injection of a painkiller, such as Demerol, will reduce labor pains without putting you to sleep. The disadvantage of analgesia is that it can't be used during the second stage of labor, when contractions are at their peak of intensity.
  • *Spinal anesthesia,* performed by injecting an anesthetic drug into the spinal canal, will also let you stay awake to witness the birth of your child. Since the area put to sleep corresponds to the area that touches the saddle when you ride a horse, it is often called a "saddle block." (See following question.)
  • *Epidural block* is similar to a spinal, except that the needle's progress is stopped just before it enters the spinal canal. The usual technique is to leave a thin tube in place at the site of the injection, so that additional amounts of anesthesia can be given without the need for sticking you again. (See following question.)
  • *Pudendal block* is done by giving two injections through or near the vagina to deaden this region just before the baby's head passes through. The length of the needle used for the injections is enough to scare you to death if you happen to see it, and many women report that a pudendal doesn't help that much anyway.
  • *Local infiltration* is the injection of a local anesthetic in the skin below the vagina just before an episiotomy is cut.
  • *Gas (general) anesthesia,* is given by mask inhalation or through an endotracheal tube. A "general" is not so commonly used as it once was, but it may be indicated when rapid anesthesia is necessary, as for an emergency cesarean section. Intermittent inhalation of nitrous oxide will help with the pain without putting you to sleep, and light amounts of this gas won't hurt the baby.

What effect does anesthesia have on the baby?   General anesthetics are capable of depressing the baby's respirations. So is Demerol, if given an hour or two before birth. When Demerol is responsible for sluggishness in a newborn, an injection that will counteract its effects can be given. To minimize fetal depression, general anesthesia should not be used unless delivery is imminent and can be accomplished within five minutes of the onset of anesthesia. Otherwise, the baby will also be anesthetized and will require resuscitation after birth.

Spinal anesthesia, epidural block and pudendal block do not depress the baby directly, but may cause a dangerous fall in the mother's blood pressure that indirectly harms the fetus. A moderate fall in the mother's blood pressure is frequently observed after the use of these methods. Another effect that has been reported recently is a severe change in the fetal heart rate, perhaps resulting from an impairment of its oxygen supply.

What are the effects of anesthesia on the mother?   General anesthesia may cause heart irregularities and may be—very rarely—fatal. The nausea and vomiting that often follow the use of gas is particularly dangerous if the woman has eaten within a few hours before induction, as she may aspirate the stomach contents into her windpipe.

Any injection into the spinal canal may cause the recipient to have severe headache lasting up to several days or longer. A more distressing long-term problem is the backache reported by some women who had spinal anesthesia during childbirth. The cause of the persistent backache is poorly understood, and long-term studies are needed to evaluate it before one can accept the frequently quoted "safety" of this method of anesthesia. Even the injection of local anesthetic into the skin at the site of an episiotomy could cause a serious or fatal reaction in a woman who is allergic to the anesthetic.

BREECH BIRTH

What is a breech birth?   This occurs when the baby's lower body, instead of its head, is the presenting part that must be delivered first.

How often does a breech presentation occur?   In about 3 or 4 percent of deliveries.

Can a breech be prevented?   This is possible if the baby's position is discovered in time. The maneuver to change the baby's position to be headfirst is known as *external version.* The physician applies pressure to the womb and gently rotates the baby's body a hundred and eighty degrees. External version can be performed during the last two months of pregnancy, but it is successful in only a small percent of cases.

Is a breech birth dangerous?   The risk is to the fetus. Headfirst, the baby's largest part comes out first and the smaller shoulders and body follow. With a breech, the buttocks are delivered first, then the shoulders and head. The umbilical cord may be compressed against the pelvic wall, thus cutting off blood flow to the fetus. Or the pressures that come to bear on the head may cause brain damage. The overall fetal death rate subsequent to a breech birth is about six times higher than for babies born headfirst.

CESAREAN SECTION

What is cesarean section?   It is the operation to deliver the baby by an incision through the lower abdomen and uterus. Popular belief has it that Julius Caesar was born this way, but it's more likely that the word came from the Latin verb *caedere* ("to cut"). Since "section" also means "to cut," *cesarean section* literally means "to cut, to cut."

When is cesarean section indicated?   The most frequent cause for a first cesarean section is that the baby can't pass through the birth canal because it is too large for the mother's pelvis, or that its position is so unusual as to make vaginal delivery impossible. Diabetes, toxemia of pregnancy, fetal distress and severe vaginal bleeding late in pregnancy are other conditions that may necessitate cesarean section. The most common overall indication for cesarean section is previous cesarean section.

Is cesarean section needed for every breech birth?   Not according to the authoritative textbook *Williams Obstetrics* (fourteenth edition), whose authors cited a large study showing that cesarean section was necessary in only one out of ten breech births. This contrasts with the current recommendation of some obstetricians that all breech babies be delivered by cesarean. Such a large increase, even in the wake of modern technology, is not indicated. The woman should first be given a trial of labor to see if she can deliver the baby vaginally.

What is a trial of labor?   It's the time allotted to a woman in labor to see if she can deliver her baby normally. The trial period varies, but is usually at least four to six hours of active labor. A trial of labor may be given for a breech presentation or other unusual presentations, or when the baby is thought, but not known, to be too large for the mother's pelvis. If progress toward delivery isn't accomplished after a reasonable trial of labor, cesarean section may become necessary.

How frequently is cesarean section done?   Until ten or fifteen years ago, cesarean section was done in about 6 percent of deliveries. Current estimates are that the rate is at least twice that now, perhaps 15 percent in some hospitals and even higher than that in others.

Why the increase? The emphasis in obstetrics has shifted from primary concern with the mother's health to a greater awareness of the factors that may harm the fetus during or just before delivery. Better equipment has made monitoring of fetal distress possible, and cesarean section has saved many babies who otherwise would have been stillborn or brain-damaged.

Other factors may also be at work having to do with the physician's convenience as well as the patient's welfare. A section can be done quickly, is well paid and entails relatively little risk.

What is the risk involved in cesarean section? About two maternal deaths per one thousand operations, though at many hospitals where thousands of sections have been done over the last decade, there have been no maternal deaths. The death rate of infants born by cesarean section depends on the condition for which the operation is done. When a cesarean must be resorted to in an emergency, such as vaginal hemorrhage, the fetal death rate is as high as 10 or 12 percent. When the section is done as an elective procedure, the chances of the baby surviving are better than 99 percent.

Can I still have a baby the natural way after I've had a cesarean? This depends on why the first operation was done. If your pelvis was too small for normal delivery, you'll probably need a cesarean for each subsequent pregnancy. If the first operation was done for a reason other than size proportions, you may be able to have subsequent children vaginally. In some hospitals half of the patients with previous sections are able to bear children the natural way.

The chances of a subsequent normal delivery are better if the doctor does the cesarean operation through a bikini-shaped cut in the lower part of the womb. Scars there heal better, with less risk of rupture of the uterus during a subsequent labor.

THE NEWBORN

What does the baby look like at birth? A normal newborn comes out wet and slippery and crying. The wetness is due to what's left of the bag of water, and the slipperiness comes from a coating of *vernix caseosa,* a greasy substance which looks like cold cream and which served to protect the baby's skin from the womb fluid during pregnancy. The crying reflects the baby's first breaths.

What is the Leboyer technique? The purpose of Dr. Frederick Leboyer's technique of "birth without violence" is to spare the newborn the usual traumatic events of being dangled by the feet, spanked and subjected to suctioning of the mouth and nose. Instead, the moment of birth is made a peaceful, loving occasion for the baby. The lights in the delivery room are dimmed. The newborn is placed on its mother's abdomen and soothed and calmed. After the cord is cut, the baby is immersed in a warm bath.

Critics of the Leboyer technique claim that the risk of an infection is higher from immersing the baby in water, and that the crucial first minutes after birth need to be given to examining the baby's heart, respiratory and other functions.

What is the Apgar rating?   It is a scoring system developed by Dr. Virginia Apgar to aid the physician in evaluating the newborn's status. The scoring, done at one minute and again at five minutes after birth, is based on awarding zero, one point or two points for each of five functions of the new baby. These are its heart rate, breathing effort, muscle tone, reflexes and skin response to breathing. The lowest possible score is zero, while a perfect score is ten.

What's the purpose of the Apgar rating?   A normal infant will have an Apgar score of seven or higher. One with an Apgar of three or less is in jeopardy. The physician must institute immediate resuscitative measures. An Apgar rating that remains low at five minutes correlates with a higher risk that the child may fail to take its first breath or may die during the first few weeks after delivery.

What are the chances that a baby will survive and be normal?   They're very good. Though the United States still ranks seventh among countries of the Western world in infant survival rate, the overall survival for liveborn babies is 98.5 percent. The chances that a normal-weight infant will survive are better than 99 percent.

What's the main cause of death among newborns?   Prematurity, defined medically as a birth weight of less than five pounds, is the most common cause of death among newborns. The chances of survival are extremely low if the baby weighs less than two and a half pounds at birth.

What's the normal weight of a newborn?   The *average* weight of newborns is about seven and a half pounds, but a normal baby may weigh between five and a half and eleven pounds. A baby weighing less than five pounds is considered premature, while a baby weighing over ten pounds is considered excessively large. Boys, on the average, weigh three ounces more at birth than do girls.

What's the normal length of a newborn?   The *average* newborn is about twenty inches long, but a normal baby may be shorter or longer than this if its birth weight is normal.

69

What is the placenta?   It is the pancake-shaped structure that draws blood from the mother's circulation and delivers it by way of the umbilical cord to the fetus. At birth, it is six to eight inches in diameter and weighs about a pound.

When will the placenta come out?   Within five minutes after the baby is born.

When will I get to see my baby?   Preferably as soon as it is born. Studies have shown that the baby benefits from immediate contact with its mother, and the trend in hospitals is away from the unnecessary practice of keeping parents and child separated. No higher incidence of infection or other complications has resulted from allowing the parents to hold the baby and cuddle it in the first hours and days after it is born.

AFTER THE BABY IS BORN

How long do you have to stay in the hospital?   The average stay is three to five days after the baby is born. A woman may enjoy having this time to rest, or she may want to leave as soon as possible. If she's doing well, the physician usually lets her be discharged when she wishes.

How quickly do you recover from childbirth?   The official recovery period is six weeks. Your breasts may engorge for a day or two, but breast-feeding, hormone therapy or the passage of time will control this. You'll have a vaginal discharge that is bloody at first, then turns brown as it slacks off in a couple of weeks. You may note an increase in urine output. You'll probably sleep better and eat better and feel more exhilarated than you've felt in a long time.

Anything special to watch for?   Infection and hemorrhage are the main postpartum complications. Let the doctor know if you have fever, chills, headache or backache. The passage of clots, bright red blood or a sudden increase in bleeding may point to retained placenta or bleeding from the stitches. Sometimes the bleeding occurs so rapidly it creates an emergency, but any amount of bleeding calls for a medical evaluation.

When is it safe to resume sexual relations?   A safe interval is three weeks after delivery, or when the doctor gives the go-ahead. Abstinence for five or six weeks postpartum is rarely necessary.

When will my periods start again?   About two months after delivery, unless you breast-feed the baby. Nursing delays the onset of menstrual

70

periods till three or four months or even a year after delivery, depending on how long you continue the breast-feeding and on how your body reacts to it.

When do I need to be seen again by the doctor? Between three and six weeks after the baby is born. This is the time for a thorough examination, and it's an opportunity for you to discuss family planning techniques with the physician.

How soon can another pregnancy occur? It can occur during the first month after delivery. Many a new mother whose periods fail to start after a baby is born finds that she is again pregnant. If repeat pregnancy is not desired, birth control must be used as soon as sexual relations are resumed.

3

SEX and
SEXUAL PROBLEMS

When does a woman reach sexual maturity? At the onset of her menstrual periods, a girl is biologically mature and capable of having children. Sexual maturity in the sense of full realization of sexual responsiveness may not occur until a woman is in her twenties, thirties or beyond.

What are the ages when a woman is most sexually active? A woman's desire for sex usually peaks between the ages of twenty-five and thirty-five —about a decade after a man's peak. Beyond middle age sex drive begins to drop off for some women. Others seem to experience a renewed interest at this time.

Does the menopause end the woman's sex life? Not at all. Menopause, which usually occurs between the ages of forty-five and fifty-five, brings an end to the menstrual periods and a decline in the production of certain sex hormones. However, freedom from worry about getting pregnant may boost sexual desire, and there is some evidence that the increase of androgen in the woman's bloodstream actually increases her sexual desire at this point in her life.

How long can a woman remain sexually active? Throughout her life. The aging woman is fully capable of having and enjoying sex, though availability of a partner is a consideration. Sexual fulfillment seems to be most dependent on good nutrition, vigorous exercise and good general health, both physical and psychic. The woman who remains sexually active despite advancing years is more likely to continue to enjoy sex than is the woman who becomes sexually inactive and then decides some years later to resume her sex life. Masturbation may provide a continuing source of sexual fulfillment, and about a fourth of women in their seventies continue this practice.

When does a man reach sexual maturity?   At the age of puberty, a boy can produce sperm and fertilize an egg to create a pregnancy. As is true for the woman, sexual maturity may not occur until a decade or more later.

How long can a man remain sexually active?   A man in good health is capable of enjoying sex throughout life. As with women, diet, exercise and general well-being are essential for a long and enjoyable sex life.

Doesn't the older man have more difficulty with sex?   In certain ways, yes. It may take longer for the man over sixty to achieve an erection, and ejaculation occurs with less force and volume than in a younger man. Also, sex drive may decrease with age. Masters and Johnson have found that the older man is more capable of putting off his sexual climax than when he was younger. He may be satisfied to have intercourse without reaching orgasm, and these factors tend to make him a slower, more sensual lover who is better able to stimulate his partner until she reaches fulfillment.

What is meant by the term "sexuality"?   It is the sexual makeup of the individual, an expression of personality, sex drive, sexual role and other qualities.

How do men and women differ in sexuality?   The traditional sex roles begin by age three. The boy is supposedly the sexual pursuer, the girl the pursued, and to varying degrees this orientation may persist throughout life. Many variations may occur. The woman may be the pursuer, the man the receptive partner. Sex drive, self-assertiveness and intelligence know no sexual boundaries, and scientists as well as informed lay people have come to the conclusion that there are no preordained norms for male and female sexuality. Those that exist seem to be molded by society, and at present they are in a great state of change.

What determines a strong sex drive?   Many factors, including physical and mental health, a normal production of sex hormones, the attractiveness of the partner, a sense of well-being and the enjoyment of sexual interactions.

What causes a weak sex drive?   Sexual behavior is a learned function, and the person with a weak drive may have grown up being taught that sex or the desire for it is wrong. This behavior can be unlearned. Some people may be more highly sexed than others, but this is an area where it is very hard to separate the physical from the psychological. Loss of sex drive when it was previously strong may be due to illness, anxiety, fatigue, fear or sexual boredom.

What are the meanings of the terms "heterosexual," "homosexual" and "bisexual"? "Hetero" means "other" or "different," so a heterosexual is one whose sexual attraction is toward members of the opposite sex. This is the most common orientation. A homosexual is attracted toward members of the same sex. Sexual orientation is not always clearly defined between heterosexual and homosexual and both qualities are to be found, in varying degrees, in everyone. Persons who are attracted sexually both to members of the same sex and to persons of the opposite sex are called "bisexual." The causes of homosexuality are poorly understood, but it is clear that with the recent liberalism of sexual attitudes, homosexuality no longer poses the severe problems it formerly did.

THE WOMAN'S SEX ORGANS

What are the woman's sex organs? The vulva consists of the pubic hair, the mons (the pad beneath the hair), and the major and minor lips, or labia. The clitoris is a hooded knob of flesh just inside the lips below the mons. The entrance to the vagina is an inch below the clitoris. The urine opening, or urethra, is just above the vagina. At the back of the vagina is the cervix, or the mouth of the womb, and the womb itself protrudes into the abdominal cavity. About four inches on either side of the uterus are the ovaries. They are attached to the womb by broad ligaments which also carry the fallopian tubes.

What is the normal appearance of the external organs? In most women the pubic hair grows in a triangular pattern with a horizontal upper border. However, it may reach to the navel or be confined to just above the main lips. The hair itself may be curly, straight, long or short. In general, Oriental women have sparse hair growth, while women of Mediterranean origin have heavier growth. The minor lips may hardly be noticeable, or they may protrude past the main lips. The clitoris may be long and obvious, or so covered by its hood that it can scarcely be located.

How do the organs respond to sexual stimulation? Sexual excitement speeds the heart rate and brings more blood to the pelvic region. The outer lips flatten to expose the vagina, while the inner lips swell to twice their usual thickness. Within ten to thirty seconds of the onset of sexual excitement, the vagina is bathed in a lubricating fluid to facilitate intercourse, and it enlarges, especially in its inner dimensions. As sexual excitement increases, the cervix and uterus are pulled higher into the pelvis to further expand the inner part of the vagina.

What causes the vaginal lubrication?   It appears in the form of individual droplets from the walls of the vagina, and represents the response of this organ to sexual stimulation. The lubricant is secreted so diffusely that its release has been attributed to a "sweating" mechanism.

What are the Bartholin's glands?   These glands, located one on either side of the entrance to the vagina, secrete a clear material that may help to lubricate the entrance to the vagina. Vaginal secretions are a far more important source of lubrication.

Does a woman have anything resembling an ejaculation?   Not really, though copious production of vaginal fluid may be mistaken for this.

Do women have wet dreams?   A woman may reach orgasm during a sexual dream, and sexual arousal may occur five or six times a night. The sleeping woman's response to arousal includes vaginal lubrication and clitoral enlargement.

What are the dimensions of the vagina?   The average length of the vagina in women who haven't had children is three inches. The average width is an inch and a half. Sexual excitement expands the depth to four and a half inches and the width to two and a half inches. The vagina enlarges after childbirth and may reach a depth of six inches in a woman who has had several children. When not in use, the vagina folds in on itself to allow for expansion of the bladder, above, or the rectum, below.

Does the size of the vagina affect a woman's ability to enjoy sex?   The vagina can expand to accommodate a large penis or tighten to ensheathe a small one. A snug vaginal opening may cause some pain at the onset of sexual relations if the woman has not worn tampons or had the vaginal opening explored during sex play. Sufficient arousal and the cooperation of the man will usually lessen the discomfort. An enlarged vaginal opening is most apt to occur in women beyond the age of thirty-five who have had two or more children.

What can be done to reduce the size of the vaginal opening?   Bringing the legs together after insertion of the penis will tighten the vaginal entrance. The woman-on-top position, by providing more clitoral stimulation, is another way of increasing sexual enjoyment. Since the size of the vaginal opening is in part related to the strength of the pelvic muscles, exercising these muscles may help.

The muscle you can most readily exercise is the pubococcygeus ("PC") muscle. Here's how to recognize it. Sit on the commode with your legs apart and begin to pass urine. Then, stop the flow. This requires use of the PC muscle, and gives a feeling similar to the way you feel when you need to urinate but have to hold it. Begin with about six PC contractions a day, and gradually work up to doing thirty contractions six times a day. Each one takes only a second, and you can do the exercises while seated, standing still or at any other time of your choosing. You should notice an improvement in sexual pleasure within several weeks. After about two months you can reduce the frequency of exercise to a hundred contractions a day once or twice a week. Continue this number of contractions to keep the PC muscle strong. (These movements are called the Kegel exercises.)

Surgery is sometimes done to tighten the vagina, but this is justified only when there are problems such as urinary incontinence.

What is the role of the clitoris in sexual stimulation?   Stimulation of the clitoris gives a woman sexual pleasure. Though there are nerve endings elsewhere in the genital area, the clitoris is largely responsible for the woman's orgasm. It enlarges slightly at the beginning of sexual excitement, then draws back into its hood inside the main lips. Here the clitoris is less available for direct stimulation, but is very responsive to indirect stimulation by way of the mons, main lips, minor lips and vagina.

What is the uterus?   It is a pear-shaped organ with muscular walls and a thin, T-shaped cavity inside. The lower end of the T is continuous with the cervix and the mouth of the womb; the upper arms of the T are continuous with the fallopian tubes. During the menstrual cycle, hormones released by the ovary cause the inner layer of the womb to grow a rich supply of blood vessels and to take on sugar, protein and minerals in preparation for the fertilized egg. If fertilization doesn't occur, the hormone secretion stops, the blood vessels wilt, and the blood-rich layer is shed as the menstrual flow.

How does the uterus respond to sexual excitement?   The uterus engorges during sexual excitement. It is pulled to a higher position in the pelvis so that the bottom of the cervix is no longer directly in contact with the vagina. At orgasm the uterus goes into rhythmic spasms that are felt as pelvic throbbings; the throbbing may spread throughout the body.

Will hysterectomy keep you from having a normal sexual response?   It shouldn't. At orgasm, you may still feel very strong pelvic contractions even after the womb is removed. However, sometimes the surgeon performing the hysterectomy removes too much of the vagina, making intercourse difficult or even impossible. If you are experiencing sexual problems after hysterectomy, you should consult another physician for a thorough examination. As in all questions of sexual response, both the physical and the psychological must be considered. Sometimes a woman who has had a hysterectomy develops unwarranted doubts about her femininity.

What do the ovaries do?   They release the eggs that allow the woman to become pregnant, and they produce the female sex hormones, estrogen and progesterone. These hormones act on the inner lining of the womb to cause the changes of the menstrual cycle, and their effects on other parts of the body include breast development and feminine body configuration.

How many eggs do the ovaries contain?   About 250,000 each, for a total of 500,000. A woman is born with all she'll ever have, though only about 400 or 500 of the eggs will ever be released. Perhaps two will be fertilized and become new human beings.

Will removal of the ovaries reduce sexual responsiveness?   Possibly so, since the woman is deprived of her source of sex hormones though there is evidence that the production of similar hormones is taken up by other glands. If she hasn't yet passed through the menopause, the operation will induce it. Replacement therapy with estrogen will slow the thinning of the vagina and retard the other changes, though this drug may present other complications. Of course, the menopause itself does not bring an end to sex drive and sexual relations.

Many women and doctors believe that hysterectomy is done too often; there has been an increase of 24 percent in this procedure since 1971. The removal of the normal ovaries of a premenopausal woman, which often accompanies hysterectomy, is usually unjustified. A woman faced with possible hysterectomy should carefully discuss the necessity for and the extent of the surgery with her physician (see p. 109–10).

What are the differences in sexual response before and after childbirth?
A woman may not reach her full sexual potential until after the birth of a child. Many women report an easier, more relaxed attitude to sexual relations after childbirth, and others have their first orgasm then. Sometimes a woman may be so absorbed in her baby, she is not interested in sex for some time after her pregnancy. Sometimes, also, the man may feel temporarily "shut out" of the bond between mother and child. Both situations are normal, and are usually temporary.

THE MAN'S SEX ORGANS

What are the man's sex organs? The penis, scrotum and testicles are the external organs. The internal organs are the vas deferens (sperm ducts), seminal vesicles and prostate gland. The urethra, the passageway from the bladder to the outside, also serves as the passageway for semen during ejaculation.

How do these organs respond to sexual stimulation? The obvious and most notable change is erection of the penis. The scrotum, or sac, thickens and constricts around the testicles. The testicles draw up higher in the sac so that during sexual excitement, their position is closer to the body.

At the height of his sexual pleasure, a man experiences strong muscular contractions in his genital passages and prostate. These culminate in ejaculation. Pelvic throbbing continues for some moments as the pleasure of orgasm slowly diminishes.

What are the dimensions of the penis? The average length of the mature, unstimulated penis is three inches. In the erect state, the penis averages six inches in length and an inch and a half in diameter. A normal man may have a penis that is larger or smaller than average. During erection, a small penis may enlarge more than a large one. This tends to even out size differences, though the large one is still bigger after erection.

Is it normal for a man to worry about the size of his penis? It's fairly common for an adolescent or young man to express concern that his penis is too small. Usually he is referring to the size of his organ compared to the penises he sees in the shower room in high school or college. Dr. Jack Annon, a sex therapist, has ascribed such fears to the "foreshortened view" each man has of his own penis. Looking down on it from above, a man sees his penis as smaller than another penis that may actually be the same size.

Does the size of the penis affect a woman's sexual satisfaction? This is a matter of personal preference. Some women do prefer a well-endowed partner, but the man's skill as a lover may be more important than the size of his penis, and the affection the couple share is of greater consequence than "perfect fit."

What is the most sensitive part of the penis? The acorn-shaped tip of the penis, or glans. It doubles in size during an erection, but remains softer than the rest of the penis. This facilitates easy entry of the penis into the vagina. The glans has a velvety texture that helps to create a slight amount of friction during vaginal thrusting.

What causes erection of the penis?   It may result from direct stimulation of the organ, from a sexually stimulating sight, or from sexual fantasies. Strictly speaking, however, the man cannot by willing it have an erection or make an unwanted one disappear. The right stimuli produce nervous and vascular reactions that result in more blood being pumped into the organ than can leave it. Two large vascular barrels become engorged, as does a smaller, midline one beneath them. The outer covering of the penis is a tough sheath that permits expansion to a certain point and no more. When the penis reaches this size, further pressure from the blood surging into it makes it hard and may cause it to throb with the pulsations of the heartbeat. The effect is not unlike inflating long balloons inside a covering of canvas. The canvas won't stretch, but it will get hard when the balloons are completely filled.

What happens to make the erection fade?   After orgasm, nerve stimuli reduce blood flow to the penis and it returns to its flaccid size. An erection also may fade without ejaculation when the physical or psychological stimulation that triggered it stops.

What is the source of the fluid that is released before ejaculation?
Preejaculation fluid is released from the Cowper's glands, two small glands at the base of the penis. It is released in response to a high degree of sexual stimulation, and its purpose is to lubricate the passageway through the penis to make it easier for semen to be ejaculated.

What is semen?   It is the ejaculate, consisting mainly of secretions from the prostate gland and seminal vesicles but also containing the sperm cells.

What are sperm?   They are the male gametes, the reproductive cells. About 100 million of them are present in each milliliter of semen.

How much semen is produced at each ejaculation?   This varies from man to man, and in the same man at different times. The average volume is about a teaspoonful, or five cc's. A normal man may produce only half this much, or his volume may exceed ten cc's. Factors that reduce the volume of semen are frequent ejaculation, dehydration (failure to drink enough fluids) and advancing age; those that favor a large ejaculation are youth, good health and absence of ejaculation for a couple of weeks or longer. Unlike a woman's sexual response, a series of ejaculations may result in diminished pleasure for a man.

Where does semen come from?   Most of it is produced in the prostate, the largest of the man's internal sex organs. The prostate is just beneath the

79

bladder, and on either side of it are the seminal vesicles, which also contribute to the volume of semen. The sperm, which are made in the testicles, account for only 5 to 10 percent of the volume of semen.

How often can a man ejaculate?   Most men experience a refractory or quiet phase lasting for a quarter of an hour or so following ejaculation. During this time another erection won't occur. The ability to have frequent ejaculations is most apt to occur in men under the age of thirty; beyond the age of sixty, some may have to wait several days or a week between ejaculations, although many have frequent ejaculations even at a quite advanced age. This seems to depend on the man's general well-being, frequency of sexual activity, nutrition and physical fitness.

What is a "wet dream"?   It is an ejaculation occurring during sleep as the culmination of a sex dream. Wet dreams are most apt to occur during adolescence or the late teens, when a man's sexual feelings are at an all-time high. They are completely normal. They seem to serve the function of clearing semen out of the genital passages when this doesn't occur through intercourse or masturbation.

What is the function of the prostate gland?   From its position at the base of the bladder, it produces the bulk of the semen that is delivered into the urethra during ejaculation. The prostatic secretion is what sets the sperm into rapid motion.

What causes prostatic enlargement?   The cause isn't known, but continuation of an active sex life into the middle years and beyond may reduce the risk of prostatic hypertrophy. This suggests that glandular inactivity contributes to the overgrowth.

How common is prostatic enlargement?   It is present in most men by the age of fifty or sixty, but causes difficulty in only a minority of them.

What are the signs of prostatic enlargement?   There may be no symptoms or the man may note increasing difficulty passing urine. At first it is more difficult to start the stream of urine, and dribbling is noted after voiding. Bladder infections may become a problem. In a severe instance of prostatic enlargement, the gland pinches off the urethra completely and obstructs the outflow of urine. Uncorrected, this may prove fatal within a matter of days.

What is the treatment for enlarged prostate?   Emergency catheterization may be needed if the man is unable to urinate. In the more common instance of partial obstruction, he may get relief from prostatic massage, regular intercourse or masturbation. The purpose is to remove prostatic secretions and relieve congestion in the gland. Treatment of a bladder or prostatic infection may also relieve the obstruction. Surgery is indicated when conservative measures fail. The surgery may be done through the urethra or by an incision in the lower abdomen.

What causes prostatic infection?   It may accompany a bladder infection which usually results from a large prostate partially blocking the urine tract.

What's the treatment for prostatic infection?   Antibiotic therapy and relief of bladder obstruction are the initial steps. Prostatic massage may be helpful. Persistent infection calls for long-term antibiotic therapy with monitoring of side effects.

What causes cancer of the prostate?   This malignancy is more likely to occur in a man whose father, grandfather or brother has or had it. It usually begins after age sixty in an enlarged prostate, and it is the third leading cause of cancer death in men, behind lung cancer and cancer of the intestine. About 64,000 men develop prostatic cancer each year.

What are the symptoms of cancer of the prostate?   There may be no symptoms with an early cancer, or the man may have trouble starting and stopping the stream of urine. Pain in the pelvis or low back may accompany advanced cancer of the prostate.

What's the treatment for prostatic cancer?   Treatment should be managed by a urologist who has been certified by the American Board of Urology. The choice of treatment depends on the extent of the cancer and the man's age and general health. Removal of the prostate is best if the cancer is confined to the gland. Radiation therapy is another choice. Radical surgery or therapy with the hormone diethylstilbestrol may control the growth of widespread cancer.

What's the outlook after treatment for prostatic cancer?   An early cancer may be cured, but the overall survival rate is about 50 percent at five years.

Will prostate surgery reduce a man's sex drive?   It may. The usual surgery, a TURP (transurethral resection of the prostate), is only occasionally responsible for a lowering of the sex drive. More often, it causes ejaculation to occur in a reverse direction into the bladder. Complete removal of the prostate is a more extensive operation. It may cause impotence, it is liable to reduce sex drive, and it will greatly diminish the volume of ejaculate.

What are the seminal vesicles?   These are two saclike structures, each sitting on either side of the prostate and contributing to the volume and nutritional content of semen.

What does disease of the seminal vesicles cause?   An overgrowth of the lining of the seminal vesicles may cause blood to appear in the ejaculate. The man with this problem should have a urologic examination to rule out cancer of the prostate, which could also be a source of bleeding. A short course of therapy with diethylstilbestrol will usually relieve bleeding from the seminal vesicles.

What are the testicles?   They are the man's gonads, comparable in size to the ovaries and producing sperm and testosterone.

What causes tumor of the testicle?   Though the cause is unknown, the peak incidence occurs between the ages of eighteen and thirty-five. An undescended testicle is more likely to become malignant than a descended one, and testicular cancer is more common in whites than in blacks, though the disease accounts for less than 1 percent of malignancies in men.

What are the symptoms of testicular cancer?   The earliest symptom is painless enlargement of the testicle; a dull ache may accompany the enlargement. Some tumors produce a hormone that causes the man's breasts to enlarge.

What is the treatment for testicular cancer?   The cancerous testicle should be removed and radiation therapy be given afterward. Cancer that has spread beyond the testicle is treated with chemotherapy.

What's the outlook after treatment for testicular cancer?   The prognosis depends on the type of tumor and varies from 50 to 95 percent survival at five years. The rarest form of testicular cancer, choriocarcinoma, is also the most malignant, and carries a much less favorable prognosis.

What can a man do to lessen the risk from testicular cancer?   Once a month he should examine himself for evidence of testicular enlargement. The examinations, which should begin at puberty and continue indefinitely, can be done in the shower or tub. A convenient time is the first day of each month—or any day of the month that can be easily remembered. Enlargement of a testicle calls for an examination by a urologist.

SEXUAL RELATIONS

Can a woman have more than one orgasm?   Yes. Continued stimulation may lead to other orgasms a few seconds to a minute apart. Some women have just one orgasm; others report great pleasure from several orgasms.

Can a man have more than one orgasm?   Yes, but men, unlike women, cannot have multiple orgasms, one after another. Ordinarily, a period of at least fifteen minutes or so must pass before a man is able to have another erection and ejaculation, though endurance and responsiveness vary.

What is the average frequency of sexual intercourse?   Two to four times a week is the most frequently quoted statistic, but such figures are open to question. The normal frequency of coitus is something each person or couple must decide satisfies them.

What is the average duration of intercourse?   On the average, three minutes and thirty to fifty thrusting movements occur between the time of penile insertion and ejaculation. However, the amount of time that may elapse during intercourse is subject to wide variation, and coitus may be preceded by a period of mutual sexual stimulation and may continue for several minutes after the man's orgasm.

Does the length of foreplay affect the woman's likelihood of having an orgasm?   Yes. If foreplay and penile thrusting are sustained for fifteen minutes, up to 98 percent of women may achieve orgasm during coitus. By contrast, three-fourths of women who masturbate can reach orgasm within four minutes.

Is lovemaking during the menstrual period unhealthy?   No. Some couples like to make love at this time, while others don't. The woman who has menstrual cramps may find that reaching orgasm relieves the pain. A diaphragm can be used to hold back the menstrual flow if this is desired, or the man may elect to wear a condom.

Do you need to douche after sex?   No. It is a matter of personal preference. In any case, wait for at least eight hours before douching if you rely on foam or the diaphragm and jelly for contraception, or if you're trying to get pregnant.

How often should you douche?   Many women never douche. Some do so daily, and others limit it to right after the menstrual period. Douching too frequently may irritate the vagina and is unnecessary. If your vaginal discharge is so heavy you feel frequent douching is called for, consult a physician to make sure you don't have an infection. In most instances, regular bathing is sufficient.

What is the best technique for douching?   Use a simple douche powder or make up your own solution by putting two tablespoons of plain white vinegar into a quart of warm water. The correct position is lying on your back in the tub. Attach the bag to something about two feet above the floor of the tub and insert the hose nozzle into the vagina. Use the other hand to close off the entrance to the vagina so that as water runs in, it can't flow back out. Then clamp the hose and let the water gush out of the vagina. Repeat this sequence until the douche bag is empty.

Is masturbation abnormal?   Certainly not. Stimulating one's own genitals is a normal part of sexual development. It may continue into adulthood as a form of sexual outlet.

Is it abnormal for a married person to masturbate?   No. Seventy percent of husbands continue to masturbate at an average frequency of twenty-four times a year. Seventy percent of wives also continue to masturbate, but their average frequency is only ten times a year.

What is "mutual masturbation"?   When two people masturbate each other. An adult couple may find it an enjoyable variation to lovemaking. Still another variation is for the man and woman to masturbate to orgasm in each other's presence.

What is oral sex?   Stimulation of the genitals by the mouth and tongue. The specific term for oral stimulation of the penis is *fellatio.* Oral stimulation of the vulva and vagina is known as *cunnilingus.*

Is oral sex abnormal?   It is much more common now than it was a generation ago, and 90 percent of husbands and wives under the age of twenty-five have engaged in oral-genital stimulation.

What techniques provide sexual gratification short of intercourse?   All sorts of experiences give different people pleasure. Two of them, oral sex and masturbation, have just been mentioned. Stimulation of the vulva with a vibrator is a way of bringing a woman to orgasm without intercourse. A man may reach orgasm from penile thrusting between his partner's closed thighs, between her breasts or in the crevice of her buttocks. Anal sex is also, apparently, more common among heterosexual couples than it was previously.

What are sexual fantasies?　　These are daydreams about sex. Men and women commonly fantasize about making love to a famous person or to someone they have seen on a street corner, and the manner of lovemaking as well as the setting may be exotic.

Is it abnormal to have such fantasies?　　No, they are the mind's contribution to each person's sexuality. Sex drive and sexual feelings are common to people of both sexes and all ages and should not cause guilt or anxiety.

SEXUAL PROBLEMS

How do you know if you have a sexual problem?　　Signs of a problem include loss of interest in sex, pain during intercourse, failure to be satisfied by sex, and inability of the man to have an erection. The shorter the duration of the problem, the easier it is to correct.

What causes a sexual problem?　　Something as mild as a vaginal infection or fatigue, or a potentially more serious condition such as guilt feelings that originate in childhood. An unrealistic view of sex is often the common denominator. Because we live in the age of orgasm, most people want and expect one with each sexual act, and when this doesn't happen, anxiety is created. One or both partners may feel a sense of failure. This puts a performance demand on them for the next sexual encounter. When that one also ends in frustration, the problem grows. Now sex becomes not so much an exchange of love as an act wherein the partners must prove themselves. Each failure creates greater fear, which may dampen sexual desire.

What is a more realistic view of sex?　　It is a body function, and like other body functions, it is subject to variation. Sexual desire ebbs and flows. A person under pressure at work may go for some time not even thinking about sex, while on a vacation the same person may want intercourse twice a day. Fatigue and physical illness also affect desire. An important consideration is that not every sexual encounter is going to be as tumultuous as every other one. Someone has said that the nice thing about sex is that when it's good it's great, and when it's bad, it's still pretty good. Someone else has said that the sexual happiness of a couple is set not in the bedroom but at the kitchen table.

What are some common sexual problems?　　The main problems for women are failure to reach orgasm and pain during intercourse. The common ones for men are failure to achieve or maintain an erection, and ejaculation before the partner reaches sexual fulfillment.

85

What causes sexual boredom?   The couple may make love in the same way at the same time in the same position for so many times that the act loses its spontaneity. Other causes of boredom are a loss of interest in the partner due to a lessening of his or her physical attractiveness, and a continuing failure to enjoy sex.

What can be done for sexual boredom?   The couple may choose alternate methods of lovemaking, change the position and timing of intercourse, or make love in unusual places. Variety may mean the introduction of oral-genital sex or a greater emphasis on foreplay. The couple should experiment with different positions for intercourse, and use several positions for each session. A short vacation together is usually helpful. Perhaps the best way to avoid boredom is to have sex when you want it and only then, not according to some predetermined time or standard of performance.

What is "frigidity"?   In the past this word was applied to the woman with orgasmic failure. It was used to describe a wide range of female sexual dysfunctions, and the term implied a coldness and lack of sexual potential. Since we now know that 99 percent of women are capable of orgasm when stimulated effectively, "frigidity" no longer has a place in describing sexual function.

What causes a woman not to have an orgasm?   The woman with primary orgasmic dysfunction has never been able to have a climax through self-stimulation, intercourse or homosexual contact. Psychological causes are the most common, and they often stem from the rigid sexual standards set for women by their families and society.

The person with secondary orgasmic dysfunction is one who was able to achieve orgasm previously but can't now. The problem may have to do with lovemaking technique, with her partner's premature ejaculation or with some newly arisen psychological problem of her own. Other causes include fatigue, worry, ill health and fear of becoming pregnant.

What can be done to help those with sexual problems?   Treatment depends on the cause and duration of the problem, since matters of recent onset are usually more amenable to therapy. The man and woman should discuss the difficulty as honestly as possible, and may elect to visit a therapist. There are people practicing sex therapy who are not qualified for one reason or another. Ask a competent gynecologist for a referral, or consult with a woman's health care center or similar organization.

Therapy may consist of exercises to strengthen the PC muscles (see p. 76) or the use of self-stimulation techniques, since the woman who can achieve orgasm through masturbation is more likely to reach orgasm during intercourse. Frequently helpful is a method Masters and Johnson have called "sensate focus sessions."

What are "sensate focus sessions"?   These are sessions centered on partners' mutual discovery of ways to give and receive sexual pleasure. The partners, nude, alternate giving and receiving pleasure. Performance demands are removed by the preset condition that the couple are not to engage in sexual intercourse or attempt to have an orgasm. They are to focus, instead, on teaching one another the tactile sensations that feel good and are enjoyable.

What causes pain during intercourse?   This problem, known medically as dyspareunia, is often due to a vaginal infection or irritation, or a vaginal opening that is too small to comfortably admit the penis. The pain is usually felt at the vaginal entrance or just below it. Pain that is deep in the pelvis and felt only during penile thrusting is more likely due to an infection in the tubes or uterus, or to endometriosis (see p. 102).

What can be done for the pain?   The first step is to determine what is causing it. If dryness of the vagina is a contributing factor, the use of a lubricant is indicated. A water-soluble jelly is preferred because petroleum-based lubricants, such as Vaseline, may trap bacteria inside the vagina. Some physicians recommend estrogen cream for vaginal dryness in a post-menopausal woman, but the hormone is absorbed into the bloodstream and most specialists now believe that it is too dangerous to warrant its use in this instance.

Vaginal infection causes discharge and itching. The pain may begin right after sex and have a burning or stinging quality. Causes of vaginitis are candidiasis and infection with trichomonas or hemophilus. Each should be diagnosed and treated by a physician.

What causes candidiasis?   Also known as moniliasis, this is the most common vaginal infection. It occurs when the normal yeast organisms on the skin and in the vagina gain an advantage and grow to an excessive degree. Especially susceptible are the pregnant woman, the diabetic, the obese individual, or the person who has had recent therapy with broad-spectrum antibiotics.

The main symptoms are itching and fiery red irritation on the vulva. The discharge is thick and somewhat like cottage cheese in appearance.

What is the treatment for candidiasis?   Women report success with yogurt used topically and added to the diet. A vaginal tablet of nystatin, used twice daily for two weeks, is curative; other antifungal drugs have been in use recently that require shorter treatment. If the skin around the vagina is irritated by the infection, antifungal cream can be used along with the vaginal treatment.

What are the symptoms of trichomonas infection?   This form of vaginitis must be considered a venereal infection because it is passed during sexual intercourse. Infection in a man is usually asymptomatic, but in a woman the infection causes a gray to greenish-yellow discharge that is copious, frothy and malodorous. The organisms also get into the urinary tract and may cause burning on urination. A fourth of women who harbor the infection have no symptoms except pain during intercourse.

What's the treatment for trichomonas infection?   Left untreated, the infection may gradually subside, and douching may help to control the discharge. Treatment with the drug metronidazole will cure the infection. The drug can be used orally or as a vaginal insert. The woman and her sex partner must be treated, but metronidazole should not be taken during pregnancy, as it may harm the fetus. The main side effect of the drug is stomach upset, though it may also cause a metallic taste in the mouth, dizziness, a lowering of the white blood cell count and allergic reactions.

What causes hemophilus vaginitis?   The bacterium *Hemophilus vaginalis,* which in some instances is transmitted as a venereal disease. The symptoms are similar to those of trichomonas vaginitis, though milder.

What is the treatment for hemophilus vaginitis?   A triple-sulfa vaginal cream will relieve the infection in most women. The cream must be instilled twice a day for two weeks. When venereal transmission is likely, both partners should be treated for a week with an oral antibiotic.

What other measures may help relieve pain during intercourse?   Venereal disease, such as gonorrhea or herpes, may cause pain during intercourse, and these conditions are discussed later in this chapter. Local irritation of the vaginal opening may give pain that is relieved by removing the source of irritation. Among the causes are bubble-bath powders, feminine hygiene sprays, perfumed soaps, colored toilet paper, contraceptive foam, or wearing tight synthetic fabrics that prevent proper ventilation of the vulva and surrounding area. Cotton fabrics are healthier than synthetics: they allow perspiration and vaginal secretions to evaporate. Pantyhose with a cotton crotch are preferable to regular pantyhose, and loose-fitting garments should be worn when possible.

What can cause tightness at the entrance to the vagina?   The hymen will usually dilate to permit intercourse without the pain one hears about. The use of vaginal tampons may reduce the likelihood that a woman will experience pain with first intercourse, and the establishment of regular sexual relations will lead to enlargement of the vaginal opening. Rarely, a woman may need a small incision of the hymen to free her from pain during intercourse.

Sexual excitement is a dilator of the vagina. Even the woman with a small vagina, provided she is sexually excited, can accommodate a large penis without pain. The most likely cause of a severe problem with tightness of the vaginal entrance is vaginismus, a psychologically induced disorder.

What can be done for vaginismus?   The treatment begins with a recognition that vaginismus is present. The woman tells of painful spasm in her pelvic area when her partner attempts intercourse, and she usually can't relax sufficiently even to allow the doctor to examine her.

Most therapists report a high degree of success in treating vaginismus when both partners work toward a solution. Psychotherapy and vaginal dilations both may be indicated. The dilations are done in the privacy of the bedroom. The woman does them or is in control of them. She may use a series of graded metal dilators or her fingers, and adequate lubrication and gentle insertion are employed. The aim is to gradually increase the size of the vagina until intercourse is possible.

What may cause a man to have pain during intercourse?   Prostatitis or a smoldering infection of the glans penis may be present. Treatment is effective. The glans of certain men is sensitive to irritation from clothing, soap or contraceptive jelly, and wearing a condom may provide relief. Gonorrhea, herpes, syphilis and other venereal diseases may cause a man to have pain during intercourse.

What about bowing of the penis?   This may create pain during an erection or during intercourse, and the cause is injury or Peyronie's disease. The latter is a progressive fibrosis of the covering sheath of the penis. The affected man, usually forty-five or older, may respond to drug treatment or to X-ray therapy or surgery. Sometimes the penis becomes so bowed that intercourse is no longer possible.

A blow to the erect organ may injure the penis, and so may a sudden change in position during intercourse. Since surgery for this problem is apt to make the condition worse, the only treatment is prevention.

What is impotence?   The inability to achieve or maintain an erection. With primary impotence the man has never been able to have an erection. Much more common is secondary impotence, where the man was previously capable of a normal sexual response. Physical disease may be at fault, but the problem is usually psychological.

89

What's the treatment for impotence?   In many instances the couple can achieve success without the need for sex therapy. An honest discussion of sexual feelings is necessary at the outset. When the impotence persists, a thorough workup is indicated to rule out medical problems, which are unlikely if the man still sometimes has erections in the shower, on getting up in the morning or at other times.

Removing performance demands on the man is important when fear or self-doubt has contributed to the impotence. One technique is to get into various stimulating situations when intercourse isn't possible. The stimulation can take the form of stroking the penis, or the couple may spend some time together with sexually exciting movies or books, or participate in oral-genital sex and sensate focus sessions. The only rule is that they do what is mutually enjoyable and refrain from having intercourse for the entire week. Therapists who instruct couples in this technique report it is not unusual for the couple to phone in a week later saying they won't be needing any more therapy. A skilled therapist is able to offer other methods of therapy as well.

What are the physical causes of impotence?   Diabetes, glandular disease, lung disease, heart disease, vascular disease—almost any serious condition affecting the man's health. Injury or disease of the spinal cord is an infrequent but serious cause. Mumps, prostate surgery, nutritional defects, severe fatigue, blood diseases and therapy with estrogen may cause impotence.

Can drugs cause impotence?   Yes, drugs such as reserpine (Serpasil), Ismelin, Aldomet, Catapres and Minipress, which are used to treat high blood pressure, may cause impotence. Tranquilizers such as Librium and Valium, antidepressants such as Tofranil and Elavil, and drugs that affect the level of consciousness, such as sleeping pills, heroin and marijuana, may cause impotence. Probably the most common drug causing this problem is alcohol, and the man who drinks heavily may be unable to achieve an erection.

What can be done when impotence persists despite therapy?   A man may be able to achieve orgasm without developing a full erection, or he and his partner may have enjoyable relations despite this problem. When the man desires surgery, two options are available. A rubberlike wedge may be placed into the penis. Though the erection is permanent, it is flexible enough to be hidden under clothing. A more elaborate operation allows the man to have a reversible erection. Two rubber cylinders are placed into the penis and connected to a fluid-filled device in the lower abdomen. By operating a small device fixed into the scrotum, the man can pump up an erection when he so desires. Release of a valve will allow the penis to return to its flaccid state.

What is premature ejaculation?   When a man ejaculates too quickly for his partner to enjoy sex. Some therapists consider premature ejaculation to exist when a man can't continue vaginal intercourse for more than a minute without reaching orgasm. Others define it as intercourse lasting longer than a minute, but still not long enough to satisfy the partner. A woman's failure to achieve orgasm frequently accompanies the man's complaint of premature ejaculation. The two conditions go together.

What can be done for premature ejaculation?   The man may be able to delay his orgasm by thinking of something other than sex or by concentrating on his breathing rather than his rising excitement. The most likely position for premature ejaculation to occur is when the man is on top. By letting the woman take the top position, the man may slow his sexual response. Having intercourse more often, or masturbating between coital episodes, is another way of reducing the level of sexual arousal. The use of a condom may reduce sensitivity and allow a longer period of penile thrusting. The squeeze technique is employed when other methods fail.

What is the squeeze technique?   A method of helping the man to delay his orgasm. First, the couple engage in sexual stimulation short of actual intercourse. When the man feels that he is nearing orgasm, he signals to his partner and she applies pressure to the penis just below the glans with her thumb and first two fingers for three or four seconds. This will stop the man's urge to ejaculate. This technique is repeated four or five times until the man is able to tolerate fifteen minutes of alternating stimulation and squeeze technique. Eventually, the couple should be able to have mutually satisfying sexual relations, though this may take several months of working together to achieve. It does not seem to be effective for the man to use the squeeze technique on himself.

VENEREAL DISEASE

What is venereal disease?   It is a disease that is transmitted by sexual relations. The infection may be passed via penile-vaginal intercourse, anal intercourse, oral-genital relations or intimate body contact.

What are the most common kinds of venereal disease?   Gonorrhea is by far the most common: it ranks just under the common cold as the most frequent communicable disease in the United States. Among the venereal diseases, syphilis follows gonorrhea in frequency, and is followed closely by genital herpes, a viral infection that has increased remarkably in frequency during the last ten years. Less common forms of venereal disease are lymphogranuloma venereum, granuloma inguinale and chancroid.

Can venereal disease be prevented?   Though the only sure way to prevent it is to abstain from sex or limit relations to one partner, there are many ways to reduce one's risk of getting venereal disease. A condom will protect against gonorrhea during sexual intercourse, though one could contract the infection during oral-genital relations. Spermicidal foam and the diaphragm and jelly offer some protection against gonorrhea. The condom protects against syphilis, but may not prevent genital herpes. Cleansing of the genitals with soap and water after intercourse is definitely indicated when a condom wasn't used, and douching after coitus may also be of value. Selectivity in choosing one's sexual partners is very important. As one caseworker put it, "Sometimes it seems like ten percent of the population spreads ninety percent of the VD."

What are the steps to take if you think you have VD?   Seek medical help from a private physician or from a VD clinic.

What's involved in the visit?   Diagnostic procedure is the same in a private physician's office and in a VD clinic where the physician is paid by the city or state. The doctor will take a history and perform a genital examination. A smear and culture are taken for gonorrhea and a blood test for syphilis. The blood test takes a day, but gonorrhea can usually be recognized immediately, so that treatment can be started. Herpes and the remaining forms of VD can usually be recognized by physical examination, and in a rare instance, consultation with a dermatologist is necessary.

What questions will be asked?   This is where a private physician may differ from one employed by a VD clinic. At the clinic the doctor or a caseworker will ask for the name(s) of sexual contacts so that the person or persons can be informed that they have been exposed to VD and should have an examination. By law, confidentiality is stressed: caseworkers do not, or aren't supposed to, reveal the identity of the individual who named the contact—merely that the person has been named and should seek treatment. Moreover, venereal disease caseworkers usually take pains to inform contacts in person when possible so that a telephone message is not transmitted to, say, a relative of the contact.

Private physicians are supposed to report all cases of VD so that a caseworker can interview the patient and obtain the names of contacts. The system often fails, however, because when the patient is someone the physician knows well and discretion is indicated, it's possible that treatment will be given and the illness recorded in the medical record as a sore throat for which penicillin was given. When the patient requests it, the physician may call a VD caseworker and report the name of the contact or contacts without revealing the name of the person who has just been treated. Most caseworkers are willing to work on this basis in the interest of public health.

Is there any way to guarantee confidentiality?   Probably not, but if discretion is desirable, it would be appropriate to call one's private physician or a competent physician in the community who may not have treated the person before. By posing a hypothetical question about an individual who might have VD and is worried about confidentiality, one can sound out the physician's views on the matter (sometimes the nurse will relay the message to the doctor or be able to provide the necessary information). Most doctors will cooperate with a person's request for confidentiality provided the individual is willing to take adequate treatment and have a follow-up blood test to rule out syphilis.

How long after treatment is it safe to resume sexual relations?   One can resume sexual relations after the symptoms of the infection are gone. Due caution should be taken to avoid reinfection, which is much more common than treatment failure, i.e., persistence of the infection despite treatment.

What causes gonorrhea?   A bacterium known as *Neisseria gonorrhoeae.* It grows readily on moist surfaces, such as the vagina, rectum or mouth. It is easy to culture, but dies rather quickly when exposed to the air. It's unlikely, though possible, to acquire it from a freshly contaminated toilet seat or item of clothing.

How do you know if you have it?   Three to seven days after contracting the infection, a man notes severe burning on urination. A pus-like discharge may drain from the penis. A culture will confirm the diagnosis.

The problem in women is that four out of five who contract gonorrhea never have symptoms of it. They may not develop the burning on urination and discharge until weeks or months later. Chronic pain in the pelvis and lower abdomen may accompany a smoldering infection. The pain is typically worse following the menstrual period. It's a good idea for a woman with discharge or symptoms referable to the pelvis to have a culture test for gonorrhea as soon as possible. The test may also be incorporated as part of the yearly gynecological checkup. A culture for gonorrhea is sometimes done by the physician during a pelvic exam without the patient's knowledge unless the test comes back positive.

What is the treatment for gonorrhea?   Penicillin is still the best drug, and the dose is 2.4 million units in each hip for a total of 4.8 million units given at one visit. The person must take a gram of probenecid by mouth to enhance the effect of the penicillin. The treatment is the same for gonorrhea occurring in the throat or rectum. The penicillin-allergic individual can be treated with tetracycline or spectinomycin.

Who should be treated for gonorrhea?   Anyone, man or woman, who has it or who has been exposed to someone proven to have it.

How do you know if the treatment has been successful?   At a follow-up exam, a culture can be taken to see if any trace of infection remains.

What can be done for treatment failure?   A few strains of gonococcus are resistant to penicillin and in this instance spectinomycin is the drug of choice, which is given by injection. The drug can't be used during pregnancy and may cause a lowering of the blood count, chills, fever and soreness at the injection site. Allergic reactions to it are fairly frequent.

A fourth of men with anorectal gonorrhea may not respond to penicillin, and tetracycline therapy is then indicated. Persistent pain and discharge may be due to nongonococcal urethritis (NGU). This infection, also known as nonspecific urethritis (NSU), is a less serious disease, though extremely common. It does not cause urethral strictures but is an inflammation of the urethra. The usual cause is *Chlamydia trachomatis* and tetracycline is generally curative, though the infection may be difficult to eradicate.

Does a resistance to gonorrhea develop?   No, as is true for all venereal diseases, you can get it again and again.

What are the complications of gonorrhea?   Arthritis, meningitis or an infection of the heart valves may occur when treatment is delayed. Stricture of the urethra is the most common complication in a man. By blocking his urine flow, the stricture may create bladder or kidney disease. The treatment is to dilate the urethra by passing a metal cylinder through the penis, and the dilations must be continued indefinitely.

Tubal infection can cause sterility, abscess formation ("pus tubes"), or an indolent condition known as pelvic inflammatory disease (PID). Though gonorrhea is often what triggers PID, other bacteria may enter the tubes and cause the disease. The woman may suffer flare-ups of lower abdominal pain, discharge, menstrual irregularities and pain during intercourse. Antibiotic therapy may help, but surgical removal of the tubes may become necessary.

How is transmission of gonorrhea to a baby prevented?   Gonococcal ophthalmia was once a common cause of blindness, but medication to prevent it is now instilled into the eyes of every baby shortly after birth. The traditional treatment, a drop of 1 percent silver nitrate solution in each eye, causes temporary eye irritation in about half of the infants who receive it.

For this reason, some physicians favor using penicillin or tetracycline ointment instead of silver nitrate. The form of treatment is mandated by law in each state.

What causes syphilis?   A spirochete, *Treponema pallidum,* is the causative organism. Its corkscrew shape gives it the microscopic appearance of a coiled hair, hence the term "spirochete."

How is it transmitted?   Through sexual relations or intimate body contact.

How does syphilis differ from gonorrhea?   It isn't as common and it's much more serious. The initial sore, or chancre, may heal on its own. By then the spirochetes have entered other body parts where they may cause secondary and tertiary forms of the disease. A skin rash may break out weeks or months after the initial infection. Anyone who touches the sores may contract syphilis. When the rash heals, the disease enters its latent phase. A pregnant woman with latent syphilis can give it to her baby, but only a third of persons with latent syphilis develop tertiary disease; the problem is that it isn't possible to say which third this will be. The late manifestations of syphilis are heart disease, aortic aneurysm (ballooning of the aorta), insanity, paralysis and severe bone destruction.

How do you know if you have syphilis?   The presence of a sore on the genitals is suggestive. This sore, the chancre, usually appears on the penis or scrotum of a man and at the vaginal entrance or on the vulva of a woman. Painless, it enlarges slowly to the size of a dime or nickel. Glands in the groin swell but do not become tender. A chancre that appears on the inner foreskin of an uncircumcised man, or inside the vagina of a woman, may go unnoticed. The sore heals in two to six weeks even without treatment.

By examining material from the sore, the doctor can tell if you have syphilis. This direct, dark-field examination method is ideal, but far more often the disease is recognized by a blood test known as a serology, or VDRL (Venereal Disease Research Laboratories), STS (Serologic Test for Syphilis) or Wassermann. The blood test is positive four or five weeks after the onset of syphilis.

Who should have a serologic test for syphilis?   Anyone who's been exposed to syphilis, gonorrhea or another venereal disease. It is routine to have the test six weeks after treatment for gonorrhea, since both infections could have been contracted simultaneously.

By law, the blood test for syphilis is required of persons wanting a marriage license. It is routine for everyone admitted to a hospital and is part of the standard workup done in the initial evaluation of pregnancy.

Does a positive serology mean you have syphilis?   Nine times out of ten, yes. Certain diseases, such as rheumatoid arthritis, lupus erythematosus and malaria, can cause a person to develop a "false positive serologic test for syphilis," but there are two special tests a physician can order to separate a false positive from a valid reaction.

What is the treatment for syphilis?   Early syphilis is treated with one injection of 2.4 million units of benzathine penicillin. Later forms of the disease are also treated with penicillin, but the dosage and type of penicillin may vary depending on the severity of the condition. Persons allergic to penicillin can be treated with tetracycline or erythromycin by mouth.

How often does treatment fail?   Relapse occurs in less than 5 percent of persons treated for early syphilis. Most such failures occur during the first three to nine months after initial treatment. This is why periodic serologic testing is indicated after therapy for syphilis. A rise in the strength of the serologic test for syphilis, or a return to a positive test after it had become negative, calls for re-treatment.

Can syphilis be contracted before birth?   Spirochetes can pass from the mother's bloodstream to the fetus's circulation and damage virtually any or every part of its body. The baby may be stillborn or severely ill at birth. Adequate treatment of the mother's syphilis is essential, and the earlier the treatment the better. Even when treatment is given relatively late in pregnancy, however, the child is usually spared from having congenital syphilis.

What is herpes infection?   Genital herpes is a venereal disease caused by a virus similar to the one that causes fever blisters (cold sores). The infection starts as a breaking out of small blisters on the vulva, penis or genital area. The virus—herpes simplex virus Type 2—may also infect the cervix. The blisters burst in a few days to form sores, which heal in a couple of weeks, but most persons who get the infection will have recurrences. The blisters may reappear after intercourse, emotional stress or an illness.

How contagious is it?   Communicability is greatest when the infection is obvious, but the virus can be passed during intercourse even when blisters or sores aren't present. Also, a person with a cold sore (caused by Type 1 herpes virus) can transmit the virus to the partner's genitals during oral sex. The Type 1 infection isn't as bad as the Type 2, but the symptoms may be just as distressing.

What are the complications of genital herpes?   A woman may pass the infection to her baby during delivery. One in four babies who contract the infection will die. One-third of those who survive will be blind or handicapped. Prophylactic cesarean section is indicated when the woman is known to have a herpes infection.

Does the infection contribute to cervical cancer?   It may. After a herpes infection, a woman is eight times as likely to have cervical cancer as a noninfected woman of the same age. Some women have developed the cancer within five years of having herpes. It's been known for a long time that girls who become sexually active early and have relations with many partners are the best candidates for herpes—and cancer of the cervix. Studies show that women with cancer of the cervix frequently have antibodies against the Type 2 herpes virus. Finally, the virus has been isolated from cervical cancer cells. Thus, while some authorities are hesitant to say it, others aren't: they insist that cancer of the cervix is a venereal disease caused by genital herpes.

What is the treatment for genital herpes?   No specific treatment is available. Local measures may relieve the pain of the blisters, but the person's best hope is that he or she will form a resistance to the virus. Many authorities now recommend that a woman with genital herpes should have a Pap smear twice a year.

Can herpes be prevented?   Avoiding intercourse when the blisters or sores are visible may lower the transmission rate. There's some evidence that the woman's use of a diaphragm and the man's use of a condom may offer protection. To prevent one form of the disease, oral sex by a partner with a cold sore should be avoided.

What about other venereal diseases?   These are lymphogranuloma venereum, granuloma inguinale and chancroid. Though uncommon, these conditions may be serious and difficult to eradicate.

Lymphogranuloma venereum is caused by a virus that enters the body during sexual relations. An ulcer develops at the site of entry, but it may go unnoticed in a woman. Fever occurs and the lymph glands in the groin swell open to discharge pus. Rectal involvement is common. Treatment is with tetracycline or a sulfa drug, but even with treatment, a rectal stricture may develop and require surgical correction.

Granuloma inguinale is caused by an indolent bacterial infection that is transmitted through sexual intercourse or intimate body contact. A sore forms on the genitals or another body part. Without treatment, it may grow slowly for years, causing scarring and mutilation of the underlying tissues. Treatment with streptomycin or tetracycline is curative, but surgery may be necessary to correct the effects of the disease.

Chancroid is caused by a rapid-acting bacterium, *Hemophilus ducreyi.* A sore on the genitals occurs one to five days after exposure, and the lymph glands on that side swell and become exquisitely tender. The disease may resemble plague. Treatment with sulfa drugs, tetracycline or erythromycin is curative.

What are venereal warts? Known as *condylomata acuminata,* these moist warts may appear on the penis, vulva or anal area. Most are discrete, single bumps, but they may become confluent to form cauliflowerlike masses. Not uncommonly, they are passed through intimate body contact, but nonvenereal passage may also occur.

What's the treatment for venereal warts? Topical application of a weak solution of podophyllin will usually cure the wart though several treatments may be necessary. To prevent skin irritation, the medicine should be washed off five or six hours after application.

4

MENSTRUAL
and
BREAST PROBLEMS

At what age do the menstrual periods begin?   The average age of onset is twelve and a half, but the periods of a normal girl may start when she's ten or not begin till she's sixteen.

What are the other changes of puberty?   The earliest change is growth of the breasts. About a year later pubic and axillary hair appears, and about a year after that, menstruation begins. The time span varies from woman to woman, of course.

What are menstrual periods?   They represent the cyclical changes that occur in the womb in response to hormone stimulation. During the first half of the menstrual cycle, several follicles in each ovary begin to grow and to make the hormone estrogen. The hormone enters the bloodstream to cause or maintain feminine body changes, and to stimulate growth of the uterine lining. Midway through the cycle one of the follicles ruptures to release an egg. Afterward the remaining follicles involute. The one that produced the egg enlarges to form a corpus luteum, and it begins to make progesterone as well as estrogen. Progesterone further stimulates the lining of the uterus, which becomes engorged with minerals, stored nutrients and blood vessels. All is now in readiness for a pregnancy to occur. If the egg is not fertilized, hormone production stops and the layer of blood and nutrients is shed as the menstrual flow. After the period is finished, the cycle starts again.

What other effects do estrogen and progesterone have on the body?   These hormones are responsible for a woman's physical and sexual development. Her breasts and hips owe their shape to estrogen. This hormone brings on the pubic and axillary hair and leads to softening of the skin over the thighs, face, neck, shoulders and abdomen. Under the influence of estrogen, the woman experiences a growth spurt coinciding with puberty. Her vagina, tubes and uterus enlarge and mature. A very specific action of estrogen is to create vaginal secretions having an acidic pH.

Progesterone promotes growth of the glands of the breasts and helps to prepare the uterus for pregnancy. The sudden drop in progesterone when pregnancy doesn't occur is what brings on the menstrual period.

How long does the period normally last?   The duration of bleeding averages three to six days. The Pill may cause short periods and the IUD may cause long ones. Some women regularly menstruate for only a day or two, some for seven or eight days. This is perfectly all right as long as there are no sudden and drastic changes in the pattern.

What's the average interval between periods?   Twenty-eight days, but the length of the cycle may range from twenty to thirty-six days in normal women. The interval between periods remains fairly constant, though it's rare for a woman to have perfectly regular periods.

What's the average blood loss during a period?   Two to three ounces.

Is iron therapy needed to make up for the loss?   You don't need iron tablets or tonic if your diet is rich in lean meat, whole grain and enriched bread and cereal, and eggs and liver. If you do want to take iron, you can get it in the form of one ferrous sulfate tablet (300 mg.) a day for about two weeks each month. The tablet should be taken with a meal (see p. 360).

Is it normal to pass clots?   A few clots may form, but a blood-thinning substance, fibrinolysin, is released along with the menstrual discharge and usually prevents clot formation. Frequent passage of large clots is abnormal and points to a problem within the uterus.

MENSTRUAL PROBLEMS

What may cause a delay in onset of the periods?   The usual cause is a family history of this pattern; if the girl's mother began late, she may too. There's no cause for alarm until the girl is sixteen, and many doctors are reluctant to say that a problem exists unless the girl is eighteen and still hasn't menstruated.

True delay in onset, known as primary amenorrhea, may be due to failure of ovarian function, damage to the ovaries by disease or surgery, endocrine conditions and a developmental defect such as Turner's syndrome (gonadal dysgenesis). Other contributing factors include general ill health, poor nutrition and severe emotional problems.

What can be done to cause the periods to start?   The first step is to discover the cause of the delay. Signs such as breast development and the presence of axillary and pubic hair point to estrogen production. Most likely the periods will start within a year. Certain bones ossify within six months before or after the onset of menstruation, and X-rays may indicate that menstruation is imminent. In these instances, reassurance and waiting are all that's necessary. Sometimes hormone therapy will cause the ovaries to begin functioning. The therapy is given for several days at the start of each month, and withdrawn after several months to see if the girl's ovaries will work on their own. There are some side effects to this treatment, and the patient as well as the physician should carefully weigh both the emotional and physiological factors involved in the delayed menstruation.

What is premenstrual tension?   It's the irritability, depression, headache, bloating and lower abdominal discomfort that may appear five to seven days before the period. These symptoms, varying in severity, occur in up to 90 percent of women and disappear soon after the onset of bleeding.

What can be done for premenstrual symptoms?   Some physicians recommend eating more leafy green vegetables, whole grains, seeds and nuts. Salt restriction and diuretics usually are not needed, but some women find that controlling water retention by restricting the use of salt does make them feel better. Some physicians prescribe a tranquilizer to be taken for the week before the onset of each period, but drugs may cause complications and should be avoided if possible.

What causes the cramps?   Menstrual pain is caused by contractions of the uterus as it expels the menstrual flow. Women bothered by cramps have stronger-than-average uterine contractions, which may be caused by excessive secretion of a prostaglandin, a smooth-muscle stimulant.

Smallness of the cervical opening may contribute to the pain. This would explain why cramps are most common in young women, occurring in at least a fourth of teenage girls, and why the pain is usually worse during the first day of bleeding, when the flow is greatest. The pain can be temporarily relieved by dilation of the cervix, and is less severe after the birth of a child —which leaves the cervical opening larger than before childbirth. Repeated menstruation without childbirth also enlarges the cervical opening, and cramps are less common in women beyond the age of twenty-five or thirty.

What can be done for painful menstruation? Taking two aspirin every three or four hours is the time-honored remedy. Acetaminophen (Tylenol) may be used in place of aspirin, and sometimes stronger analgesics may be necessary. Some women get relief from special exercises, warm baths or the use of hot water bottles or heating pads. Activity—even including jogging —has been known to relieve menstrual cramps.

What causes severe pain with menstruation? About 10 percent of women have menstrual pain that is bad enough to cause them to miss work or school, and this is probably the best indication that the pain warrants the designation "dysmenorrhea."

If the pain has been present since soon after the onset of menstruation, it's called primary dysmenorrhea. Usually, no specific abnormalities can be found. Secondary dysmenorrhea involves pain occurring in a woman who previously did not have it or had much less severe cramps. Among the causes of secondary dysmenorrhea are endometriosis, uterine fibroids and pelvic inflammatory disease.

What's the treatment for dysmenorrhea? The treatment for primary dysmenorrhea is first a workup to make sure that the pain does not represent pelvic disease, and then the use of aspirin and similar products. At times a codeine-containing painkiller may be necessary. Birth-control pills may sometimes, for various reasons, relieve the pain of primary dysmenorrhea. Because the Pill is contraindicated for many women, its use as a treatment for this problem should be carefully considered before it is attempted.

The treatment of secondary dysmenorrhea is to correct the cause. Antibiotics may cure pelvic inflammatory disease, though surgery may be necessary to remove a tubal abscess. The treatment for endometriosis or uterine fibroids is more difficult and depends on the extent of disease and the amount of the woman's discomfort.

ENDOMETRIOSIS AND FIBROIDS

What is endometriosis? The endometrium is the lining of the womb that is shed during the menstrual period, and endometriosis is the presence of endometrial tissue in sites other than the womb. A small bit of endometrium may be propelled upward during a menstrual period and enter the tubes. There it passes out to the ovaries and is deposited on them as well as on other parts of the pelvis and lower abdominal cavity. Like seeds, the endometrial cells grow into clumps varying in size from quite small to as large as a tennis ball—the so-called chocolate cyst. Very rarely the endometrium may be carried through the blood to the kidneys, lungs or skin.

102

Who is most likely to have endometriosis?   It is most common between the ages of thirty and forty and is said to have a predilection for women in the middle and upper socioeconomic groups. Teenagers are rarely affected. The incidence is difficult to estimate, but it may account for the problems of 10 percent of women who visit a private gynecologist for treatment.

What are the symptoms of endometriosis?   The most common symptom is secondary dysmenorrhea, the onset of painful menstruation beginning in the late twenties or early thirties. Endometriosis may also cause irregular or prolonged menstrual bleeding and is sometimes responsible for pain during intercourse. In some women it causes infertility.

What is the treatment?   The best treatment may be no treatment, since endometriosis often subsides spontaneously. Symptomatic therapy and observation are indicated initially. One event that usually brings relief is pregnancy, though symptoms may return after the baby is born. Since the endometrial implants do respond to hormone therapy, cycling of the periods with birth-control pills is another way to relieve the pain. A form of progesterone such as the mini-Pill is usually given. Surgery to remove the endometrial implants is necessary when symptoms are severe or the implants are large. The surgeon should make every effort to spare the ovaries and leave the uterus in place.

What are fibroid tumors?   A fibroid tumor is a benign growth of the muscle of the uterus. Also known as a myoma or leiomyoma, the tumor is five times more common in black than in white women. Several fibroid tumors may appear in the same uterus, and at times the tumors may grow large enough to mimic pregnancy.

How can you tell if you have fibroids?   Most of the time the tumor is diagnosed during a pelvic examination. The woman may have noticed few or no symptoms. When symptoms occur, these may consist of excessive or irregular bleeding, painful menstruation or pelvic discomfort due to pressure of the tumor on the rectum or bladder.

What's the treatment for fibroids?   No treatment may be indicated, or the person may need to have the fibroids or the entire uterus removed.

Do fibroids ever turn into cancer?   Yes, degeneration of a fibroid into a cancer (sarcoma) sometimes occurs. It is much more likely that the fibroma will regress spontaneously, remain benign or turn into a wombstone.

What is a wombstone?   Over the course of many years, a fibroid may absorb calcium from the bloodstream and take on a rock-hard consistency that feels to an examiner very much like a stone. An X-ray will reveal the calcium deposits within the fibroid and confirm that it is a wombstone.

IRREGULAR OR EXCESSIVE BLEEDING

What causes irregular menstrual bleeding?   The two main causes are hormonal imbalance and structural disease of the uterus or ovaries. Endometriosis, fibroids and uterine cancer are examples of structural disease. Hormonal imbalance is a far more frequent basis for irregular bleeding, and failure to ovulate (anovulatory cycles) is usually responsible.

What is an anovulatory cycle?   It's a menstrual cycle occurring without ovulation and resulting from an imbalance between the regulatory hormones of the brain and the estrogen produced by the ovaries. When an egg isn't released, progesterone is not secreted and the great endometrial growth that is characteristic of the last two weeks of a normal cycle doesn't occur. Instead, bleeding is irregular because the uterine lining grows in a patchy, unpredictable layer that is as apt to be shed as it is to continue growing.

How can you tell if you're having anovulatory cycles?   One clue is that the bleeding is not associated with menstrual pain (cramps). Anovulatory cycles occur most commonly in teenage girls who have just begun to menstruate, and in women over the age of thirty-eight who are nearing the menopause. The bleeding itself is characteristic. It's irregularly irregular. You may skip a period and then have several periods only a couple of weeks apart. Sometimes the bleeding is excessive and lasts over a week, and at other times it's slight and lasts only a day.

What's the treatment for irregular bleeding?   The woman in her thirties or forties may need a D & C (dilatation and curettage) or a biopsy of the endometrium to make sure she doesn't have uterine cancer. For reasons not understood, the D & C may correct the irregular bleeding even when no abnormality is found. Tablets or an injection of progesterone can serve to diagnose and treat anovulatory cycles. By stimulating endometrial growth, the progesterone brings on a normal period within several days. Sometimes it's necessary to give the progesterone each month for several months, though this treatment isn't always successful.

Most teenage girls have some anovulatory cycles, which are considered normal in the first few years of menstruation. Birth-control pills may be taken for three to six months if the irregular cycles persist or cause excessive or troublesome bleeding. Usually, ovulatory cycles begin after the birth-control pills are stopped.

What causes spotting?   Periods that are light enough to be called spotting occur normally in some women. When this is the regular pattern, further workup is not necessary unless the woman has trouble getting pregnant or stops having periods altogether. The user of birth-control pills is apt to have scant menses. The light flow is related to the relative amounts of estrogen and progesterone in the Pill. Choosing another Pill with higher estrogen content or lower progesterone content will usually allow heavier bleeding, if this is desirable.

Spotting between periods may occur in a normal woman, and it's estimated that over 90 percent of women have had at least a small amount of spotting at mid-cycle. The slight staining may be noted right after the pain of mittelschmerz, which coincides with ovulation. Anything that gives rise to irregular bleeding may cause spotting between periods. The user of birth-control pills or an IUD is more likely to have spotting at mid-cycle. Anovulatory bleeding, uterine cancer, cervical cancer and endometrial polyps are other sources of spotting between periods, and the treatment is directed toward the specific problem.

What are polyps?   A polyp is a stalklike growth on the lining of a body cavity. Endometrial polyps are seen in women beyond the age of forty who have irregular bleeding due to anovulatory cycles. Prolonged estrogen stimulation in the absence of ovulation seems to contribute to the polyp's growth. Some endometrial polyps are cancerous, but most are not. Cervical polyps are unlikely to be cancerous, but they bleed easily and may cause spotting.

What's the treatment for polyps?   They should be removed, either in the doctor's office or in the operating room.

What causes flooding?   Among the sources are endometriosis, fibroids, uterine cancer, anovulatory bleeding and an IUD. Endocrine disease and a blood disorder are other possibilities. An isolated instance of heavy bleeding may occur in an otherwise healthy woman and is not necessarily an indication of disease unless the bleeding recurs.

How do you know if you're flooding?   For normal menstrual bleeding, three to six pads or tampons a day are sufficient. Bleeding that requires more than these is excessive. Bleeding that requires you to change every hour or two is definitely excessive, and so is bleeding that leaves you feeling dizzy or as if you may faint.

What's the treatment for flooding?   The treatment is directed toward the underlying problem. A trial of birth-control pills may be indicated in a young woman when anovulatory cycles are suspected, and an IUD should be removed if one is present. Hypothyroidism (thyroid failure) may produce flooding, and the treatment is thyroid hormone. The resultant iron deficiency may be corrected with iron tablets. When the woman is over forty, a D & C may be indicated, and the curettage itself may halt the excessive bleeding. Hysterectomy is done when the bleeding is due to fibroids or when the hemorrhage proves refractory to other methods of therapy.

What may cause the periods to stop?   Pregnancy is the most common cause, but anything that affects a woman's health, nutrition or hormonal balance may bring her periods to a stop. Some of the possibilities are:
  · Obesity
  · Rapid weight loss from dieting
  · Chronic illness such as tuberculosis
  · Severe emotional disturbance
  · Birth-control pills—after they're stopped
  · Hormone therapy with estrogen, Depo-Provera or a similar agent
  · Drug therapy with tranquilizers, such as Mellaril, Thorazine or Stelazine
  · Use of narcotics
  · Endocrine disease, such as diabetes, hypothyroidism or adrenal hyperfunction
  · Failure of ovarian function from disease or surgery
  · Menopause

What's the treatment?   When a drug is at fault, stopping it will usually cause the periods to start. The woman who has recently gone off the Pill should resume her normal periods within six to twelve months at the latest. Clomiphene therapy can be given if she wants to get pregnant but there are potential complications that should be carefully considered. Loss of weight for an obese person, or gain of weight for an undernourished individual, may allow the periods to start. Specific therapy for an endocrine problem or ovarian failure may restore the menstrual periods. Menopause is the normal end to the menstrual cycles, and does not require therapy.

What causes bleeding after intercourse?   The appearance of small amounts of bright red blood after coitus or douching points to a disease of the cervix. Cervicitis, an inflammation of the mouth of the womb, is suspect until ruled out. This condition occurs in most women who have had children, though it's not usually bad enough to cause bleeding. Other sources of postcoital bleeding are cervical polyps, cervical erosion and cervical cancer.

What's the treatment?   Bleeding after intercourse calls for a medical examination to detect the cause. Cervical polyps can usually be removed in the office, and cervicitis may clear up after using a sulfa-containing vaginal cream or freezing or cauterizing the cervix. Caught early, cervical cancer can be cured.

GYNECOLOGIC CARE

How do you find a good gynecologist?   Select a Board-certified specialist in obstetrics and gynecology who is courteous but not condescending, and interested in you—but only professionally. Do the selecting before you develop a specific problem so that your needs are not urgent.

How do I know if the doctor is any good?   Even though certified specialists share much the same training, they obviously differ in skill, experience and intelligence. Some physicians exercise better judgment than others. Some are warmer, friendlier and more perceptive than others. Some are more likely to operate than others; a few may be more interested in making money than in providing good patient care. If you can find a gynecologist who counts among his patients women doctors, nurses and the wives of doctors, you probably won't go wrong in choosing this physician for your own care. You can learn a lot from talking to other women the doctor has cared for, and you can see for yourself if you like the office, the nurse and the examination.

What are the signs of a well-run office?   First, the signs of a poorly run office: a crowded waiting room with ashtrays and magazines strewn about; a rude nurse; and a hasty examination by a physician you believe you saw but aren't sure because he or she was gone so quickly. This is assembly-line medicine at its worst, and you should avoid it if you have a choice.

The doctor with the most crowded office is not necessarily the best. More likely the appointment system has failed, or the doctor has no one to cover for him or her in the event of a delivery or emergency. You can find out many things from the nurse who usually reflects the doctor. If she's courteous, warm and honest, the doctor is apt to be, too. The old routine of undressing and getting into the stirrups before you even see the doctor is no longer acceptable. The examination should be conducted after the doctor has taken a history, and the findings should be discussed with you. The exam itself should cause a minimum of discomfort. The doctor should tell you what is going to happen at each stage of the exam, and insertion of the speculum shouldn't be painful. The doctor should keep a careful record of the exam and treatment.

What is the problem-oriented medical record? It is a record-keeping system that is built around you and your problems. It begins with a data base workup; the doctor records your medical history, examines you, and orders a blood count, blood chemistries, urinalysis, chest X-ray and Pap smear. (Bear in mind that health insurance doesn't always reimburse for this workup.) Then your problems are listed in order of importance in the chart and a plan of therapy is made out for each one. At subsequent visits your progress is noted and the problem list is kept current as new conditions arise.

What difference does record keeping make? Medical excellence and good record keeping go hand in hand. The medical record is an instrument for your treatment. You have the right, in many instances, to see it and to know how it is being kept. A good doctor won't object to your asking if he or she uses the problem-oriented method. If this method is not used, which method is being used, and how effective is it?

How often should you be seen? Though less frequent examination is now being considered, especially for older women, many physicians recommend that you should have an annual Pap smear beginning after the first intercourse or no later than age twenty. Of course, you should see the doctor during the year if you notice anything unusual (see p. 112–13).

GYNECOLOGIC SURGERY

What's a D & C? It is a *d*ilatation and *c*urettage of the uterus. The cervical opening must be dilated before the curette, an elongated instrument with a scoop on its end, can be inserted and used to scrape out the uterine lining. The scraping is done in a clockwise manner in a regular pattern so that the entire endometrium can be removed. The physician can tell when the lining is gone by the gritty sensation that can be felt through the curette and heard as a sandpaperlike scratching sound.

How often is the D & C done? Each year an estimated 1.5 million women have a D & C. It is the most common gynecologic procedure, and at a cost of $350 per operation, it accounts for half a billion dollars a year of medical economics. Many feel that the operation is done too frequently.

What are the indications for a D & C? It may be used in diagnosis, as in determining the cause of heavy or irregular bleeding, or in therapy, as in removing retained pieces of placenta when bleeding persists after a miscarriage or an induced abortion. It's not uncommon for the procedure to be both diagnostic and therapeutic. For example, D & C may stop a woman from having heavy bleeding while at the same time showing that the lining of her uterus was not cancerous and did not contain polyps. The indications include:

· *Workup of heavy or irregular bleeding*
· *Diagnosis of suspected cancer* of the cervix or uterus
· *Evaluation of bleeding* that occurs after the menopause
· *Treatment of an incomplete miscarriage or an induced abortion* when bleeding persists or increases

When is D & C not indicated?   D & C is not usually indicated in the workup of missed menstrual periods, scanty periods, slight spotting at mid-cycle or spotting just before the onset of the period. It usually isn't necessary to diagnose anovulatory cycles in a woman under the age of thirty-five. It won't help in the evaluation of bleeding from the rectum or bladder.

What should you ask the doctor before submitting to a D & C?   If the procedure is to be done for anything but the above indications, ask the doctor how necessary it is. This question may cause him or her to reconsider. Since the D & C is usually an elective operation, it can be put off while alternate methods of therapy are tried. For example, hormone therapy will usually stop the bleeding from anovulatory cycles. If the bleeding becomes troublesome later on, a dilatation and curettage can be done.

Doctors who do the D & C too often may justify it because of its known usefulness in diagnosing uterine cancer. When cancer is mentioned, it is difficult for most persons to remain rational: the urge is to do whatever is necessary to rule out this dread disease. Nevertheless, if you're under forty, have a negative Pap smear and haven't had heavy or very troublesome bleeding, you're not likely to have uterine cancer (though you could). It might help, in weighing a decision, to ask the doctor how likely it is that you might have uterine cancer, how often D & C is needed to make the diagnosis and what the dangers are in delay.

Don't hesitate to seek an opinion from a second doctor. You may ask the first doctor to refer you to someone, but it's probably better to find the second specialist yourself. The first doctor is obligated to supply the consultant with copies of your medical records.

What is a hysterectomy?   It is the operative removal of the uterus (womb). It may be done through the abdomen (abdominal hysterectomy) or through the vagina (vaginal hysterectomy). It may be partial (only the womb is removed) or total (the womb, the tubes and the ovaries are removed).

When is hysterectomy indicated?   It may be needed to treat:
· Cancer of the cervix, endometrium or ovary

· Severe uterine bleeding that cannot be stopped by more conservative measures

· Serious pelvic infection or abscess that doesn't heal with antibiotic therapy

· Fibroids or endometriosis when these cause severe bleeding or pain that is unresponsive to other therapy

· Serious pelvic relaxation when it is accompanied by prolapse of the uterus

When is hysterectomy not indicated?   It is not needed to control excessive or irregular menstrual bleeding when tumor or endometriosis is not present and when conservative measures have not been attempted. It is not indicated as a means of sterilization or of ending the menstrual periods when no uterine abnormality exists. It is never indicated as a treatment for nervousness, depression or menstrual cramps. A type of hysterectomy that constitutes malpractice is to remove the abdominal part of the uterus and leave the cervix in place. No qualified specialist will perform this operation, since to leave the unnecessary cervix behind is to risk cancer developing in it.

Should the ovaries be removed during a hysterectomy?   For years the practice was to take out the ovaries along with the uterus on the chance that the woman might later develop ovarian cancer if these were left in. This approach still has its proponents. If your gynecologist is one of them, find another surgeon. To remove healthy ovaries on the outside possibility that this will prevent cancer is no more reasonable than to remove the breasts or thyroid to prevent cancer in these organs. When a woman beyond the menopause needs hysterectomy, the ovaries may be removed, though many doctors believe that the ovaries continue to function slightly and should be left in.

When is surgery on the pelvic muscles necessary?   This surgery, known as anterior and posterior vaginal repair (A-P repair) is justified when a woman has marked weakness of her vaginal muscles that can't be corrected by performing Kegel's exercises (described in Chapter 3). Among the specific indications are a prolapsed uterus, urinary incontinence, or a bulging of the bladder or rectum through the vagina. Wearing a pessary is an alternate means of therapy, though it is not very effective in holding back a bulging or fallen rectum. A pessary may serve as a temporary means of pelvic support while a decision about surgery is being made. A-P repair is often combined with a vaginal hysterectomy, but the muscle-strengthening surgery can be done, in many instances, without removing the womb.

GENITAL CANCER

What exactly is a Pap smear?   The test is named for Dr. George N. Papanicolaou, who developed it as a screening test for cancer of the cervix. The examiner first exposes the cervix, then scrapes cells from around its opening, from the vagina just behind the cervix, and, often, from the cervical canal. These scrapings are smeared onto two or three glass slides and placed in a fixative—a solution to prevent the cells from deteriorating while they are en route to the pathologist. The pathologist examines the smears microscopically and sends a report to the physician.

What preparation is needed for the test?   It can be done at any time, but it's best not to have it during the menstrual period, as the bleeding makes interpretation of cervical cells more difficult. Also, the woman should not have douched or used vaginal cream, foam or suppositories within two days before the test. Lubricating jelly that would ordinarily be applied to the speculum to facilitate its insertion can also interfere with the Pap test. For this reason, the physician must lubricate the speculum with warm water when a Pap smear is to be done.

What does a positive Pap test mean?   The pathologist will report the test as one of the following: negative (Class I), atypical cells (Class II), suggestive of malignant cells (Class III) or definite for malignant cells (Class IV). A positive test is any class but a Class I. A Class II Pap is no cause for alarm, though it should be repeated every six months until it reverts to normal or becomes a Class III. A Class II Pap is sometimes caused by conditions such as cervical irritation or trichomonas infection (see p. 88), which should be treated. A Class III or a Class IV Pap suggests that a malignancy may be present. Further investigation and therapy are indicated.

How accurate is the Pap smear?   Experience has shown that it is 95 percent accurate in detecting cancer of the cervix. It is falsely suggestive of malignancy about 5 percent of the time. It is also falsely negative about 5 percent of the time, meaning that a negative Pap test does not ensure that you don't have cancer of the cervix. The Pap, after all, is a screening test. A change in the appearance of the cervix should prompt a biopsy or one of the other studies used to diagnose cancer of the cervix.

What are the other tests for diagnosing cancer of the cervix?   A repeat Pap smear is done when the test is reported as positive. At the second exam a thorough visual examination of the cervix is made, and any area that appears suspiciously different from the surrounding tissue is biopsied: a piece of tissue is removed for microscopic examination and examined by the

111

pathologist. The accuracy of the pathologist's report for the biopsy is higher than that for the Pap smear.

Colposcopy is a diagnostic method that originated in Europe and has become popular in the United States in the last ten or fifteen years. Through a microscope-like instrument, the specialist examines the cervix close up. Details that can't be seen with the naked eye are visible, and suspicious areas can be biopsied.

Conization amounts to a biopsy of the entire rim of the cervix. After anesthetizing the womb, the operator cuts a circumferential, cone-shaped wedge of tissue from the end of the cervix. The specimen is submitted for detailed pathologic examination for evidence of cancer.

What are the symptoms of cervical cancer?   The early ones are bleeding after intercourse or douching, spotting between periods, and a slight, blood-tinged discharge that may not seem significant. Pain is a late symptom and occurs when the tumor has invaded the rectum, bladder or pelvic wall.

How common is this form of cancer?   It accounts for 85 percent of all pelvic malignancies in women, and about one in every sixty-three women can expect to develop cervical cancer during her life.

Who is most likely to get cancer of the cervix?   The least likely person is one who has never had sexual intercourse. The cancer is also uncommon in a woman who's never had children. Factors that increase the risk of cervical cancer are:
 · Early age of first intercourse
 · Intercourse with many different partners
 · Herpes infection
 · Having first child before age twenty
 · Having several children
 · Lower socioeconomic group
 · Age forty or older

What is the treatment for cancer of the cervix?   It depends on the stage of the cancer, which is determined by physical examination, staining tests and X-ray studies after the cancer is diagnosed. Stage I cancer is still confined to the cervix, and Stage IV cancer has spread beyond the pelvis. Stages II and III are intermediate. The treatment for the early stages is usually hysterectomy, and the treatment for Stage IV is radiation therapy. (At some medical centers, radiation therapy is the method chosen to treat all but the earliest stages of cervical cancer.) Advanced or recurrent cancer is sometimes treated with cell-killing drugs, a procedure known as chemotherapy.

What's the survival rate from cancer of the cervix?   As is true of any malignancy, the earlier the cancer is detected, the better the survival rate. The five-year cure rate from a Stage I cancer is 70 to 80 percent. The five-year survival from Stage IV disease is about 15 percent. The survival rates of Stages II and III are intermediate between these extremes.

Is uterine cancer different from cervical cancer?   Yes. Though the cervix is the lower part of the uterus that protrudes into the vagina, cancer of the uterine lining is considered a separate disease, "endometrial carcinoma." The two cancers differ in cell types and growth patterns, and respond differently to therapy. Sometimes, however, it's impossible to tell whether an advanced malignancy began in the cervix or in the lining of the uterus.

How common is uterine cancer?   It's less common than cervical cancer, but one out of a hundred women can expect to develop it during her life. The onset is usually after age fifty.

What factors predispose to uterine cancer?   Diabetes, high blood pressure and obesity are said to predispose to endometrial cancer, though the association is disputed by some authorities. A predisposing factor that seems hard to dispute is estrogen therapy. Women who take estrogen replacement therapy beyond the menopause are much more likely to develop uterine cancer than are women who don't take estrogens.

What are the symptoms of uterine cancer?   The main one is bleeding, especially when it recurs a year or more after the menstrual periods have stopped. In a woman whose periods haven't stopped, the cancer may cause spotting between periods and irregular bleeding.

How is the cancer diagnosed?   Because cancer cells may spill into the vagina, the Pap smear is positive in 65 percent of women with uterine cancer. (In taking the Pap smear, the doctor also gets material from a small pool of secretions behind the cervix.)
   The cancerous uterus may be enlarged and softened in ways somewhat similar to the changes of early pregnancy. Confirmation of the diagnosis depends on the obtaining of tissue by endometrial biopsy or D & C.

What's the treatment?   Hysterectomy and radiotherapy, though the radiotherapy is usually given before surgery. Advanced cancer may be treated with further radiation, hormone therapy or chemotherapy.

What's the survival rate from cancer of the uterus?   The average five-year survival rate is 55 percent. When the treatment is begun while the cancer is still in its earliest stage, the survival rate after five years is 85 percent.

What about cancer of the ovary?   Though it is less common than cervical or uterine cancer, ovarian cancer is more deadly. It ranks fourth as a cancer killer in women—behind cancer of the breast, colon and lung—and three-fourths of women found to have it don't survive beyond five years. The main reason for the poor survival is that there's no easy way, such as the Pap smear, to screen for ovarian malignancy.

What are the symptoms of ovarian cancer?   Early signs are minimal. Pain may occur during intercourse or the woman may note a feeling of heaviness or vague discomfort in the lower abdomen. Abdominal swelling accompanies growth of the cancer. In some instances the cancer causes fluid accumulation that can lead to massive abdominal distention. Tumors that are hormonally active may cause the growth of facial hair, an enlargement of the clitoris or a reduction in the size of the breasts. Fifty-two is the average age when the cancer is diagnosed, and women in the upper socioeconomic groups have the greatest risk of developing it.

How is the cancer diagnosed?   It is suspected by the discovery of an enlarged ovary during a pelvic examination. Four out of five ovarian tumors are not malignant, and X-ray studies and ultrasound may help to establish whether cancer is present. Surgery is done when the initial studies are completed, and the diagnosis is confirmed during exploratory laparotomy.

What's the treatment?   The tumor, the opposite ovary, the uterus and tubes are removed when the cancer has not spread to the pelvic or abdominal wall. Radiation therapy may be given after surgery, and in far-advanced cancer, chemotherapy is used. In the case of a benign tumor in a young woman, the opposite ovary and uterus may be preserved so that she can bear children.

What about cancer of the vulva and vagina?   These cancers account for less than 5 percent of malignancies in women, and vulvar cancer is three times as frequent as vaginal cancer. The woman with cancer of the main or minor lips, usually older than fifty-five, seeks help because of a lump or ulcer that itches or bleeds. Sometimes vaginal cancer represents an extension of cancer of the cervix, but it may arise in its own right. Pain and bleeding are the main symptoms.

What factors contribute to these cancers?   Venereal disease such as granuloma inguinale and, rarely, venereal warts (condylomata acuminata)

114

may contribute to vulvar cancer. Often, the woman with cancer of the vulva has or has had another malignancy, such as cancer of the cervix.

The association between therapy with diethylstilbestrol (DES) during pregnancy and the occurrence of vaginal cancer in a girl born of that pregnancy is well established, though it is not as common as originally feared. The cancer has occurred in such persons between the ages of seven and twenty-nine, usually in association with a condition known as vaginal adenosis. In vaginal adenosis, islands of cells that ordinarily would occur only in the cervix appear in the vagina. Maldevelopment of the vagina is another side effect that may occur in the daughter of a DES-treated mother.

What's the treatment for vulvar or vaginal cancer?   Surgery to remove the tumor and the surrounding tissue is the preferred treatment for vulvar cancer. Radiation therapy may be used to treat far-advanced malignancy.

Unless the cancer has extended from another organ, surgery is the treatment of choice for vaginal cancer. Radiation therapy is preferable if the cancer began in the cervix. The woman or girl with vaginal adenosis should be cared for by a specialist with experience in treating this condition. Removal of the islands of abnormal tissue may be indicated, and vaginal surgery may become necessary.

MENOPAUSE

What is menopause?   It's the time in a woman's life when her ovaries stop functioning. Her periods cease, and when she's been without bleeding for a year, menopause is complete. This usually occurs between the ages of forty-five and fifty-five.

Does it occur abruptly?   No. Menopause is a gradual process that begins before the end of the reproductive years and stretches to about five or six years after the periods have stopped. It's a time of transition to a new phase of life.

What are the symptoms of menopause?   Symptoms occur in about 60 to 70 percent of women, and include hot flashes, fatigue, nervousness, headache and difficulty in sleeping.

The hot flash is the most characteristic symptom, and it is created by a sudden rushing of blood to the skin. Flushing and a stinging warmth may occur. The attacks happen day or night and may last a few seconds or half an hour. The symptoms, which are most noticeable in the face, neck, chest, arms and back, may be followed by profuse sweating and a clammy sensation. Hot flashes may begin a year before the menstrual periods end and may continue for several years after the periods stop.

What is early menopause?   It's menopause occurring before age forty. Not uncommonly a woman in her late thirties will go through the menopause, and premature menopause has occurred as early as age seventeen. The most frequent setting for early menopause is removal of the ovaries, known by doctors as "surgical menopause."

What causes menopause?   The ovaries contain a "clock" that tells them when the woman's reproductive years are over, but like other changes that come with aging, it's poorly understood. The age for menopause does seem to be inherited: the daughter of a woman who went through menopause early is liable to do so as well.

Does estrogen production stop completely at the menopause?   No. The hot flashes and cessation of menstruation are due to a decline in the amount of estrogen produced by the ovaries, but these glands continue to make small amounts of estrogen for many years. The adrenal glands also make estrogen. Forty percent of women continue to show evidence of estrogen production to age eighty and beyond.

How can you tell if you're entering the menopause?   You may develop the symptoms mentioned above, which are very suggestive if you are between the ages of forty-five and fifty-five. The menstrual periods lessen in amount and may occur irregularly.

   By examining a scraping taken from the vagina, a doctor can tell if estrogen effect is diminishing. A more expensive test is to measure the quantity of follicle stimulating hormone (FSH) in the blood or the urine. Released cyclically by the brain, FSH initiates the menstrual cycles during the reproductive years. After menopause the brain produces more FSH as if trying to stimulate the ovaries to continue functioning. FSH output remains elevated for the rest of the woman's life, and the presence in the urine of large amounts of it indicates that a woman is entering or has passed through the menopause.

What are the other changes of menopause?   These symptoms vary from woman to woman. The vaginal walls may become thinner and lose their acidic pH. The main lips and mons may diminish in size. The woman's breasts, hips and waist may lose their previous shape. A reduction in the protein and mineral content of bone may lead to osteoporosis, which is more prominent in some women than in others, and may give rise to back pain, stooped posture and a reduction in height. All these factors seem to be dependent upon general good health, nutrition and regular exercises to a larger degree than was previously understood.

Do you need treatment for menopause?　Menopause has been a cause of concern to women down through the years. They have visited physicians and been given tranquilizers, psychotherapy, minerals, hormones and vitamins.

Much of the emphasis in recent years has been on the use of estrogen therapy. Since menopause is a time of decreasing estrogen production, the reasoning went, why not reverse the possible changes brought by osteoporosis and the increased risk of heart disease by giving estrogens? An estimated 5 million American women were taking estrogens in 1978. Recent evidence has indicated that such widespread use of estrogen therapy is unjustified because of the risks involved.

What are the risks of estrogen replacement therapy?　The biggest risk is an increased likelihood of developing cancer of the uterus. This form of cancer has been growing in frequency during the last decade, and estrogen replacement therapy may be responsible. The estrogen user is five to ten times as likely to develop it as the woman who doesn't take estrogens. The risk rises to fourteenfold when estrogens have been used for seven years or longer. The chances of getting breast cancer are much greater for the woman who takes estrogens, and she runs a higher risk of developing gall bladder disease, vascular disease and possibly other problems, such as high blood pressure and diabetes.

Is one form of estrogen safer than another?　No. "Natural," "synthetic," "conjugated" and "unconjugated" forms of the drug appear to be equal in their incidence of side effects. Estrogen creams used in the vagina are absorbed, so that the same effects of the hormone occur as with the oral form of the drug.

What's the cancer risk after stopping estrogen therapy?　Six months after going off estrogen therapy a woman's risk of uterine cancer falls to about that of one who never took the drug.

Who should not take estrogen replacement therapy?　You shouldn't take estrogens if you have a family history of cancer of the breast or uterus, or if you have lumps or nodules in your breasts. Avoid this drug if you have had clotting in the legs or elsewhere, stroke, heart attack, angina pectoris, or liver or gall bladder trouble. Vaginal bleeding of unknown cause, uterine polyps and fibroid tumors are additional contraindications for estrogen therapy. *Estrogen therapy is never indicated during pregnancy.*

What are the benefits of estrogen therapy?　Estrogen may relieve hot flashes, but it is not usually effective in treating depression, irritability or

117

nervousness. To some extent it will reverse the menopausal changes in the vagina. It helps in some instances of osteoporosis, when other measures, such as taking calcium supplements, are also employed. Replacement therapy may be useful when a woman's ovaries are removed before she is forty, or in the rare instance when a girl doesn't develop feminine body changes because her ovaries are unable to produce estrogen.

How is estrogen therapy taken?   At the lowest possible dose, and cyclically to mimic the action of the ovaries. This means taking it for three weeks each month, then waiting a week before resuming therapy. The cream should be used cyclically in the same way as the pills. The woman taking estrogen for the relief of menopausal symptoms should restrict the course of therapy to three to six months. Longer therapy is more likely to cause side effects.

Is there anything else that can be used for the symptoms of menopause? A tranquilizer may help to relieve nervousness, but it should be taken for only a short time so that it doesn't create a physical or psychological dependence. Dr. Louise Tyrer, a gynecologist with the Planned Parenthood Federation, has found that vitamin E helps to relieve hot flashes. The dose is 400 to 1,600 international units a day, taken in divided doses with meals. To date, this beneficial role for vitamin E has not been substantiated scientifically. Other things that may help are a good diet and regular exercise. Certainly a positive, open-minded attitude about this normal time of life is helpful in keeping symptoms to a minimum.

Do men go through a "menopause"?   Many do experience a male climacteric in their late forties or early fifties. A fall in production of testosterone is responsible, and among the symptoms are hot flashes and nervousness. Also important in this condition are the psychological reactions to aging.

THE BREASTS

What are the breasts composed of?   Most of a breast is fat, but milk-producing glands are distributed evenly throughout the fatty tissue. These glands are joined by a network of small ducts that end in the nipple. Sheets of tissue radiate inward from the nipple. By passing through the breast and attaching to the chest wall, these suspensory ligaments maintain the breast in its characteristic shape.

How do the male and female breasts differ?   The male breast contains the same structures as the female breast, but it doesn't develop because it isn't exposed to the female sex hormones.

How do hormones affect the breasts? Estrogen causes fat deposition and growth of the ducts that drain the breast glands. Progesterone stimulates growth of the milk glands.

What determines the size of the breasts? The girl whose mother and grandmothers had large breasts may inherit this feature, and vice versa. Pregnancy causes breast growth, and the enlargement may be permanent. Birth-control pills and estrogen therapy will stimulate growth of the breasts, but some reduction in size usually occurs when the therapy is stopped. A woman's nutrition and general health may affect the size of her breasts.

For poorly understood reasons, some women develop extremely large breasts. Most such women have not taken the Pill or used any form of estrogen therapy. It's thought that they are extremely sensitive to their own, naturally produced estrogen. At times surgery is requested to reduce the size of the breasts.

What causes one breast to be larger than the other? Most women vary up to 10 percent in the size of the two breasts. The right is apt to be larger in a right-handed person, the left in a left-handed individual. More than a 10 percent difference in size may also be normal.

Can women have extra nipples? Accessory, or supernumerary, nipples occur in one out of every two hundred Caucasians; the incidence is higher in Orientals. The extra nipples appear below the breasts in the "milk line" on one or both sides as either a complete nipple or a small spot that may pass for a mole. Sometimes two accessory nipples are present on both sides, but almost never more than this. Breast tissue doesn't usually develop beneath the extra nipples, which may occur in men as well as women.

What's the cause of nipples turning in? Inversion of the nipples is a variation in breast development that occurs in 1 or 2 percent of women. It affects both breasts, and is not abnormal. By using a breast pump, the woman with inverted nipples can still nurse her baby. When a turned-in nipple occurs in a breast where the nipple was previously everted, the cause may be an infection, injury or cancer of the breast.

Will going without a bra harm the breasts? No, the braless way is the natural way, though jogging without a bra is said to hasten sagging. Since the ligaments that support the breast tend to stretch, the breasts may sag with the passing years and the pull of gravity, but this tends to happen with aging whether or not you wear a bra.

BREAST DISEASE

What causes breast pain?   A common source of pain is the engorgement that occurs before the menstrual period. Birth-control pills, estrogen therapy and pregnancy may produce pain and tenderness in the breasts. Injury, infection and cystic disease of the breast may cause breast pain. Cancer of the breast is usually painless in its early stages.

What can be done for breast pain?   Wearing a bra will help to relieve pain from any cause. The bra should be well-fitted and worn both day and night. Aspirin or acetaminophen may give symptomatic relief. The user of birth-control pills may need a Pill that is lower in estrogen content; the woman on estrogen therapy may need a lower dosage.

How does breast injury occur?   Because of its position, the breast may be injured in a fall or when it is struck in a crash injury or by a direct blow. A bruise is usually followed by quick healing. Sometimes a painful collection of blood requires aspiration for relief. Occasionally an injury destroys some of the breast tissue and causes a condition known as fat necrosis. A lump may develop at the site of injury and one may not be able to distinguish it from breast cancer. A mammogram (breast X-ray) may help in the workup, and biopsy of the lump is sometimes necessary. Injury to the breast is not a cause of cancer.

What causes infection of the breasts?   It may occur after breast-feeding when a slight injury to the nipple becomes infected. Usually the baby can be nursed at the opposite breast until the infected one has healed. Infection may occur after an injury to the breast, and on rare occasions the infection may reach the breast from other body parts. The worst infections follow a human bite. The mouth contains germs that, when injected beneath the skin, can cause severe infection.

What's the treatment for breast infection?   The breast should be put at rest by support with a bra. A wound should be kept clean and allowed to drain. Application of heat in the form of a hot water bottle or warm water may help to speed healing. Antibiotic therapy is frequently necessary, and the choice of drug is based on a culture of the breast effluent. A nursing mother may prevent infection by washing the nipples with soap and water after each feeding.

What is cystic disease of the breast?   This condition is also known as fibrocystic disease, chronic cystic mastitis and mammary dysplasia. It occurs in six out of ten women in the reproductive years and is characterized by the presence in the breasts of cysts that may be painful and tender before the menstrual period. The cysts vary in size from month to month. They contain brown, black, green, gray or clear fluid, and have a ropy, irregular feel on palpation. They occur in the upper, outer parts of both breasts, and in other areas as well. Though cystic disease is benign, the woman who has it is twice as likely to get breast cancer as a woman of the same age whose breasts don't contain cysts.

What causes cystic disease? The cause is unknown. The condition is related to the hormones produced by the ovaries, and it regresses after the menopause.

What's the treatment for cystic disease? The pain and tenderness may be relieved by applying heat to the breasts or by taking aspirin or acetaminophen. The person should have an annual breast examination by a doctor, and should go sooner if her own examinations reveal a suspicious change in a breast. A cyst that contains fluid may be aspirated and this will relieve the pain and may cause the lump to disappear; the fluid can also be examined microscopically.

What causes reddening and irritation of the nipple? This may occur during breast-feeding, and it calls for temporary cessation of use of that breast. An antibiotic ointment should be applied to the nipple until it is healed.

Erosion of the nipple in an older woman is known as Paget's disease. A thickening and slight enlargement of the nipple may occur, followed by irritation and formation of a sore that doesn't heal. This condition occurs in association with an underlying cancer of the breast, and it should be reported to the physician for appropriate therapy.

What causes a discharge from the nipples? A small amount of milky discharge may appear normally when a woman is in her reproductive years. Vigorous manipulation of the breasts is apt to produce it. A greenish to grayish discharge may come from cystic disease of the breasts. A usually benign tumor of the breast known as a papilloma may produce a bloody or clear discharge. The tumor can be removed in a relatively simple operation. About one in ten women who have a bloody discharge will have cancer of the breast. The source of the discharge can be determined by physical examination, mammography and lab studies.

BREAST EXAMINATION

How often should the breasts be examined by a physician?   The breasts should be examined yearly, in conjunction with the taking of the Pap smear. An immediate examination by an internist, a gynecologist or surgeon is indicated when a woman discovers a lump in her breast.

What's the purpose of self-examination of the breasts?   Experience has shown that 85 to 90 percent of breast cancers are discovered during self-examination of the breasts. This method clearly yields earlier diagnosis of cancer than waiting for a routine medical exam.

When should self-examination be done?   It should be done right after the menstrual period, when tenderness, thickening and other hormone-induced changes are at a minimum. The woman beyond the age of menopause should examine her breasts the first day of each month because this is a day that is easy to remember.

What is the technique for self-examination?   Begin by studying the breasts in the mirror with your hands behind your head, your hands at your sides, and your hands behind you while leaning forward. Look for a turning in of a nipple, the drawing to one side of a nipple, dimpling or irregularity in the skin of the breast, scaling or irritation of a nipple, or any dissimilarity between the two breasts that was not present previously.

Lie on your back and place a pillow or folded towel under one shoulder. Use the opposite hand to feel this breast. Employ the sensitive undersides of your fingers to feel for lumps or irregularities. Use a moderately firm pressure (about the same as the doctor uses) against the chest wall. Make sure the examination includes all parts of each breast as well as the armpits. Squeeze the nipples to see if there is any discharge. Some physicians advise their patients to do the palpation in the shower or tub while the breasts and hands are soapy. This may make it easier to detect a lump in the breast, but it is not a necessary or usually recommended part of self-examination. An excellent pamphlet on self-examination is available from the American Cancer Society.

What do you search for during self-examination?   By destroying the normal architecture of the breast, a cancer may cause retraction or inversion of a nipple. The skin over the cancer may become adherent to it, producing a dimpling of the skin. Sometimes the skin over a breast cancer takes on a thickened, irregular appearance not unlike the peel of an orange. Any of these changes should be reported to the doctor.

If you have cystic disease, you may note irregularities in both breasts. The irregularities have a rubbery consistency and are freely movable. They may change in size from month to month, and are especially tender just before your period. View with suspicion a hard, firm mass which doesn't move freely and which isn't tender. It may be isolated or attached to another part of the breast, may be small or large, and is especially suspect if it increases slowly in size. Report it or any unusual lump to the doctor.

BREAST CANCER

What does a lump in the breast mean?   Though it could mean that you have breast cancer, chances are good that you don't. Most lumps turn out to be cystic disease of the breast or a benign tumor.

What is a benign tumor?   A tumor that isn't cancerous. "Tumor" is the medical term for swelling. A collection of blood or a swelling from an infection is a tumor. A lump from cystic disease is a tumor. A benign tumor is generally taken to be a noncancerous breast lump that isn't caused by cystic disease.

What are the benign tumors of the breast?   Papilloma, fibroadenoma and lipoma are three that occur frequently:
· *The papilloma* calls attention to itself by producing a clear to bloody nipple discharge. The tumor is so small that it usually can't be felt. The diagnosis rests on finding the area of the breast in which pressure produces the discharge; the area is then removed via a wedge resection of the breast.
· *The fibroadenoma* is a discrete nodule occurring in one breast. Often found in young women, it is the most common benign tumor of the breast. It may enlarge rapidly during pregnancy and regress afterward. Removal of the nodule serves to both diagnose and treat it.
· *A lipoma* is a tumor of fatty tissue. Soft, movable and painless, it occurs as an isolated nodule. The treatment is sometimes excisional biopsy, though because lipomas are so easily diagnosed and are benign, they are often left in place.

What may cause one part of the breast to enlarge during pregnancy?
Aberrant breast tissue is usually responsible. This tissue may occur near or in the armpit on both sides, and may go unnoticed until pregnancy, when the high levels of hormone cause it to enlarge. It disappears after pregnancy. A fibroadenoma may enlarge during pregnancy and shrink afterward. Since 1 percent of breast cancers begin during pregnancy, this possibility must always be considered when a lump appears in a pregnant woman's breast.

How dangerous is breast cancer?   It is the number one cause of cancer and cancer death in women. About 35,000 women die from it each year, and about one in fourteen women (7 percent) can expect to develop it in her lifetime. The peak incidence is between the ages of forty and sixty, but a woman's risk of developing the cancer increases with her age. The cause of breast cancer is not known, but because of certain risk factors, we do know that some women are more likely to develop it than others.

What are the risk factors for breast cancer? Factors that favor the development of breast cancer are:
- Age fifty-five or older
- History of breast cancer in the mother and grandmother. The presence of the disease in sisters or aunts is a less important risk factor.
- Previous cancer in one breast, since there's a 10 percent chance of cancer developing in the opposite breast
- No pregnancies, or first pregnancy occurring after age thirty-five
- Menstrual periods beginning at age eleven or earlier
- Menopause occurring after age fifty
- Estrogen therapy
- Middle or upper socioeconomic group
- Previous cancer of the uterus or ovary
- Cystic disease of the breast

What factors mean a lower risk of breast cancer? A woman who does not have any of the risk factors given above has less chance of developing breast cancer. The factors associated with low risk are:
- First pregnancy by age eighteen
- Three or more pregnancies by age thirty-five
- Breast-feeding of each baby
- Neither she nor her family has a history of cancer

Does breast cancer occur in men? Yes, and it is especially dangerous, though it is one hundred times less common than in women.

What steps should a woman at high risk take? She should examine her breasts monthly, and report any changes to her doctor (even women who are not at high risk should do this). Medical examination is indicated every year or twice a year. Mammography may be done periodically to look for early breast cancer.

What is mammography? It is an X-ray study of the breasts. A cancer may show up on the films as an area of increased density containing a finely stippled pattern of calcification, though other patterns may also indicate cancer.

How accurate is mammography? It detects up to 90 percent of cancers that have characteristic X-ray features, but not all cancers have these features. In one study, mammograms were interpreted as negative in almost half of women with a lump in the breast that was later found to be cancer. Though a negative mammogram does not rule out breast cancer, the X-ray can sometimes detect lumps that are too small to be felt during a breast examination.

When is mammography indicated?   To assess a lump in the breast or to follow a woman whose risk of breast cancer is higher than average. A person over fifty who has large breasts may also benefit from mammography, since it's difficult by palpation to detect a cancer in a large breast. The use of mammography in asymptomatic or low-risk women under fifty is not recommended, as the X-ray increases the risk of developing breast cancer about 0.07 percent for each mammogram.

Isn't mammography useful as a screening test?   Yes, but the yield is low. Of 20,000 women who had mammograms, only 55 breast cancers were detected (an incidence of 0.27 percent). The difficulty is in deciding whether a great many women should be exposed to possibly harmful radiation in order to diagnose relatively few cancers. The pendulum now has swung toward greater emphasis on breast self-examination.

What other tests are used to diagnose breast cancer?   Xerography, or xeroradiography, is a recent modification of mammography that employs much lower doses of radiation. It is safer than the original form of mammography and will probably replace it in a few years. Thermography is a method of detecting breast cancer through analyzing the differential heat patterns of the breast. The heat study misses four out of ten cancers, and in 40 percent of the women where it's positive, no breast cancer is found. Ultrasound is being employed in the diagnosis of breast cancer. It doesn't apparently harm the breast, but we don't yet know its accuracy. The best test when a suspicious lump appears is to do a biopsy and examine the breast tissue under the microscope.

How is breast biopsy done?   The skin is opened and a part of the lump or the entire lump is removed and sent to the pathologist for examination. The biopsy can be done under general anesthesia, so that further surgery can be done immediately, or it may be done as a separate surgical procedure, sometimes under local anesthesia. After the report is back, a decision can be made about further surgery.

What if the lump is cancerous?   Efforts are made to see if the cancer has spread. The surgeon will order blood tests and X-rays, and will have an idea about local spread from examination at the time of the biopsy. The degree of spread determines treatment, for it would be foolish to perform radical surgery for breast cancer that had already spread to the liver, lung, brain or other organ.

What is the treatment for breast cancer?   Stage I cancer is limited to the removed lump, and the chance of surgical cure is excellent. Stage II cancer has spread to the lymph glands, but these are only minimally involved; surgery is again the initial treatment. Later stages exist when the tumor has reached the chest wall, the skin of the breast or distant sites, such as the lungs and brain. Cancer that has spread beyond the breast and armpit is not usually treated with surgery, though removal of the primary tumor may be indicated for cosmetic and psychological reasons, as well as to decrease the total "load" of tumor cells on the body and to prevent the possible break-down of the primary tumor. The treatment of advanced cancer is with cell-killing drugs. Hormonal therapy is also employed in advanced cancers.

What about radiation therapy?   Radiation will selectively kill cells that are dividing rapidly—cancer cells—and the idea is to destroy any residual malignant cells that were not removed by surgery. The treatment is given by a radiotherapist who, by taking into account the size and type of tumor, its extent and the surgery that's been done, can calculate an amount of radiotherapy that will increase the likelihood of a cure.

The therapy is given with a cobalt machine several times a week for a couple of months starting after the mastectomy wound has healed. Though painless, radiotherapy may cause nausea lasting for a day or more after each treatment. It's not unusual for the person to lose weight during the therapy. A skin reaction that is like a bad sunburn may form at the site of the irradiation and give a permanently darker tint to that part of the body.

What type of surgery is usually done for breast cancer?   Radical mastectomy is most often done. This involves the removal of the breast, the chest muscles below the breast and all the fat and lymph glands from the breast to the armpit. In many parts of the country a modified form of surgery has replaced the traditional radical mastectomy.

What are the drawbacks of radical mastectomy?   The operation produces deformity, disfiguration and disability. The arm on that side swells, aches and is difficult to move. Sometimes so much tissue is removed that the skin around the removed breast will die and slough off. Skin grafts from the thighs or buttocks become necessary. The incision itself extends up over the shoulder, so that it is hard to hide, and since all the flesh beneath the collarbone is removed, the defect is difficult to conceal with anything but a high-necked dress.

126

What are the alternatives to radical mastectomy?   A less extensive operation, modified radical mastectomy, may be done. The breast and the glands in the armpit are removed, but the chest muscles remain in place. The woman is left with an arm that is stronger and less likely to swell than after a radical mastectomy, and it's much easier for the plastic surgeon to construct a new breast, if this is desired.

An even less extensive operation, simple mastectomy, is sometimes done for very early breast cancer: the breast alone is removed. Removal of just the cancerous lump—lumpectomy—is advocated by a few surgeons, but it remains a very controversial form of therapy. The disagreement stems from the possibility that small but removable amounts of cancer may have spread beyond the main lump of tumor, and without removing more than just the lump itself, it may not be possible to detect these areas of cancer.

Which form of surgery offers the best chance of a cure?   For early breast cancer (Stage I or Stage II), the modified radical mastectomy offers the same five-year survival rate of 80 percent as does the more radical surgery. In selected instances simple mastectomy offers a high cure rate. Limited experience with lumpectomy has shown that in some instances it may cure early cancer when combined with radiation therapy, but again, it is still a controversial method of treatment.

Why is radical mastectomy still done?   It's been in use for over a century, ever since Dr. William S. Halsted of Johns Hopkins popularized it after the Civil War. Surgeons who have learned it as *the* method believe it is the safest. Radical mastectomy certainly has a place in the treatment of breast cancer that has advanced beyond Stage II, and certain studies show that it offers the best ten-year cure rate for early disease. Studies are currently under way to examine further whether there is a continuing need for it.

What questions should the woman with breast cancer ask the surgeon?
In times past, a woman signed a consent for radical mastectomy before she knew she had cancer. She was put to sleep, the biopsy was done, and the surgeon stood by her side poised to do a radical mastectomy if the pathologist reported the lump as cancerous. Now more and more women are choosing to have the initial biopsy done as a separate procedure from the actual surgery. This way, there is time for a decision about the type of surgery to be done after the results of the biopsy are known. The first question to pose to the surgeon is whether this arrangement would be agreeable to him or her. The drawbacks to doing the surgery in two steps are that this procedure not only is more expensive but exposes the patient twice to anesthesia. The risk from anesthesia is very low, and many women feel the extra expense is justifiable.

If you don't want radical mastectomy, you may wish to explore the possibility of obtaining a modified operation. Doctors tend to be dogmatic about their ability, based on training, to select a form of cure for a particular patient. They are often right, but many surgeons fail to take into consideration the desires of the patient. A woman may prefer to take her chances with a more limited operation that leaves less disfigurement. The decision will naturally be affected by the extent of the disease, because the more advanced the cancer, the less likely that modified surgery will be effective. For early cancer a strong case can be made for modified surgery. If the surgeon refuses to discuss this possibility, seek a second or a third opinion.

Radiotherapy will be used postoperatively in most instances after either radical or modified surgery, and it is simpler to have the radiotherapy at the same hospital. Inquire about this before the surgery. If time permits, visit the radiotherapist and ask to look at the equipment, which should include a cobalt unit. Since you'll be going back frequently for treatments, accessibility is a consideration that may affect your choice of where to have the surgery.

What happens after mastectomy?   If you've had radical surgery, you can perform exercises that will strengthen your arm and reduce the amount of swelling. You can be fitted for a prosthesis that will be similar in appearance and consistency to your other breast. A choice that has become available in recent years is breast reconstructive surgery.

How is breast reconstruction done?   A plastic form, filled with silicon gel, is made exactly to your size and shape. It is placed beneath the skin to form a new breast. A nipple can be constructed from the outer labia, or the original nipple can be saved and sewn onto the skin of the leg at the time of the mastectomy and then returned to the new breast after reconstructive surgery. This is one reason why it's desirable to discuss the possibility of reconstruction with the surgeon before the initial surgery. The incision for mastectomy can be placed in a way that will make reconstruction easier.

A plastic surgeon performs the surgery. You can get the names of qualified individuals in your area by writing the American Society of Plastic and Reconstructive Surgeons, 29 East Madison Street, Suite 807, Chicago, Ill. 60602. Ask to see before-and-after photos of the doctor's previous patients. Most physicians wait a year after the mastectomy before doing a reconstruction. There's no time limit beyond which you cannot have the operation, and women have had reconstructive surgery as long as twenty years after a mastectomy.

5

SICK BABIES
and CHILDREN

When is the best time to select a pediatrician? Since pediatric care begins at birth, you need a pediatrician before your first child is born. The ideal is to have the child specialist present in the delivery room so that the baby can be examined immediately.

How do you find a pediatrician? Your obstetrician may be able to recommend several good ones. The local medical society will supply the names of pediatricians, and the *Directory of Medical Specialists,* available in many libraries, is another place to start. Probably the best way to find a good pediatrician is to rely on the recommendations of friends who have children.

What questions should you ask the pediatrician? The most important thing is to find someone you trust. You'll be calling and visiting this physician over a period of years, and a lot of the treatment will be in the way of advice given over the phone. It pays to choose not only a well-qualified individual, but one who has the intelligence to make decisions and give you practical advice, as well the patience and courtesy to respond to your concerns.

Make an appointment to see the doctor at his or her office and begin by asking about the doctor's training. A qualified pediatrician has finished a residency in this specialty and is certified by the American Board of Pediatrics. Those from large, well-known teaching hospitals are generally better trained, because they have been exposed to more of the things that can go wrong in infants and children. Many pediatricians have subspecialty training. There are pediatric allergists, cardiologists, endocrinologists, hematologists, rheumatologists and so forth. An important new subspecialty is pediatric neonatology, or the care of the newborn. Your doctor needn't have a subspecialty, but he or she should have a knowledge of the subspecialists to whom your child might be referred if this becomes necessary.

Ask about office procedures. How much does a visit cost? A phone call? (Yes, this may cost something.) Ask about the schedule for well-child visits and immunizations. Usually the shots can be given without the child having to be checked each time by the doctor. This saves money—and time. Find out how long it will take to get an appointment if your child needs one right away. Most pediatricians allot an hour or two a day for call-in appointments —generally the first and last hours of the day. An important thing to know is how the doctor handles night calls. Are calls shared by other physicians? How many, and how well qualified are they? What hospital or emergency room does the physician use? What record system does he or she favor? The problem-oriented medical record is best, with a system of notifying you when immunizations or booster shots come due. Make a tour of the office if possible, and meet the phone receptionist and nurses. You'll be talking to them more than to the doctor, so form an impression of their competence. It will sometimes be hard for a really good and really busy doctor to take the time away from a sick patient to answer all these questions. You may decide that the doctor's reputation for caring for his or her patients is so good that you can rely upon it.

How often should the normal child be seen by the pediatrician?   The pediatrician should examine the child immediately after birth and before the infant is released from the hospital. A two-week or four-week follow-up visit is advisable. At this time you can ask questions about the baby and obtain a copy of the immunization schedule. A brief exam by the doctor or nurse is usually done before the immunizations are started at the age of two months. Well-child visits should occur five times during the first year, three times during the second year and about once a year thereafter until the child is six. School-age children can be seen less often, but well-child visits are advisable at least every three years until age eighteen. Additional visits will be needed to evaluate the progress of children with special problems.

What is a well-child visit?   It's an evaluation of the child's growth and development in order to spot and treat problems before they become serious. Among the aspects of development that are checked are head circumference, weight, height, posture, gait, vision, hearing, blood pressure, tooth development and eating habits. An important well-child visit is the preschool examination done at age five.

130

THE NEWBORN

What may cause the baby's head to be misshapen?   Since they are not fused at birth, the bones of the skull may overlap one another in the tight passageway of the birth canal. This is nature's way of facilitating the birth process. Mild changes in the symmetry of the head are common, and sometimes the back of the head is bullet-shaped. This molding of the head is temporary, and within several weeks the baby's head will be rounded and symmetrical.

What's the cause of a large bump on the back of the head?   Known as *caput succedaneum,* this condition may accompany a long and difficult labor. The bump corresponds to the part of the head that was wedged against the cervix during the first part of labor. The inequality of pressure forced fluid into this spot between the scalp and the skull. The caput won't harm the brain, and usually disappears in several days.

What may cause a bump on the side of the baby's head?   Bleeding into the space between the brain and the skull gives rise to *cephalhematoma,* which may cause an enlargement on one or both sides of the baby's head. The bump may not appear until several hours or days after delivery, and it may continue to enlarge during the first week of life. Damage to the inner lining of the skull is the cause. The damage is incurred by forces brought to bear on the head during labor or delivery, or by the use of forceps. A defect in the baby's blood-clotting system may contribute to cephalhematoma. The bump usually disappears spontaneously.

Do forceps injure the head?   Not if they are used properly, which means applying them during the last part of delivery to help ease the head out of the birth canal. Sometimes the forceps leave marks that appear as bands on either side of the head from the crown to just above the ears. These marks usually disappear in a few days or a week.

What is the soft spot on the baby's head?   It is the gap between four skull bones that haven't yet grown together. It may be an inch and a half both wide and long. In babies with little hair, it can be seen as well as felt. It pulsates with the heartbeat and sinks in slightly when the baby is held upright. The growth of the head and skullbones causes this soft spot to close within eighteen months to two years or during the first year in some infants.

What other newborn conditions will change in time?   About a third of babies become jaundiced during the first days of life. The yellowish skin tint is temporary and reflects immaturity of the baby's liver. If the jaundice is severe, exposing the skin to a special form of light (phototherapy) will

131

hasten its clearing up. When jaundice is a symptom of a blood incompatibility such as Rh disease, blood transfusions may be needed.

Markings that are flat, red or mottled may appear on the back of the head, neck, eyelids or forehead. These will fade within a year. Strawberry marks usually also fade in a year. A blue-green splotch near the base of the spine is known as a Mongolian spot. It appears frequently in Oriental, American Indian and black babies, as well as in many Caucasian babies having olive skin color. It will fade within the first few years of life, though a part of it may persist to adulthood.

An umbilical (navel) hernia is present in one in five newborns. It is more common in black and in premature infants. The navel protrudes in a bump that may contain a small bit of intestine. The defect usually closes on its own within the first few years of life, but persistent hernias may require surgery.

Absorption of hormones from the mother may cause a baby's breasts to enlarge slightly a few days after birth. A small amount of milk ("witch's milk") may ooze from them. This will soon cease; no attempt should be made to squeeze the milk out, as to do so may cause a breast infection. Girl newborns sometimes develop a temporary vaginal discharge that is due to the effects of the mother's hormones.

When will the umbilical stump heal?   The cord will dry up during the first day of life and will be shed a week to ten days after birth. If it is kept clean, it should heal completely in another week.

What causes a baby's feet and hands to turn a darker color?   The circulation through a baby's arms and legs is not sufficient to keep them as warm as the rest of the body, so a mottled discoloration may be noted when the limbs are exposed to the air. The hands and feet may feel colder than the rest of the body. These normal findings are no cause for concern.

What are the white dots on the baby's nose and face?   These are tiny cysts known as *milia.* They may appear on the forehead, face and scrotum, but disappear during the first few weeks of life.

Will the amount or color of the baby's hair stay the same?   No. A normal baby may have little or no hair, or the hair may be so abundant it reaches to eye level. Baby hair will be replaced by permanent hair, which is apt to have a different color and texture.

Are the newborn's eyes the same color they will be as an adult?   Not necessarily. Eye color is determined by the presence in the iris of pigmented granules, the same spots of pigment that determine skin color.

What about skin color?   Skin color is determined by the interaction of several genes. The color of a black child at birth may be misleading, since many black babies are born very light. Within a few days or weeks the baby's skin begins to darken to its permanent appearance.

When will the baby have its first bowel movement?   Usually the first day or two of life.

When will the baby pass urine the first time?   Sometimes right after birth, or not till a day or two. The first few urinations may contain a pink staining from uric acid crystals.

How many hours a day does the baby sleep?   About eighteen to twenty hours at first, but by six months the baby will stay awake for six to eight hours a day.

What's the best position for sleeping?   The baby should sleep on its stomach. Most babies prefer this position, which is desirable because any spit-up or secretions will drain out of the throat and not get into the lungs.

What is the startle reflex?   A loud noise or sudden movement may cause the baby, even when asleep, to throw its arms out and begin crying. This is a normal reflex—the baby's response to being startled.

What does crying mean?   Crying right after birth is the baby's way of aerating its lungs to begin the respirations that will last throughout life. After that, crying is the baby's main way to communicate. A baby learns to cry when it wants to be held, is hungry, wet, frightened, too hot or too cold. The crying will stop when the stimulus for it is removed. The parents must learn to pick the baby up when it obviously needs comfort, and yet to restrain themselves from responding to every little cry. Causes of prolonged crying include colic, bad dreams and various illnesses that require a doctor's attention.

Why doesn't the baby have tears when it cries?   The tear glands do not begin to function until several weeks after birth.

FEEDING

What are the advantages of breast-feeding?   It is the natural way, and it gives satisfaction to the mother and her baby because of the very close, warm experience they share. Mother's milk is always available, always sterile and already warm. It is easier for the baby to digest and less likely to cause an allergy than cow's milk. The nutrient content of mother's milk and present-day commercially prepared formulas is about the same, but the biologic availability is much greater in mother's milk than in cow's milk. An important benefit of breast-feeding is the passage of the mother's antibodies to the infant. These breast-milk antibodies afford protection against various illnesses and may be responsible for the fact that breast-fed babies have a lower incidence of diarrhea, ear infections and other problems than do bottle-fed babies.

What are the disadvantages of breast-feeding?　It may be difficult, but not impossible, for a working woman to breast-feed her baby. Some infants aren't able to nurse well, and in a very few women a good supply of milk doesn't develop. A relatively unimportant disadvantage is that the breast-fed infant has more frequent bowel movements than the formula-fed baby. Some few women seem to dislike the idea of breast-feeding and it is probably not wise for them to force themselves to do it. As long as the baby is held close to the mother's body during feeding and allowed to suckle as long as it likes, bottle feeding is all right.

How do you know if your breasts are big enough to produce milk?　The size of the breasts is not related to the amount of milk you can produce. A relaxed attitude, plenty of rest and good nutrition are far more important factors in determining milk supply.

How much extra should you eat if you're breast-feeding the baby?　An extra thousand calories a day. You also need to drink three quarts of fluids a day, and your diet should be balanced among the four food classes. Many mothers find they can lose weight gained during pregnancy, even while they are nursing, by judicious calorie restriction.

What preparations do you need for breast-feeding?　Begin two months before delivery to rub your nipples with hydrous lanolin once or twice a day. Then gently pull the nipple several times. This helps to soften and condition it for the baby's mouth. To prepare the breasts for nursing, grasp the pigmented, outer part of the nipple between the second and third fingers. By pressing against the chest and then sliding the fingers forward, you should be able to express a few drops of colostrum each day.

What is colostrum?　It is the thin, white or yellowish secretion that precedes the production of milk. High in protective antibodies and protein, it lasts for two to four days after birth, when it's replaced by regular milk.

How long does it take to get a good milk supply?　It may take two weeks before an ample supply of milk is produced, but only rarely are supplemental feedings needed during this time. Successful breast-feeding depends on relaxation, good nutrition and a commitment to nursing. The sucking reflex is the strongest stimulus to milk production, and the baby should be offered both breasts at every feeding.

Why doesn't milk come out of the breasts as soon as the baby begins sucking?
Milk production and milk release are two different matters. The breasts make milk and store it for release at the right moment. This moment arrives when the baby's sucking triggers a reflex known as "milk letdown." A hormone is released by the mother's brain in response to the sucking; it enters the circulation and passes to the breasts, where it stimulates smooth muscle cells to squeeze out the milk. It takes a minute or two from the onset of sucking to the release of milk, and then the milk may flow out so rapidly that the baby has trouble swallowing it. The letdown reflex affects both breasts at the same time.

How long should the baby nurse? Ninety percent of a breast's milk is delivered during the first five minutes of nursing, but the baby has a need to continue sucking for longer than this. Also, both breasts should be given at each feeding. One way is to allow nursing on the first breast for ten minutes, then to switch to the other breast for the rest of the feeding; the sequence is reversed at the next feeding. Another way is to allow feeding for fifteen or twenty minutes on the first breast, then about half this interval on the second breast—also reversing the sequence at the next feeding.

How often should the baby be nursed? A baby can digest mother's milk more completely and quickly than it can formula, so nursing may be desirable every two to three hours until a regular feeding pattern is established. After ten days the baby will usually go for three to four hours between feedings, and maybe six to eight hours at night. Many infants continue to want frequent feedings for the first six weeks; at the other extreme is the baby who has to be awakened for feeding.

When can the nighttime feeding be omitted? By the age of six to eight weeks the baby should sleep through from 10 or 11 P.M. to 6 A.M.

How long should I continue nursing the baby? Four to six months is average, but you may be able to continue breast-feeding till the baby is a year or eighteen months of age.

How is weaning accomplished? Replace one feeding with a bottle, and three or four days later, replace another feeding with a bottle. Continue this until the baby is weaned. Older infants can often be weaned directly to the

135

cup. Begin the replacement at the feeding the baby enjoys least, such as in the afternoon; wait till last to replace the first morning feeding. With slow weaning, you don't need hormone therapy to dry up the breasts.

What care do the breasts need during nursing?   The breasts and nipples should be gently washed with soap and water after each feeding, or at least three times a day. The purpose is to prevent a tiny fissure from forming in either breast. The fissure could serve as the entry site for an infection known as mastitis. Should this infection occur, it can be treated with antibiotics, and nursing can be continued at the other breast until the infection has healed.

Do breast-fed babies need iron supplements?   Studies indicate that beyond six months the breast-fed baby may need iron supplements, and some pediatricians start them as early as four months.

Will my baby be all right if fed on the bottle?   Yes, bottle-feeding has stood the test of time. It's more expensive and more likely to cause side effects than breast-feeding, but it's more convenient in many instances and certainly acceptable to the baby.

What are the side effects of bottle-feeding?   Babies fed from the bottle have a higher incidence of skin problems, colic, diarrhea and respiratory infections than do breast-fed babies.

Why do these effects occur?   Cow's milk in a formula is not the natural food for human infants. It is harder to digest, and the baby may react to it with colic. Infectious diarrhea is more frequent because of the greater chance for germs to get into the bottle, the milk or the nipple. Ear infection may occur when the baby is propped on its side to take a bottle, for this position favors the entry of germs from the throat to the middle ear through the open Eustachian tubes. These tubes normally open each time the baby swallows, but the upright position keeps milk out of them.

What formula should I choose?   The American Academy of Pediatrics now recommends that all bottle-fed babies receive an iron-fortified formula. You can select one of these, or let the pediatrician make a recommendation. Sometimes it's necessary to make a change if the baby doesn't tolerate a certain type of formula.

Is whole milk a satisfactory formula?   Milk straight from the dairy is not a good formula for infants under three months of age. It is low in iron and doesn't contain enough water for the amount of calories that are in it. Its protein is not as easily digested as that in breast milk. A baby may be

136

switched to whole milk after three months if supplemental water feedings and iron are supplied.

Is it all right to use skim milk as a formula? No, it doesn't contain enough calories to nourish the baby.

How much at a time should the baby be fed? The rule is to offer three more ounces than the baby's age in months till age six months. Most babies will take only two or three ounces a feeding during the first week or two, and beyond the first six months, won't take more than eight ounces a feeding.

Fill the bottle with an ounce more than the baby usually takes. This is to prevent the baby from sucking air and to make sure that the feeding is sufficient. Under no circumstances should you try to get the baby to take more milk than it wants. Fat babies aren't healthy babies. Don't try to save milk left over from a feeding. Throw it out and wash the bottle.

How often should the bottle be given? At first the baby may want the bottle every two or three hours. By the end of the first week, feedings every three or four hours will probably satisfy most babies; a four-hour schedule is usually established by the baby by the age of one month. The baby will usually begin to sleep through the nighttime feeding between the ages of six and eight weeks. The frequency of feedings will diminish when the baby begins to take cereal, juices and other foods.

When should you give water? Give it right from the first if the baby is hungry between feedings. A thirsty baby will take some water; a hungry baby will let you know it wants milk.

Do you need to add sugar to the water? No, it's better to give it straight.

Do you have to sterilize bottles and nipples? No. They should be washed and rinsed thoroughly, and the milk should be kept in the refrigerator. It may help to sterilize the equipment if the child has recurring bouts of diarrhea or if the water comes from a well, cistern or spring and there is some doubt about its purity.

Do you need to warm the milk? Full-term infants can tolerate milk at room temperature, though it is common practice to warm the milk during the first few months; thereafter babies will take it cold or at room temperature. The bottle containing water can be given at room temperature.

What's the best position for bottle-feeding? With the baby cuddled in your arms to simulate breast-feeding.

How long should bottle-feeding continue?   Usually not beyond a year and a half. The baby will be drinking from a cup by then and bottle-feedings can be transferred to cup-feedings. Do not, however, rush the cup. Babies need to suck and to be cuddled, and it is wise to follow each infant's lead as to when he or she is ready for the cup.

When should solid foods be started?   You can begin offering baby cereal at about three to six months, followed by fruit, vegetables and meat a month apart in that order. New foods should be introduced one at a time several days apart. This way, if the baby doesn't tolerate a particular food you will know what food caused the trouble and you can try something else.

When do you start table foods?   By eight to ten months of age, the baby will eat small portions of mashed potato, banana and other finger foods. Feeding at table should not be rushed, and the foods should always be broken into small portions so that the baby won't choke. Consumption of table foods will progress as dental development occurs.

SPECIFIC PROBLEMS

Why does a newborn tend to lose weight?   It takes several days for a good feeding pattern to get started. Meanwhile the infant is burning calories and eliminating wastes. The normal weight loss is about 7 percent. A loss of more than 10 percent of birth weight is abnormal.

When is the weight regained?   By the fifth day, weight gain begins and a normal baby will regain its birth weight by ten to fourteen days of age.

What are the symptoms of a feeding problem?   A baby should take nourishment readily, gain weight steadily, and not have loose stools or excessive spitting up. A feeding problem may exist when any of these conditions is not met. Other symptoms include irritability and crying, constipation, colic and abdominal distention.

What can be done for a feeding problem?   It depends on the cause, which may be underfeeding, overfeeding, infection, a birth defect or some other problem. Premature infants tend to have more feeding problems than children of normal birth weight; bottle-fed babies have more problems than breast-fed children.

How much spitting up is normal?   Some spitting up after a feeding is not unusual. It can be kept to a minimum by burping the baby, whether breast or bottle fed, during and after feeding. Spitting up becomes vomiting when it occurs forcefully, repeatedly or between feedings.

What causes vomiting in a newborn?   Persistent vomiting beginning in the first day or two of life suggests a congenital obstruction of the stomach or intestine. Often the vomit is propelled some distance from the baby. The suspicion of an intestinal obstruction calls for emergency medical evaluation; surgery to correct the defect must be performed as soon as possible.

Pyloric stenosis is another cause of projectile vomiting in a newborn. Because the obstruction between the stomach and intestine is only partial, vomiting may not begin until a week or two after birth, and only occasionally at first. Within several weeks, vomiting may follow every feeding. The condition occurs most commonly in boys and the treatment is surgical correction.

Overfeeding is the most common cause of vomiting in a newborn. It can be distinguished from the above conditions in that it doesn't cause persistent or projectile vomiting. The baby simply takes so much milk, or the formula is so rich, that vomiting occurs. Failure to burp the baby may contribute to the vomiting. Also important is the baby's position after feeding. A baby is more likely to vomit if placed on its back or left side. Lying on the stomach or right side promotes normal emptying of the stomach.

How many bowel movements does a normal baby have?   The breast-fed baby may have six to eight a day, sometimes one after every feeding. A formula-fed infant will have three or four stools a day. The number of bowel movements begins to diminish in the first few months of life, and by the age of three months the breast-fed baby will have three or four stools a day, while the bottle-fed baby will have one to three stools a day.

What do the stools normally look like?   At first the infant passes meconium, the residual of intestinal secretions during fetal life. Meconium is green to greenish-black and pasty in consistency. After four days, a breast-fed baby's stools turn yellow and have a loose or seedy consistency. The stools of a formula-fed baby are yellow to golden in color and have a salve-like consistency.

How can you tell when diarrhea is present?   The frequency of stools may double. Watery and smelling worse than usual, the stools may be passed with explosive forcefulness. The most frequent color change is to green or brown. Serious diarrhea is a life-threatening illness in infants, and a physician should be consulted at once. (See below.)

What causes mild diarrhea in an infant?   Among the possibilities are overfeeding, cow's milk allergy, giving a formula that is too rich in sugar, or the mother's taking a laxative that is passed to the baby through her milk. Changing formulas, switching from breast to formula or from formula to whole milk, or introducing a new food may cause diarrhea. Frequently a mild infection is responsible, especially in bottle-fed babies. A "bad" germ reaches the intestine and multiplies faster than the "good" bacteria already there. Diarrhea is the body's way of flushing out the intestinal contents so that the normal bacterial balance is restored.

These instances of diarrhea are less serious than those that accompany malabsorption, immunologic deficiency, inflammation of the bowel or a serious infection, such as epidemic diarrhea of the newborn. (See the discussion of serious diarrhea below.)

What's the treatment for mild diarrhea?　　Stop all feedings of solids and milk. Give the baby sugar water made up by adding two tablespoons of white Karo syrup or cane sugar and a half teaspoon of salt to a quart of boiled water. Feed the baby as much of this as it wants. Leave the remainder in the refrigerator, and make up more as necessary. The sugar water works by putting the intestinal tract at rest so that the baby's natural processes can stop the diarrhea. Pedialyte, a commercial preparation of sugar water and electrolytes, is available in drugstores. The use of patent remedies, such as Kaopectate, or prescription drugs, such as paregoric, is *never* indicated in the initial management of diarrhea in an infant.

When the diarrhea has stopped, usually after twenty-four to forty-eight hours of the sugar water formula, you can offer a weak dilution of milk. Make it by adding a half cup of non-fat powdered skim milk to a quart of boiled water. If the baby tolerates it without diarrhea, increase the strength to a cup of dried skim milk per quart of water. After a day or two you can return to giving the regular formula, but dilute it with two parts of water to one part of milk. If this is tolerated, you can return to giving the formula at usual strength. Reintroduce solids one at a time several days apart. Take extra precautions to make sure that the bottles, nipples, pans and water are clean.

What are the signs of serious diarrhea?　　Diarrhea which is unusually severe and accompanied by fever or which continues for more than a day in spite of the above treatment is serious. A baby hasn't the reserves to tolerate diarrhea for long, especially if there is also vomiting and fever. The signs of infectious diarrhea are fever, irritability, lethargy, dehydration (sunken soft spot, sunken eyes, dry mouth and tongue) and the appearance of blood or pus in the stools. Diarrhea in a breast-fed baby is presumed to be infectious until proven otherwise.

What's the treatment for serious diarrhea?　　A doctor must give treatment based on the cause of the diarrhea, and hospitalization may be indicated.

The need is to replace the baby's deficit of fluid and minerals, to take stool cultures, and to look for noninfectious causes of diarrhea.

Certain instances of serious diarrhea occur in babies already in the hospital. Epidemic diarrhea of the newborn is due to pathogenic varieties of the ordinary colon bacteria, *Escherichia coli*. It is spread by hand contamination in the newborn nursery, and has caused mortality rates of up to 40 percent. Though not usually so dire an infection, serious diarrhea contracted outside the hospital is always an urgent situation requiring immediate medical attention.

What else may cause diarrhea in an infant? Poor absorption of milk or sugars present in the formula may lead to diarrhea. One problem is a deficiency of the enzyme lactase, and such infants may develop frothy, loose stools within a few days of birth. It is imperative that the cause of the problem be recognized early so that an appropriate formula can be given. With increasing age the child may overcome the milk intolerance.

What is "failure to thrive"? This means that a baby's weight and height lag far behind the average for that age. The usual cause is undernutrition: failure to feed the baby enough food or the right kinds of foods. The baby is skinny. Its abdomen may be swollen with fluid, its eyes may sink in and its hair may fall out—a condition known as kwashiorkor. Diarrhea is common. Paradoxically, the baby may show little interest in feeding.

What is the treatment for failure to thrive? The baby must be given adequate nutrition, beginning with intravenous therapy and progressing to milk formula, vitamins, minerals and solid foods. Since failure to thrive is often set against a background of ignorance and want, the treatment becomes as much social as medical.

When underfeeding is not present, a workup may show that the cause is an endocrine disease, an inborn error of metabolism, a genetic disease or some other rare condition. Treatment is aimed at the underlying problem.

What is colic? It is abdominal pain that comes on suddenly, is accompanied by crying and is due to excessive gas formation, which distends the intestine and thus causes the pain. The baby may appear to be doing well but will suddenly begin crying loudly. The crying may last for hours or may stop within a few minutes if the pain eases. During an attack the colicky baby's face is congested, the abdomen is distended and the legs are drawn up. The passage of gas or stool may give relief.

Colic affects many infants, but to varying degrees. The attacks usually begin at two or three weeks of age, occur most frequently in the evenings or at night and may persist till the baby is three months old.

141

What causes colic?   Among the causes are:
· *A feeding problem,* such as giving too much milk, failing to burp the baby or positioning the child on its back or left side rather than on the stomach or right side after feeding. Underfeeding can also cause colic.
· *A formula problem,* such as a milk that contains too much sugar or fat. Colic is more common in bottle-fed than in breast-fed babies.
· *An allergy to cow's milk.*
· *Something in the mother's diet of a breast-fed baby.* What the mother eats may affect the baby within several hours, and the upset may last a day or two.
· *Tension* from the increase in household activity that occurs around the supper hour. The infant may be overly reactive to the extra noise and stimulation it gets at this time of day.

What's the treatment for colic?   A feeding problem should be corrected. The mother of a breast-fed baby should avoid spicy foods, beans and other gas-producing foods. Switching to a different formula or diluting the formula with more water may help. An infant with an allergy to cow's milk may be given a soybean formula or goat's milk. (Check with the pediatrician before switching.) When tension is thought responsible, provide a quiet, soothing environment for the baby. Hold the baby half an hour at each feeding, and don't express anger or frustration in the baby's presence.

What are the symptoms of constipation?   The stool is firm or nodular and difficult to pass. Even three stools a day, when very firm, represent constipation.

What causes constipation?   The usual cause is a lack of enough fluid. Sometimes the formula is too high in fat or protein and doesn't contain enough sugar. Feeding whole milk to a baby may cause constipation. An infant who has been ill may pass hard or firm stool until it recovers. Constipation is rare in breast-fed babies.
A newborn who doesn't pass stool should be checked for anal atresia (failure of the anus to open). Aganglionic megacolon (Hirschsprung's disease) is a more serious cause of constipation in an infant. It is inherited, more common in boys, and may cause other problems such as vomiting and failure to thrive.

What's the treatment for constipation?   Give the baby more fluid in the form of water or sugar water. A change in formula may be indicated. The infant who can take solids should be given foods with more bulk, such as cereals and fruits. Prune juice, apple juice and other juices may help.

Surgery is indicated in the rare instance of anal atresia or Hirschsprung's disease.

GROWTH AND DEVELOPMENT

How much weight should a baby gain in its first months of life?   The average is an ounce a day during the first three months. By five months the baby will have doubled its birth weight. By the end of the first year the baby should weigh three times its birth weight. It won't quadruple the birth weight till the age of two and a half.

How fast does growth occur during childhood?   A child gains about five pounds a year between the ages of two and nine. At three the average child is three feet tall. At four an average child will weigh forty pounds and be forty inches tall. At age seven the average child will weigh seven times its birth weight.

Do boys grow faster than girls?   Yes, in the first year of life. After that, growth occurs at the same rate in both sexes till age nine. The adolescent growth spurt occurs a year or two earlier in girls than in boys, but a girl usually reaches her adult height by age eighteen. The average boy tends to grow taller than the average girl because he doesn't stop growing as soon.

What are some ways to predict the baby's adult height?   Birth weight is of no help in the prediction, but a baby over twenty inches long will probably be a tall adult. Birth length doubles by age four and triples by age thirteen. An estimate of adult height can be obtained by doubling the height at eighteen months for a girl, and by doubling the height at two years for a boy. This rule is subject to individual variation.

How much does the head grow?   At birth the head is two-thirds as big as it will ever be; it accounts for a fourth of the baby's length. By age six it will have grown to almost adult size. The skull bones are not completely fused until early adulthood, when the head accounts for an eighth of body length.

What if my child is bigger or smaller than the average size?   The child is probably normal. "Average" is a theoretical size determined by measuring a great number of children and dividing the sizes by the number of children measured. Were this same group of children lined up from the smallest to the largest, a continuum of sizes would be seen. The ones in the middle would be about the same size, but those at the larger or smaller ends would be just as normal. Size is determined by many factors, especially heredity.

143

What if I'm concerned about the size of my child?   Ask the pediatrician to examine the child and keep a growth curve for several months. This will show if there's anything to worry about. Periodic measurements of the head are indicated when it appears too small or too large.

Is hormone therapy indicated to stimulate a small child's growth?   Not unless the child has a thyroid deficiency, pituitary dwarfism or one of the other endocrine conditions discussed in Chapter 13. Indiscriminate use of hormones to stimulate a child's growth may cause serious side effects.

When do the teeth appear?   The first two teeth, the lower central incisors, appear at about six months of age. Next come the upper central incisors about a month later. The remaining primary (deciduous) teeth make their appearance in the next two years. These come out, and the secondary, or permanent, teeth begin to appear at about school age and continue to develop up through the teenage years. The wisdom teeth appear in the late teens and may not be completely erupted till the mid-twenties.

What if the first tooth doesn't appear at six months?   It may not appear until a year of age, which doesn't mean the baby is abnormal. Dental development, like other forms of development, is subject to individual variation. The teeth don't necessarily appear in the sequence given above, either. (In a rare normal person, secondary teeth never appear.)

When does the average child crawl, walk and speak?   The average child will crawl at eight to ten months, walk alone at twelve to sixteen months and say a few words by fifteen months. Individuals vary considerably. Many children walk before a year and say words before fifteen months. First children speak earlier than subsequent children, and girls may speak sooner than boys.

When should the child get out of diapers?   By the age of two, most children can begin using training pants. Toilet training is usually accomplished by age three, though accidents and bed-wetting may still occur. Girls adapt to toilet training more quickly than boys. It is important not to be too concerned about a timetable for training. Your child will obviously be toilet-trained before school age, and putting pressure on a youngster who isn't ready may cause problems a lot more serious than soiled diapers.

How long will bed-wetting last?   Usually not beyond the age of four to six, but occasionally it may last till adolescence. The frequency of accidents will diminish after the age of eight or nine.

When do the self-help skills appear?   These skills, consisting of feeding, toileting and dressing, appear between the ages of two and five. Most children can handle finger food at the age of one and use a spoon by the age of one and a half or two. By the age of two to four, a normal child can feed himself or herself. A three-year-old can generally figure out the mystery of a button and knows how to shed clothes and take off shoes. By the age of four or five, the child can dress himself or herself except for tying shoes.

How do I know if my child's development is delayed?   Because there are enormous variations in when children develop various skills, these guidelines should serve only as signals to seek consultation and should not cause you to become overconcerned. Signs of delayed development arc:
 · Failure to sit up by age one
 · Failure to walk by age two
 · Failure to say words by age two
 · Failure to say short sentences by age three
 · Failure to develop any self-help skills by age four or five
Seizures, spasticity, paralysis, hydrocephalus, or a history of head injury at birth or afterward are medical signs pointing to possible developmental delay. A delay in physical growth often accompanies a delay in mental development.

What should I do if I suspect my child has a developmental delay?   Let the pediatrician help judge that a delay is present: X-rays and lab tests may uncover a cause. Psychologic testing is the next step. The tests, which include hearing and visual examinations, may be administered in a private facility (cost: about $200) or, if the child is five or older, through the school administration.

Isn't it best to wait and see if a child will outgrow a delay?   No, the earlier treatment is begun, the more effective it is apt to be. People who tell you it's "something he'll grow out of" mean well, but fail to realize that recognizing a problem for what it is doesn't make it any worse. Attributing slow speech to a normal delay won't help the child who shows up at kindergarten unable to speak and is subsequently found to have a hearing impairment. A child who isn't walking and talking by age three should be tested.

What if a delay is found?   Treatment is given by the physician, speech therapist, hearing therapist and/or education specialist. This team will make the appropriate recommendations regarding school placement and specialized training if these are indicated.

BIRTH DEFECTS

What are birth defects?   A birth defect may be one that is hereditary and that may have been present from the moment of conception, or it may have been acquired during the months in the womb, during labor and delivery or the weeks immediately after birth.

How serious are birth defects?   The defects range from those that are relatively mild and correctable, such as a harelip or a hernia, to a devastating condition such as Tay-Sachs disease or a chromosomal aberration involving multiple congenital abnormalities. As a rule, the defects occur in groups. A child with mongolism may also have an obstructed intestine; a baby blind from German measles may also have a heart condition. The victim of an inborn error of metabolism, such as phenylketonuria, may have mental and physical retardation as well as convulsions.

How frequently do birth defects occur?   About 4 percent of babies have birth defects that are serious enough to require medical attention. The incidence is higher if one includes umbilical hernias that eventually close, undescended testicles that descend in the first few years of life, and skin blemishes and birthmarks that either go away or do not cause problems.

What tests are done routinely to screen for birth defects?   Physical examination is a screening test, for most defects are obvious to the naked eye. Gonorrhea infection of the eye is treated prophylactically by instilling silver nitrate solution or another agent into the newborn's eyes. A blood test for phenylketonuria (PKU) is done on newborns throughout the United States. In Massachusetts, Oregon, California, New York and other states, the blood of newborn babies is screened for a panel of detectable birth defects.

What can be done to prevent birth defects?   Major defects that can be prevented or reduced are:
· *Tay-Sachs disease.* This disease causes blindness, retardation and a progressive deterioration of the nervous system resulting in death by the age of three to five years. It is passed as an autosomal recessive trait, meaning that one in four children will have it when both parents carry the trait. The disease occurs most commonly in children whose parents are both Jewish, and one in thirty Ashkenazic Jews carries the trait. A blood test can now be done to screen for the Tay-Sachs trait. Persons of the Jewish ethnic group should be screened. When the husband and wife both have the trait, they may choose not to have children, or to have every pregnancy monitored by amniocentesis. Tay-Sachs disease can be diagnosed from examining the amniotic fluid, and an abortion can be done if this is what the parents wish. Before the test is performed, the risks should be evaluated and the parents

146

should consider what they will do if the fetus does have the disease.

· *Phenylketonuria.* This disease, also an autosomal recessive trait, occurs about once in every 10,000 births. These children lack the enzyme needed to break down phenylalanine, an essential amino acid. They may develop mental retardation, hyperactivity and seizures. Present screening programs detect about 200 PKU children each year. The treatment, a diet limited in phenylalanine, must be continued at least till age six and possibly until adolescence. Normal development is possible when the diet is followed.

· *Rh incompatibility.* Hemolytic disease of the newborn may cause death before birth or soon after. It involves an attack on the baby's red blood cells by antibodies which may destroy the cells and cause jaundice. Children who survive because of exchange transfusions may be mentally retarded. Present techniques have the potential to eliminate this condition. Every Rh-negative woman should receive an injection of a medication that prevents the formation of active antibodies after having a baby or an abortion (unless the child's father is also Rh-negative). The woman should be monitored during pregnancy so that her level of anti-Rh antibodies can be followed. If necessary, a baby who develops Rh incompatibility can be transfused while still in the womb or shortly after birth.

· *Mongolism (Down's syndrome).* This condition begins at conception when the egg or the sperm introduces an extra chromosome into the zygote so that each cell in the resulting fetus will also get one too many chromosomes. The extra genetic material slows cellular activity, thus causing mental and physical retardation.

Mongoloid children have stubby fingers and hands, a flat face, slanted eyes and a sweet disposition. Usually the extra chromosome comes from the mother, for the risk of having a mongoloid is proportional to her age at the time of conception. A woman under age thirty has a one-in-1500 risk of having a mongoloid baby. The risk rises to one in 280 for women aged thirty-five to thirty-nine, one in 130 for women forty to forty-four, and one in 65 for women over forty-five. The way to reduce the incidence of mongolism is to have the pregnancy monitored by amniocentesis for every woman who becomes pregnant beyond the age of forty. Mongolism can usually be detected by sampling the amniotic fluid so that an abortion can be performed if the fetus is affected. It's especially important for a woman who has a mongoloid child to have future pregnancies monitored by amniocentesis, for she has a higher risk of having another child with this condition. Parents of a mongoloid should have chromosome testing. One or the other may carry the extra chromosome without showing any signs of mongolism, and the carrier state greatly raises the risk of having another affected child.

What are some other ways to lower the risk of a birth defect?   Prenatal care is very important. Prematurity is a leading cause of mental retardation, and a woman who's had no prenatal care is two or three times as likely to have a premature baby. Diabetes, high blood pressure and hypothyroidism may affect the baby, and it's essential that these and other diseases be treated. The pregnant woman should avoid drugs, X-ray studies and unnecessary exposure to viral illnesses, as, for example, going to a crowded theater during a flu epidemic. Smoking and alcohol have been shown in recent studies to have adverse effects on the fetus and should be avoided (see p. 43). When the mother or father knows of any hereditary disease in the family, genetic counseling by a specialist may be indicated before conception.

What exactly is genetic counseling?   It means discussing with a specialist your chances of having a child with a birth defect. The specialist may or may not be a physician, but he or she should be thoroughly knowledgeable about hereditary and congenital diseases and have the facilities for testing chromosomes and biochemical patterns in blood, urine and amniotic fluid.

How do you find a genetic counselor?   Your physician can refer you to one. Sometimes the physician will serve as the counselor when backup information is obtained through a nearby medical facility.

The National Genetics Foundation can offer information. The address is 250 West 57th Street, New York, N.Y. 10019; the telephone number, (212) 265-3166. The National Foundation and March of Dimes puts out a directory giving the addresses of genetic counselors. A copy is available to medical professionals who write the Professional Education Department, National Foundation—March of Dimes, P.O. Box 2000, White Plains, N.Y. 10602.

Are there birth defects that can't be predicted?   Certain defects are inherited in a complex way or occur when inherited factors act in concert with environmental factors. Among the conditions that fall into these categories are:
  · Hydrocephalus
  · Congenital dislocated hip
  · Clubfoot
  · Congenital heart murmur
  · Cleft lip and cleft palate
  · Anencephaly and spina bifida
  · Pyloric stenosis
Increased risk is established once the defect occurs in a family. For instance, brothers and sisters of a person with a cleft palate are more likely to have a child with this condition. Parents of a child with the most common type of cleft palate have a 3 to 6 percent chance of having another child with this condition. A very rare type of cleft palate is inherited through a domi-

nant gene and the parents have a 50 percent chance that any subsequent child will be affected.

What about brain injury? This is by far the most common cause of mental retardation, and the brain damage may occur before birth, at the time of birth or shortly thereafter. Probably the most frequent cause is failure of the baby to begin breathing immediately and the lack of oxygen damaging the brain. For poorly understood reasons, a premature baby may develop brain damage. Meningitis, head injury and cerebral hemorrhage are other causes. Many brain-injured children are paralyzed or spastic and have been classified under the term "cerebral palsy." However, not every brain-injured child is spastic, and not every cerebral palsy victim is mentally retarded.

What can be done to prevent brain injury? Early prenatal care is indicated in every pregnancy. Treatment can be given when a woman has a medical condition that may cause a difficult delivery. Diabetic babies tend to be bigger than average, so in many instances labor will be induced several weeks early. The woman whose pelvis is too small can make plans for cesarean section. Delivery by a skilled obstetrician will minimize the risk of brain injury.

What should be done for a retarded child? Everything possible! The management begins with an early diagnosis of the problem. Psychologic testing is indicated if a child is not walking and talking by age three. Once retardation is diagnosed, management is shared by the pediatrician, a speech and hearing specialist, a teacher and others as indicated. Most retarded children can live at home, attend public school and learn a skill that will enable them to work as adults.

Public Law 94-142, passed by the Congress in 1975, entitles every handicapped child to a public education. Known as the Education of All Handicapped Children Act, the law provides for yearly evaluation of each retarded child and placement in an appropriate educational setting till age twenty-one. Parents can find out about special education facilities in their community by contacting the local school administration or education agency.

Literally dozens of parent organizations have been formed to help parents cope with caring for and educating a retarded child. Perhaps the best known is the National Association for Retarded Citizens. Each state has a chapter of this organization. You can obtain the address of your chapter by contacting the national organization at 2709 Avenue E East, P.O. Box 6109, Arlington, Tex. 76011. The telephone number is (817) 261-4961.

IMMUNIZATIONS

What is a good immunization schedule?   The one shown in the accompanying chart is a slightly modified version of the standard schedule of the Infectious Diseases Committee Report of the American Academy of Pediatrics.

IMMUNIZATION SCHEDULE

Basic Series
2 months—DPT and oral polio
4 months—DPT and oral polio
6 months—DPT and oral polio
15 months—measles, German measles,
        mumps (triple vaccine)
18 months—DPT and oral polio

Boosters
4–6 years—DPT and oral polio
10–12 years—German measles vaccine for
      a girl whose rubella titer is
      negative or less than 1:16
14–16 years—T (d)
Every 10 years—T (d)

D=diphtheria
P=pertussis (whooping cough)
T=tetanus (lockjaw)
(d)=adult diphtheria (small dosage)

Who should receive shots?   Every youngster who doesn't have a condition that might render the shots ineffective or dangerous. The pediatrician is the judge in these instances, which is one reason for having the child examined by the doctor before the immunization program is undertaken.

When should inoculation not be given?   It should not be given to children who have an immunologic disease that makes them unable to respond to the shots. It is not a good idea to inoculate a child who is sick, has fever or is just recovering from an illness. The injection can be given after the child is well. A minor infection, such as a cold without fever, is not a contraindication.

What are the side effects?   Fever and soreness at the site of the injection (usually the thigh or buttock in infants and the upper arm in older children) are the main side effects. The fever is ordinarily less than 101° F. Fever of more than 103° F. or severe lethargy or convulsions should be reported to the pediatrician immediately. A severe reaction calls for caution with future injections. Small doses of the individual toxoids are given at wide intervals to minimize the chance of a future reaction.

What if the child misses a shot?   It makes no difference in the child's immunization program. The shots do not have to be started over, but the next one in the series should be given when possible, and the same number of doses should be taken at comparable intervals.

Is immunization really necessary?   It certainly is. People still die from lockjaw because of a failure to obtain immunization. Diphtheria outbreaks still occur—with fatalities. Polio is a dread disease that once ran rampant across this nation. Even measles, usually a mild disease, may cause brain damage and death. The reason for controlling rubella is to prevent it from damaging the fetus of a pregnant woman. Numerous deaths and untold misery and suffering are prevented by the immunizations.

Are the boosters necessary?   Yes, the body may lose its "memory" for a disease unless it is reminded by way of a booster injection. Resistance to polio is thought to last a lifetime after the first booster, but boosters for tetanus and diphtheria must be given periodically.

Is it best to get a tetanus booster after a cut or stepping on a nail?   A child previously immunized to tetanus may not need a booster if one has been given in the last year. An adult may not need a booster if one has been given in the last five to ten years, but this depends on the cut, its depth, and whether it is soiled or treatment is delayed for more than a few hours. Good surgical care of the cut is essential, and the surgeon should make the judgment about the need for additional tetanus prophylaxis.

Is smallpox vaccination necessary?   After it was determined that the risk of naturally contracting smallpox was less than the risk imposed by the vaccination, routine immunization was stopped. The World Health Organization considers the disease eradicated, but some countries are not so optimistic; persons traveling to these nations may need smallpox vaccination to gain entry. Information about the immunizations needed for foreign travel can be obtained by writing for the booklet *Health Information for International Travel* (Publication 76-8280) from the Center for Disease Control, Atlanta, Ga. 30333.

What other precautions should be taken?   Testing for tuberculosis is usually done at nine months to one year, before the child enters school and periodically thereafter. The usual screening is a skin test (see p. 171).

CHILDHOOD ILLNESSES

What are the signs of serious illness in a child?   Failure to eat when the appetite was previously good is a sign of illness, though loss of appetite doesn't imply that the illness is serious. Lethargy and sleepiness may accompany both mild or serious conditions. Persistent crying in a previously happy youngster points to illness. Blueness about the mouth and under the fingernails is a danger signal that there is insufficient oxygen in the blood. Other signs of a serious problem are trouble with breathing, persistent vomiting or diarrhea, cessation of urination, fever above 103° F. (39.5° C.), stiff neck, twitching, jerking or a convulsion. A more complete list is given in the accompanying chart.

SIGNS OF SERIOUS ILLNESS IN A CHILD

- Difficulty in breathing
- Loss of consciousness or extreme lethargy
- Convulsion or muscle twitching
- Fever of 103° F. (39.5° C.) or higher
- Chest pain, wheezing or rapid breathing
- Persistent headache or stiff neck
- Severe abdominal pain or persistent abdominal pain
- Persistent vomiting, diarrhea or loss of appetite
- Bloody urine, very dark urine or blood in the stool
- Severe pain in the testicle

What should be done in the event of serious illness?   Notify the doctor and ask for advice. If the child appears to be in need of immediate attention, take him or her to the nearest emergency room or call the Emergency Medical Service for transportation.

What if my doctor can't be reached?   An emergency-room physician will treat your child if you consent, and at the same time, the hospital will attempt to contact your doctor. If hospitalization is indicated, the doctor on call will take responsibility until your physician can be reached.

Wouldn't it be better to watch the child at home rather than rushing him to the emergency room?   The best plan is to have the child taken care of by the physician who knows and regularly cares for him or her. But children may get sick a lot quicker than adults, and the only way to rule out a serious problem is to have a medical evaluation. So if your doctor is unavailable, don't hesitate to ask for another doctor's opinion when you feel it's indicated. That's what the emergency room is there for. Still another point is that if you want help, it's better to get it early in the evening than to wait till the middle of the night. Being human, doctors function better at 8 or 9 P.M. than at 2 A.M. Many emergency rooms are better staffed prior to 11 P.M. than afterwards.

How can you tell if a child has fever?   You may suspect it by feeling the forehead. Lethargy, sleepiness, sweating and a lack of appetite may accompany fever, or a child may appear relatively normal and go outside and play in spite of a fever of 103° F. (39.5° C.). The only sure way of knowing is to measure the body temperature.

What's the best way to take a child's temperature?   Until a child is of school age, a rectal temperature is preferable. Shake the rectal thermometer until the column is below 98.6° F. (37° C.), lubricate the end and insert it into the rectum. Keep the thermometer in place by holding the buttocks together with your hand. After three minutes remove it and read the temperature. Since the rectal thermometer is not used for oral readings, you need only wash it with soap and water before putting it away for future use.

Oral temperature can be taken when a child is old enough and careful enough to follow instructions. Wash the thermometer and wipe with alcohol, shake it down and place it under the tongue for three minutes. A cold drink within the previous half-hour may give a falsely low reading.

What's the normal temperature?   The average oral temperature is 98.6° F. (37° C.), but a given individual's normal temperature may be one degree higher or lower than average. The rectal temperature is one degree higher than the oral temperature, so a rectal reading of 100° F. (37.7° C.) or more must be present before fever can be said to exist. The axillary temperature (taken under the arm) is notoriously inaccurate, and tends to run at least a degree lower than the oral temperature.

What degree of fever is significant?   A rectal reading of 100.4° F. (38° C.) or greater is significant. While not necessarily dangerous, fever in the range of 103° (39.5° C.) is serious enough to warrant a call or visit to the doctor.

Is low temperature ever significant?   A temperature of less than 97° F. (36° C.) may point to a serious problem. To get a low reading, you have to shake down the thermometer to 95° F. (35° C.). Among the causes of a low temperature are an overwhelming infection, prolonged exposure to cold weather, or circulatory failure from a serious illness. Low temperatures sometimes occur in a "rebound effect" after a high fever and are not serious.

What causes fever?   Ninety-nine percent of the time an infection such as strep throat, a cold or infected ears is responsible. Other causes are the flu, kidney infection, pneumonia, bone infection and childhood illnesses, such as measles. (Infections are discussed in Chapter 6.)

Fever lasting for more than two weeks may be due to an indolent infection such as TB or to a noninfectious disease. Among the latter are rheumatoid arthritis, childhood leukemia and autoimmune conditions, such as lupus erythematosus.

153

Is high fever a sign of the severity of an illness?   To a degree, yes, though there are exceptions. Some children will run 103° F. (39.5° C.) with a cold, while others may not have much fever in spite of severe tonsillitis. Cough, sore throat and earache point to a respiratory infection even if the fever is mild, and the child should be seen by the doctor. Fever accompanied by persistent headache, or fever that continues for more than a day or two without apparent cause, should be evaluated by a physician.

When and how should the temperature be lowered?   It may be lowered when the child is uncomfortable and the cause of the fever is known, when the fever is over 103° F. (39.5° C.) in a child prone to have febrile convulsions, or when the fever is of recent onset and thought to be due to a cold or the flu. The three ways to lower temperature are to give aspirin, to give acetaminophen or to use a sponge bath. Acetaminophen irritates the stomach less than aspirin, and it can be given as drops, liquid or tablets. A warm bath at about 96° F. (35.5° C.) for ten to fifteen minutes will lower temperature comfortably and can be used in conjunction with aspirin or acetaminophen therapy.

You can give the bath in the tub, but do not fill it with water. The idea is to soak a towel or rags, lay these across the trunk and legs and keep them wet. As the water evaporates, it will lower the temperature. Rub the skin to stimulate the circulation and continue sponging until the temperature is less than 100° F. (37.7° C.) rectally.

If the child is dehydrated or begins to twitch in convulsion, a cool (55°–60° F., or 13°–15.5° C.) enema of 1/2 teaspoon of salt in a quart of water may be given slowly. Try to persuade the child to hold the water in as long as possible.

What are febrile convulsions?   These seizures may be brought on by fever over 103° F. (39.5° C.) in a child six months to five years of age, and seldom occur beyond the age of seven. Suddenly the child loses consciousness and has jerking motions of the arms and legs. The seizure usually lasts only a few minutes. Boys are twice as susceptible as girls, and many such children have parents who also had febrile convulsions.

The main danger is that, untreated, these convulsions may progress into the continuous seizure activity of status epilepticus. The child may literally convulse for many hours and brain damage or death could occur. The other danger of convulsion in a febrile child is that it could signal meningitis or encephalitis. Most children who are treated adequately for febrile convulsions do not suffer serious consequences.

What is the treatment for febrile convulsions?   The child should be seen immediately by a physician and treated for the infection as well as for the seizure. Phenobarbital is usually given to prevent further seizures. Infections should be treated promptly, and aspirin, acetaminophen or sponging should be used to lower a high fever and prevent the convulsions.

Do febrile seizures mean a child has epilepsy?   True epilepsy may begin as febrile seizures, but the great majority of children who have seizures only with fever do not have epilepsy.

What is croup?   It is an infection of the voice box (larynx) or the tissue around it that creates mild to severe respiratory obstruction. A "croupy sound" is characteristic of the infection. Caused by swelling of the larynx, it is similar to the sound made when you draw a breath in very quickly. Coughing and difficulty in breathing are the main symptoms.

How dangerous is croup?   One form can be extremely dangerous, but the most common form is a relatively mild infection that tends to occur again and again in a susceptible child. It is caused by a virus. A child three months to three years old develops a cold that persists for several days and gradually progresses into croup. Coughing, respiratory obstruction and gagging or vomiting may appear. Fever is mild or not present, and the child may seem all right during the day.

The dangerous form is much more abrupt in onset. Caused by *Hemophilus influenzae,* it may produce serious respiratory obstruction in only a few hours in a child who was previously well. Children three to seven years of age are most likely to be infected. Fever of 103° F. (39.5° C.) or more is present. Speech is difficult and the child may drool or complain of sore throat. Blueness about the mouth and fingernails is a serious sign pointing to oxygen deficiency.

What's the treatment for croup?   The dangerous form is an emergency requiring immediate hospitalization and intensive antibiotic and airway therapy. Sometimes a child with viral croup must be admitted to the hospital. More often, the mild form can be treated by using a cool mist vaporizer at the bedside. The child must be watched closely so that serious breathing difficulty can be reported to the physician. For a sudden worsening of the croup, take the child into the bathroom and turn on the hot shower. As the room steams up, the child's breathing should improve. Some physicians elect to treat even mild croup with an antibiotic such as ampicillin to prevent the more severe form from occurring.

What is asthma?   It is an allergic disease of the airways found in both children and adults. During an attack the smooth muscle around the bronchi squeezes down to partly shut off the flow of air in and out of the lungs.

155

Wheezing, coughing and shortness of breath are the symptoms. An attack may last an hour or persist for more than a day.

How common is asthma?   It affects 7 percent of American children, and is twice as common in boys as in girls. Improvement during adolescence is typical, but the disease may persist into adulthood.

What's the treatment for asthma?   A bronchodilator may be taken by aerosol to abort a mild attack. Epinephrine, terbutaline or a cortisone preparation may be needed to treat severe asthma. Theophylline, which relaxes smooth muscle in the lungs, is the mainstay of most oral medicines. Theophylline and similar drugs stimulate the central nervous system and may cause nervousness, insomnia or an irregular heart rhythm. Convulsions have occurred after use of these drugs. More frequent side effects are nausea, vomiting, rapid heartbeat and an increase in urine output. These effects are rarely troublesome when drug dosage is kept at a minimum.

Prevention of asthma attacks may be possible following the daily inhalation of cromolyn sodium. It doesn't work for all asthmatics, and its long-term side effects aren't yet known. Desensitization to specific allergens may be helpful. A more practical approach is to test for the offending allergens, such as a pet whose dander triggers wheezing, and have the child avoid them.

Must the asthmatic child avoid outdoor activities?   No, activity should be encouraged. Most children learn the degree of activity they can tolerate without developing wheezing.

What is hay fever?   It is an allergic condition causing nasal obstruction, sneezing and runny nose. It may occur as early as one or two years of age and may accompany asthma. The two types, perennial and seasonal, are really gradations of the same condition.

How do you know if a child has hay fever?   The child sneezes and seems to have a cold all the time. Doctors look for the "salute sign," made as the youngster rubs an itching nose by passing the palm straight up over the face. Children with established hay fever have nasal speech, breathe through the mouth and tend to snore loudly while asleep. Hay fever in an infant may cause trouble nursing or eating.

A history of allergic disease in the family and the finding of eosinophils on a smear of the child's nasal secretions is very suggestive of hay fever. Skin testing will establish what allergies exist (see pp. 274–75).

What is the treatment for hay fever?   Desensitization shots are the best form of treatment. Symptomatic agents include antihistamines and nose drops, though the latter should be used sparingly because of the tendency to develop a dependence on them.

What are the symptoms of a heart murmur?   Ninety-nine percent of childhood heart murmurs don't indicate disease, and the child has no symptoms. The murmur is an incidental finding by the examining physician and should be followed at regular visits. It usually disappears by the teenage years or adulthood. Another type of murmur can be more serious and may indicate problems with a heart valve or other conditions requiring medical treatment.

What signs point to heart disease in a child?   Heart disease may be congenital or acquired. Septal defects and other malformations may occur during fetal development and are present at birth. Rheumatic fever is the most common cause of acquired childhood heart disease. The signs of heart disease are listed below, although each of these signs may also indicate some other illness:
  · Shortness of breath or rapid respiration
  · Cyanosis, a blue discoloration of the nails, lips and other body parts
  · Swelling of the feet or the most dependent part of the body
  · Enlargement of the heart as detected by physical and X-ray examinations
  The specific defect can be diagnosed by electrocardiogram or other techniques done in the doctor's office or in a hospital setting by a heart specialist.

What is rheumatic fever?   It represents a reaction of the body to a streptococcal infection, and the disease has been said to "lick the joints and bite the heart." Following a long bout of strep throat, a susceptible child continues to have fever and develops pain and swelling in the joints. The inflammation may involve the heart to produce valve damage and a heart murmur.

How common is rheumatic fever?   Not nearly as common as it once was, it strikes one in ten thousand persons a year. One out of a thousand school-age children has rheumatic heart disease. Peak susceptibility occurs between the ages of five and fifteen.

What's the treatment for rheumatic fever?   The strep infection must be eradicated with penicillin. To prevent heart damage, the child is treated with aspirin and other anti-inflammatory agents and kept relatively inactive. He or she must stay home from school for two to four months, though complete bed rest is not necessary.

A strong program to prevent future strep infections, which could initiate or worsen heart damage, is necessary. This usually requires monthly injec-

157

tions or oral administration of penicillin. The treatment must be continued for at least five years after the first attack, and some physicians believe the therapy should be continued for life.

What may cause abdominal pain?   A common cause is the stomach's revolt against junk food, unripe fruit or other disagreeable items. Other sources are the intestinal flu, constipation and colic. Injury to the abdomen from a blow or a fall is fairly frequent and may or may not be serious. Other causes include appendicitis, kidney infection, pneumonia, food allergy, peptic ulcer, colitis, intestinal parasites, intussusception (see question below on severe pain in a child under two), twisted ovary, pelvic infection, pancreatitis, regional ileitis (inflammation of the small intestines) and kidney stone.

How can you tell if the pain is serious?   A sick child wants to remain in bed, won't eat and can't be distracted from the pain by an offer of a treat. Other serious signs are:
 · Vomiting or diarrhea
 · Blood in the urine
 · Blood or blood-tinged mucus in the stool
 · Pain that doubles the child up
 · Pain that radiates to the back or to another body part
 · Persistent pain
 · Pain that is made worse by sitting up or standing up
 · Pain that is accompanied by fever and chills

What are the symptoms of appendicitis?   They usually begin in the early morning with abdominal pain and loss of appetite. At first the pain is around the navel and is mild. It may even let up, but keeps coming back. Mild fever may occur, and vomiting once or twice is an early symptom. Within several hours the pain shifts to the right lower abdomen, where it persists and worsens. As the infection progresses, the child notes pain during a cough or any movement. A classic history is for the child to complain of every bump the car passes over en route to the hospital. Getting onto the examining table brings a grimace from the pain of stepping up and twisting around.

How common is appendicitis?   One in fourteen persons will develop it during their lifetime, and about 200,000 appendectomies a year are done in this country. The disease is most common in teenagers and young adults, but may occur any time from infancy to old age.

How is the diagnosis made?   Examination shows tenderness localized in the right lower abdomen. In particular, after the abdomen is pressed, there is a sudden increase in pain when pressure is removed. The white blood cell count is elevated, and other studies show that the pain is not caused by pneumonia, gastroenteritis, kidney infection or, in a girl, tubal infection or a twisted ovary. A definite diagnosis cannot be made until the time of surgery.

What is the treatment for appendicitis?   Surgical removal of the appendix.

What may cause severe abdominal pain in a child under two?   Intussusception, a protrusion of one part of the intestine into another. This most often involves a telescoping of the last part of the small intestine into the first part of the large intestine. Obstruction and gangrene of the bowel are the complications. The child, usually under the age of two, suddenly screams and doubles up the legs from severe pain. It's not uncommon for the pain to let up for several minutes and the child to appear well. Soon the spasm returns accompanied by vomiting and diarrhea. At first the stools contain mucus, then blood. Fever, sweating and abdominal distention are other symptoms.

What is the treatment for intussusception?   A suspicion of this condition calls for emergency evaluation of the child by a pediatrician and/or surgeon. The diagnosis must be confirmed by X-rays and a barium enema; the enema itself will reduce the intussusception in over half of the infants. When the enema is not successful, the condition must be relieved surgically.

Do children develop ulcers?   Yes, and this condition is on the increase, perhaps because of the stresses of our highly competitive society. Teenagers are at highest risk, and boys are affected twice as often as girls. Ulcers also may occur in infants and small children.

What are the symptoms of an ulcer?   In an adult, the symptoms are recurring upper abdominal pain that is relieved by eating or by taking antacid. The child is apt to have different symptoms. Vomiting after eating is the main sign in a child under six, and vomiting blood or passing a bloody stool is often the first sign of ulcer in older children.

What's the treatment for ulcer disease?   The child should be hospitalized. Suctioning of the stomach's contents will relieve vomiting, and antacids may stop bleeding. At times surgery is necessary. Preventive measures include a healthy diet and the avoidance of foods that cause difficulty. Stress must be lessened and the individual shown how to deal with it in a more constructive manner.

What causes blood in the stools?   A hard stool may scratch the lining of an infant's anus or rectum. The blood appears on the outside of the stool and is bright red. In an older child a hemorrhoid may bleed in a similar manner. Blood that is mixed in with the stool may be a sign of bacillary dysentery, an infectious diarrhea due to Shigella bacteria. Wine-colored stools indicate bleeding in the large intestine. Bleeding from the stomach or upper intestine gives grayish black or tarry stools, which are typical of an ulcer. Certain foods, such as beets and red peppers, may turn the stool red, and so will the pinworm medicine, Povan. Iron therapy may darken the stool but is not a cause of tarry stools.

What should be done for bloody stools?　If the stool is in a diaper, save it in case the doctor wants to see it. Look at the child's anus for signs of bleeding or the presence of a foreign body. Take the child's temperature. Then, phone the pediatrician, describe what happened and ask for advice. The child who has more than one bloody stool should definitely be evaluated by a physician.

What are pinworms?　They are intestinal parasites of the species *Enterobius vermicularis.* The adults live in the large intestine, but the females crawl to the anus to lay eggs, which hatch to produce the pin-sized white worms. Scratching the anus gets the eggs under the nails, where they can reach the mouth and be swallowed for reinfection.

How do children get pinworms?　They get them from other children who have them or from coming in contact with eggs that are attached to soiled linens or clothing. Because the eggs are so light, they can blow across the room when bed sheets are shaken. It is not unusual for all the members of a household to become infected.

What are the symptoms?　Itching of the anus, grinding of the teeth, difficulty sleeping, general irritability and short attention span in school.

Are they dangerous?　Not usually, though the worms are capable of causing appendicitis, ulcers of the intestinal lining, and, possibly, perforation of the wall of the intestine.

How is the infection diagnosed?　During the night you may be able to see the tiny worms swarming around the anus. Apply the sticky side of a piece of transparent tape to the anal skin then or first thing in the morning, before the child has had a bowel movement. Take the tape to the physician; the eggs and adult worms will be visible under a microscope.

What's the treatment for pinworms?　The best drugs are Povan, Vermox or Antepar. The child's nails should be cut, and he or she should sleep in two pairs of pajamas or other protective clothing to keep the fingers from scratching the anus. Sheets and covers should be handled gently and laundered frequently.

What causes blood in the urine?   In a girl under twelve a bladder infection is usually responsible. The more likely cause in an older girl is for menstrual blood to get into the toilet and make the urine appear bloody. Kidney infection and kidney stones may cause bloody urine in either sex.

What should be done for blood in the urine?   The doctor should be notified. A urinalysis and urine culture are indicated, and further treatment is based on the findings and other signs of illness.

What causes increased urine output?   Bladder infection may do this in a girl. It's not that so much urine is actually produced, but that the irritation causes frequent urination and burning on urination. Increased urine output in either sex may be due to diabetes, which will be discussed in Chapter 13.

What can be done for persistent bed-wetting?   When bed-wetting reappears in a child who was dry, or continues as a nightly problem in a school-age child, urinary infection may be responsible. A pediatrician should be consulted. Rarely, a defect in the structure or function of the bladder is discovered. Sometimes emotional problems may trigger bed-wetting in an older child.

The best parental approach is a calm and tolerant one. It may help to restrict fluid at supper and afterward and to wake the child at night to urinate. A reward system emphasizing praise for dry nights is often helpful.

What may cause vaginal bleeding during childhood?   The most common cause is a foreign body which the child has inserted into the vagina. Unfortunately, child abuse is another common cause. Vaginal tumor is a rare cause of bleeding that should be considered when the child's mother took estrogen during the pregnancy.

What is an undescended testicle?   One that hasn't slipped into the scrotum as it normally should (in the fetus the testicles normally migrate from the abdomen into the scrotum). The condition occurs in three or four percent of boys, but the testicle will usually descend on its own within several months after birth.

What is the treatment?   Treatment is usually given if the testicle hasn't descended on its own by the age of one. The first step is to try chorionic gonadotropin injections or testosterone by mouth to see if these will induce descent. If hormone therapy fails, surgery is necessary. Some urologists recommend early surgery, but others do not operate unless nondescent persists till age five.

What's the purpose of treatment?   An undescended testicle is more vulnerable to injury during play. The body temperature is two degrees higher than the scrotal temperature, which prevents the testicle from producing sperm. The boy who reaches puberty with two undescended testicles will usually be sterile. Cancer of the testicle is more likely to occur in an undescended testicle than in a descended one.

What may cause severe pain in the testicle?   Infection, injury and torsion of the testicle are the three main causes. Kidney stone is sometimes the source of pain that is referred to the testicle. The important distinction to be made is between twisting of the spermatic cord and an infection. Pain and swelling occur in both. Gentle upward lifting of the testicle may give relief from the pain of infection, but not from the pain of torsion, which persists and worsens. Gangrene may occur when the twisting shuts off blood supply to the testicle. Lack of blood flow can be shown with a Doppler ultrasonic stethoscope.

What's the treatment for severe testicular pain?   A urologist should see the child. Antibiotics are used to treat infection, but surgery is the treatment for torsion. Rarely, the doctor is able to untwist the testicle, but surgery may be needed to prevent a recurrence.

CHILDHOOD INFECTIONS

What causes measles?   Three distinct types of measles are recognized, and each is caused by a virus. These are roseola infantum, rubeola and rubella.

Roseola infantum (baby measles) occurs in children between the ages of six months and two years. Fever in the range of 103° to 104° F. persists for three or four days, and a generalized measles rash appears on the same day that the fever suddenly disappears. The rash fades in a day, and the child is well.

Rubeola ("big red measles") is the disease most people mean when they speak of measles. Nine to fourteen days after exposure to it, a susceptible child develops high fever, lethargy, cough and red eyes. The cough is harsh and worst at night. The rash appears within three days. It consists of small red dots and slight bumps that may become so extensive from head to foot that the entire body seems to be covered. The rash lasts a week to ten days.

Rubella (German measles, or three-day measles) is a serious disease not because of what it does to a child who has it, but because it may be contracted by a pregnant woman and infect her unborn baby. The incubation period is two or three weeks. Though fever may occur at the outset, it is usually mild. The most typical feature is a painful enlargement of the lymph glands behind the ears and along the back of the neck. The rash begins on the face as small pink spots. It spreads to the trunk and extremities, but rarely lasts longer than two days. The neck glands may remain enlarged for several days to a week.

What are the complications of measles?   Some children with roseola infantum have febrile convulsions. The worst complication of rubeola is encephalitis, which occurs in one out of a thousand children infected with big red measles. Forty percent of those developing encephalitis die or develop permanent brain damage. Rubella infection in the first three months of pregnancy may cause the baby to be mentally retarded, blind or have heart disease and other defects.

What's the treatment for measles?   A child prone to have febrile convulsions should be treated by sponging and the use of aspirin or acetaminophen to keep the fever down. Bacterial infection occurs as a complication in 5 to 15 percent of children with rubeola and may require antibiotic therapy. The child with signs of encephalitis, such as coma and convulsions, should be admitted to the hospital. Anyone, child or adult, with German measles should be treated symptomatically and kept away from women in the reproductive-age group who have not yet had the illness.

The ideal treatment for rubeola and rubella is prevention. Immunization according to the schedule given on p. 150 will protect against these diseases.

Can you get measles twice?   You can get each type only once. The three kinds of measles—roseola infantum, rubeola and rubella—do not recur after one has had them or received immunization for the last two. Confusion about having the same type of measles twice arises because other viral illnesses may cause a rash resembling that of measles.

What causes mumps?   It is caused by a virus.

What are the symptoms?   Many children have no symptoms, but painful swelling of one or both parotid glands, at the sides of the face, is the classic feature of mumps. Fever is mild or absent. Abdominal pain and vomiting may occur.

What are the complications of mumps?   The virus may cause a mild form of meningitis from which recovery almost always occurs. Involvement of the pancreas or ovaries may cause abdominal swelling or pain. The mumps virus may infect one or both testicles if the disease occurs after puberty. Swelling and pain in the testicles occur, but, contrary to popular belief, the testicular infection very rarely causes sterility.

163

What's the treatment?　　Specific therapy is lacking, so bed rest and supportive measures are indicated for the six or seven days of illness. Fever, headache and stiff neck call for admission to the hospital for observation. Nausea and vomiting may require medication for relief. An athletic supporter will help to relieve the pain of an infected testicle. A man who contracts mumps may lessen his risk of testicular involvement by taking a shot of mumps hyperimmune gamma globulin. The best treatment is to prevent the infection by immunization during childhood.

What causes chicken pox?　　It is caused by a virus and is one of the most contagious of childhood illnesses. In an adult, the same virus may cause shingles (herpes zoster).

What are the symptoms?　　Two or three weeks after exposure to the disease the susceptible person develops crops of small blisters on the trunk and face. These continue to appear for several days and may even occur inside the mouth. The blisters rupture, crust and slowly heal. At a given time, some of the blisters are in the process of healing or are festered while others are just breaking out. This is how one can distinguish the infection from smallpox, where all the sores are at the same stage of development. Fever is not usually severe, but the chicken pox sores may cluster around the nose, causing pain and irritation.

What are the complications?　　Pneumonia and encephalitis may occur, but are rare. Secondary infection of the skin is a fairly common but not usually serious problem.

What's the treatment?　　A specific form of gamma globulin can be given to treat chicken pox pneumonia or encephalitis. The gamma globulin may also prevent an extensive case of chicken pox from occurring in a child with an immune deficiency or a severe burn. Antibiotics are given when secondary bacterial infections occur.

How is whooping cough treated?　　Erythromycin is specific for the infection, but antibiotic treatment is not always successful. Childhood immunizations started at the age of two months will prevent the disease. This bacterial disease is most severe in children under two, in whom it causes severe coughing spasms, following which the child suddenly gasps for air and whoops. An infant may die from the cough or a complicating pneumonia.

Does diphtheria still occur?　　Yes, though most physicians have never seen a case and would never have to if everyone were to take routine immuniza-

164

tions. When an outbreak does occur, the disease is highly contagious. The initial symptoms are sore throat, cough and fever; difficulty in breathing, heart irregularities and pneumonia then occur. Diphtheria can be fatal and the recovery rate is largely dependent on early detection and treatment.

What is the treatment for diphtheria?　Penicillin therapy will eliminate the germs, but severe heart damage may result from diphtheria toxin. Antitoxin must be given as early as possible, preferably within the first two days of the disease. Carriers must also be treated with penicillin, and an intense immunization program is indicated once the outbreak is over.

What is the treatment for skin diseases in children?　See the discussion on pp. 228–31.

6

INFECTIONS

What causes an infection? It's caused by a tiny organism, or germ, that invades a part of the body, grows and attempts to survive by using the body as a host. In order of descending size, the germ may be a protozoan, fungus, bacterium or virus.

How do these agents enter the body? Most are passed from one person to another via respiratory droplets, unwashed hands or direct body contact. Other ways of transmission are through contact with infected urine or feces, or from the bite of an insect or animal.

What are the signs of infection? The common denominator of all infections is that the body resists the invasion in a kind of cellular warfare, creating tumor, rubor, dolor or calor:
  · Tumor is the swelling that accompanies infection of the skin, bone or other organ.
  · Rubor is the redness occurring from heightened blood flow at the site of infection.
  · Dolor is pain at the site of infection or, as in the case of the flu or similar infections, throughout the body.
  · Calor is the fever created by breakdown of white blood cells.

Does a viral infection differ from a bacterial infection? Yes, since they are a hundred times smaller, viruses create a different body response than bacteria do. The common cold is caused by a virus. Fever is minimal, and the white blood cell count stays the same or may go down. On the other hand, flu is a viral infection which may cause severe illness and high fever. A strep throat is caused by bacteria. Fever tends to be high, the white count is elevated, and the onset is somewhat more sudden than with a cold.

Bacterial infection tends to be localized, such as in one area of the skin, while a viral infection is more likely to be diffuse, such as the many sores .of chicken pox. Unlike bacteria, viruses rarely infect the kidneys, bones or bladder, but they do infect the liver, heart and brain. Body sites such as the throat, lungs and intestinal tract are commonly infected by both viruses and bacteria.

Does immunity develop to both kinds of infections?   Yes, but how long it lasts depends on the infection. Immunity to the common cold protects you for the rest of the season against that specific virus, but you're still susceptible to other cold-causing viruses. Resistance to viral illnesses such as measles, chicken pox and polio is thought to last a lifetime. Immunity from a strep throat may last for several months. Immunity to diphtheria, whooping cough and other bacterial infections tends to be longer-lasting, but not usually for a lifetime.

What specialist should treat you for an infection?   For an ordinary infection the pediatrician should treat a child, and the internist or general practitioner should treat a person over age twelve to fourteen. An infectious-disease specialist should be called in when the infection is serious, as in meningitis, of uncertain origin, as in septicemia, or baffling as in Legionnaires' disease. Hospitalization is indicated when an infection is serious or persists despite initial therapy as an outpatient.

A gynecologist should treat pelvic infections in a woman, and a urologist or general physician is qualified to treat venereal disease in a man. A surgeon's help may be needed when an infection of the arm or leg is so severe as, for example, to cause gangrene or require surgical drainage. An orthopedic specialist should participate in the care of a bone infection or an infected joint.

RESPIRATORY INFECTIONS

What causes strep throat?   It is a bacterial disease caused by Group A beta-hemolytic streptococci. These are the most virulent and potentially serious streptococci, but other forms may also cause throat infection.

What are the symptoms of strep throat?   The onset of fever and sore throat is sudden: it's possible to feel well one hour and be sick the next. Fever reaches 102° to 103° F. (38.8° to 39.5° C.). Pain is felt on swallowing and the glands beneath the jaw swell and become tender. Cough is often present, but runny nose is not usually a symptom of strep throat.

What is scarlet fever?   Some children with strep throat break out in a rash a day after the onset of fever. The rash consists of tiny dots and is accompanied by a generalized flushing that resembles sunburn. This rash is scarlet fever, and without treatment it may last for two or three weeks. It need not be feared if the child is treated promptly, for penicillin will cure the strep throat as well as the rash.

What are the complications of strep throat or scarlet fever?   The infection may spread to the ears or sinuses. A pocket of pus may appear in one or both tonsils (streptococci are the most common cause of tonsillitis). The two dread complications are rheumatic fever (see p. 157) and glomerulonephritis (see p. 425). These may damage the heart or kidney, respectively, and represent an immune reaction of the body to the strep infection.

What's the treatment?   Penicillin should be given by mouth or injection. In older children or adults, a single injection of benzathine penicillin or two injections given at the same time may end the infection. Erythromycin or cephalothin may be used when the person is allergic to penicillin. Oral antibiotic therapy must be given for a full ten days to make sure the infection is eradicated.

What causes the common cold?   It is caused by any of about a hundred different viruses. Not one of these viruses is susceptible to the action of antibiotics, which is why penicillin is ineffective in treating a cold.

How common is the common cold?   It's the most prevalent of all infectious diseases. Children are affected more often than adults, but adults have an average of three colds a year.

What are the symptoms?   Scratchy throat, runny nose, mild fever, aches, cough, stuffiness and generalized misery. The worst symptoms last only a few days, but the cold may drag on for two weeks.

What's the best treatment for a cold?   A child or infant may need nose drops to relieve nasal obstruction. Rest and aspirin or acetaminophen usually bring relief in an adult. Though they help to dry up secretions, patent remedies may cause unpleasant side effects, as may prescription cold preparations. In well-controlled studies, continuous vitamin C therapy did not prevent the common cold, but some studies indicated that vitamin C, taken from the outset, may shorten the duration of a cold.

What is the difference between a cold and the flu?   It's a matter of degree. Since both are caused by similar viruses, a severe cold may be indistinguishable from mild flu. If you're sick enough to stay in bed and have more than one degree of fever, chances are you have the flu. If you feel well enough to keep going, it may be a cold. The symptoms overlap, and you may have a very severe cold or a very mild flu.

What about flu epidemics?   Epidemic influenza may be much more serious than a cold. Cough, headache, muscle aches and fever of 102° to 105° F. (38.8° to 40.5° C.) occur. Persons over the age of sixty may develop a complicating pneumonia and die.

What are the worst strains of flu?   The flu pandemic of 1918 was attributed to swine flu. In recent years, Hong Kong flu and Russian flu have been more troublesome.

Are flu shots of value?   In the wake of the swine-flu vaccination program of 1976, many people, including doctors, are not enthusiastic about widespread immunization programs. It is clear that flu outbreaks occur almost every winter and that immunization will prevent the infection; the problem is having to anticipate a year in advance which strains will occur and thus which vaccines are needed. Persons who should consider having the flu shots are those over sixty-five and those who have lung problems or a chronic medical condition.

What are the chances of getting Guillain-Barré syndrome from a flu shot?
This syndrome of progressive paralysis occurred once after every 100,-000 injections of swine flu vaccine. Only 5 percent of affected individuals died, but another 5 or 10 percent were left with some degree of paralysis. The swine flu vaccine is no longer in use.

What's the treatment for flu?   Bed rest, fluids, aspirin or acetaminophen, and good nutrition. Antibiotics are ineffective unless a complication such as bacterial pneumonia occurs.

What is bronchitis?   It is an infection of the bronchial tree, the passageway through which air reaches the lungs. The infection may be caused by a virus and is a frequent accompaniment of a cold ("chest cold"). Viral bronchitis in a child under the age of two can be a serious illness. Known as bronchiolitis and caused by the respiratory syncytial virus, the infection

169

causes fever, gradually worsening cough, excessive secretions, and difficulty in breathing. The child must be treated in the hospital, where antibiotics and airway assistance are given. Some infants develop asthma after an attack of bronchiolitis.

Bronchitis may be caused by bacteria, but the bacteria usually invade the lungs and the condition becomes pneumonia. Bronchitis in an adult is often a chronic condition caused by smoking. It may create enough damage to cause a type of lung failure known as chronic obstructive respiratory disease —CORD—which is discussed in Chapter 15.

What is pneumonia?　　It is an infection of the lungs caused by bacteria, viruses, tuberculosis or fungi. The characteristic feature of pneumonia is that it causes an outpouring of fluids, pus or very thick inflammatory material into the lungs.

How serious is pneumonia?　　Viral pneumonia may not be serious, but bacterial pneumonia usually is. A common form, pneumococcal pneumonia, is fatal in one out of fifteen persons who develop it; it kills 13,000 to 66,000 people a year in the United States. Bronchopneumonia, a more extensive form of pneumonia that occurs most commonly in children and old persons, may be fatal when treatment is not started early.

What are the symptoms of pneumonia?　　Fever, chest pain and cough are the classic ones, but in an elderly or bedridden person, fever may be the only sign. In a child, fever, irritability, failure to eat and vomiting or diarrhea are frequent symptoms. A previously well adult who suddenly develops pneumonia usually has pneumococcal pneumonia. The onset is sudden, with a shaking chill that may last half an hour. The fever climbs rapidly to 103° to 105° F. (39.5° to 40.5 C.). Cough productive of rusty sputum and pain in the chest are early but not universal symptoms. Lack of appetite, vomiting and difficulty in breathing in any but a sitting position may develop as the infection progresses.

How is pneumonia diagnosed?　　The doctor may hear the characteristic sounds (rales) created by fluid or exudate in the lungs, and the pneumonia will show up on chest X-ray. The specific type of pneumonia is determined by culture tests of the sputum.

What is the treatment for pneumonia?　　Penicillin and other antibiotics are given for bacterial and certain viral pneumonias. Other measures include adequate hydration, positive pressure breathing, and suctioning to remove bronchial secretions.

Can pneumonia be prevented?　　A vaccine has been developed to prevent pneumococcal pneumonia. A single injection provides 80 percent protection for up to three years. The immunization is indicated in older persons and those at high risk of pneumonia because of chronic lung disease or other medical condition. The vaccine can't be taken during pregnancy and isn't effective in children under two years of age. Soreness at the injection site and low-grade fever occur in most persons who receive the vaccine. Persons who are allergic to any component of the vaccine run the risk of a severe or life-threatening reaction, and for this reason it must be used with caution in one with a history of allergic reactions.

What causes tuberculosis (TB)? A red-staining, brick-shaped germ known as *Mycobacterium tuberculosis* causes TB. It grows slowly, is resistant to ordinary antibiotics, and causes a cheesy type of tissue death as it destroys the lungs or other organs.

What are the symptoms of TB? Fever, night sweats, weight loss, chills, cough and blood-tinged sputum are the main ones. Before effective therapy was available, TB caused such marked wasting that it literally seemed to consume the victim, hence the designation "consumption."

Who is most susceptible to TB? Conditions that predispose to TB include mental and physical stress, poor nutrition, diabetes and lung disease, such as silicosis. American Indians are more susceptible to this infection than persons of European or African ancestry.

How is TB diagnosed? Most cases are diagnosed through screening tests, such as the tuberculin test that is required of schoolchildren, schoolteachers, food handlers, health professionals and others. A positive screening test leads to an X-ray, which may show the infection in the lungs. Subsequent sputum tests are positive for *M. tuberculosis.* Tuberculous infection of the kidneys is diagnosed by urine tests.

What is the treatment for TB? Infection limited to the lungs is usually treated with a combination of the drugs isoniazid and ethambutol for eighteen months. Streptomycin injections may be given when the infection is severe. Some specialists prefer to begin therapy with a combination of rifampin and isoniazid. Each of these drugs has side effects. Streptomycin may damage hearing or harm the kidneys. Isoniazid may cause liver damage, and so may rifampin. The most serious side effect of ethambutol is a usually reversible reduction in vision. The drugs are, however, effective in treating TB so that the trade-off between side effects and benefits is usually acceptable when therapy is carefully monitored.

What if your skin test is positive and your X-ray is negative? A positive skin test means that you have come in contact with the TB germ in the past.

If the X-ray is negative, the chances are good that your body formed a resistance to TB without developing a full-blown infection.

Conversion from a negative to a positive skin test in someone under thirty-five usually calls for a year of therapy with isoniazid. The treatment may prevent the development of overt TB later on, though the isoniazid poses the risk of causing liver damage. When one member of a family develops a positive skin test, other family members should be checked for skin test conversion or active TB.

Will a positive skin test become negative? If you remain in good health, you can expect your skin test to remain positive. For this reason, you don't have to have a repeat skin test every year for job purposes, provided your physician has a record of the positive reaction and fills out the necessary papers.

What is histoplasmosis? It is a fungal disease that can cause many of the symptoms of tuberculosis. The disease may spread throughout the body, but most commonly remains in the lungs. A natural resistance may develop to a mild infection, but a severe case of histoplasmosis can be treated with an antifungal agent.

What is coccidioidomycosis? It is a fungal disease most prevalent in the San Joaquin Valley of California (hence the name "valley fever"). It may affect the lungs, skin, bones and other organs, and amphotericin-B, a toxic but usually effective drug, is used in the treatment. Skin tests can be done for histoplasmosis or coccidioidomycosis.

What is Legionnaires' disease? It's a type of pneumonia caused by a bacterium known as the agent of Legionnaires' disease. The infection came to light in the summer of 1976, when an outbreak occurred among persons attending the American Legion Convention in Philadelphia. Twenty-nine of 182 persons with the disease died. In 1978 an outbreak of the disease occurred in the garment district of New York, and fatalities were noted.

Studies by the Communicable Disease Center have shown that the infection is passed through the air (possibly through air-conditioning systems), though not from person to person. Retrospective studies indicate that Legionnaires' disease was responsible for mysterious outbreaks of pneumonia in 1965 and 1968. The infection has occurred in most states and in foreign countries. Many persons carry antibodies to it, indicating an asymptomatic infection in the past.

What are the symptoms of Legionnaires' disease? It begins like the flu, but progresses more rapidly. Two to ten days after exposure to the infecting agent, the victim has a generalized sick feeling with muscle ache, headache and dry cough. Chills and fever of 103° to 104° F. (39.5° to 40° C.) occur on the second day. The cough worsens, and some victims develop chest or abdominal pain. Later, the person may become short of breath or lose consciousness. Death may occur within a few days to a week of the onset. More likely, the fever will break within three days and recovery will occur over the next two weeks.

Who is most likely to develop Legionnaires' disease?   Elderly persons, those with lung disease and those receiving immunosuppressive therapy are most susceptible, but the disease may also strike able-bodied younger persons.

How is Legionnaires' disease diagnosed?   The chest X-ray is positive for pneumonia in nine out of ten persons with the disease. The infection can be confirmed by a blood test.

What is the treatment?   A person with suspected Legionnaires' disease should be admitted to the hospital for oxygen therapy and other supportive measures. Erythromycin and tetracycline have proven useful in treating the infection.

MENINGITIS AND ENCEPHALITIS

What is meningitis?   It is an infection of the lining of the brain, the meninges. This thin layer forms a watertight covering beneath the skull, and inside it the brain is cushioned on all sides by fluid. An infection of the lining soon involves this cerebrospinal fluid, which is why a spinal tap to sample it is a useful diagnostic procedure.

What causes meningitis?   It may be caused by bacteria (bacterial meningitis), viruses (aseptic meningitis), fungi (cryptococcal meningitis) or tuberculosis (tuberculous meningitis).

Bacterial meningitis is the most common form. The germ responsible for it in children is usually *Hemophilus influenza.* In adults, *Neisseria meningitidis* is a more likely cause. It's thought that the germ enters the body through the upper respiratory passages, and is carried by the blood to the meninges. Less than 1 percent of people who carry one of these germs in the nose or throat ever develop meningitis, however.

What are the symptoms of meningitis?   After a day or two of what seems to be a cold, the person develops high fever, headache and gradual stiffening of the neck. Vomiting, lethargy, confusion and stupor may occur. Some persons go into a coma within twenty-four hours of the onset of meningitis.

Sometimes a rash of pink to red or dark-colored dots appears on the skin. The rash may be scarcely noticeable or as prominent as that due to measles.

How dangerous is meningitis?   Untreated bacterial meningitis is almost always fatal. Even with treatment, the mortality rate is 10 percent. Delay in diagnosis and treatment worsens the prognosis. Viral meningitis is rarely fatal.

How is meningitis diagnosed?   It may be suspected by clinical examination, but must be confirmed by a spinal tap. In bacterial meningitis, white blood cells (pus cells) are present in the normally cell-free spinal fluid. The spinal-fluid protein is elevated. The glucose in the spinal fluid is low. A smear and culture of the spinal fluid reveal the causative bacteria. Viral meningitis elevates the spinal-fluid protein content but doesn't affect the glucose and produces a much milder cellular reaction.

How does the doctor know when to do a spinal tap?   In medical parlance, the indication for a spinal tap is just to think of possibly doing it to evaluate the patient's illness. Anything remotely suggestive of meningitis—unexplained fever, vomiting, convulsion or headache—is justification for a spinal tap. Obvious indications include fever and headache in association with a stiff neck and a reduction in the level of consciousness.

What is the treatment for meningitis?   Penicillin administered intravenously is used for the most common form of meningitis, but ampicillin, chloramphenicol and other drugs may also be employed. Antibiotics are not indicated for viral meningitis, and amphotericin-B and antituberculous drugs are used to treat fungal and tuberculous meningitis, respectively.

Should contacts be treated?   Household contacts of a person who develops bacterial meningitis should be treated with a sulfa drug or rifampin to prevent him or her from developing meningitis. The nursery-school contacts, siblings and playmates of a child who gets meningitis should also receive prophylactic therapy. The amount and type of preventive therapy are determined by the doctor treating the patient for meningitis.

What is encephalitis?   It is an infection of the brain that causes headache, fever, nausea, vomiting, stiff neck, drowsiness and coma (hence the term "sleeping sickness"). It occurs in epidemics. The usual cause is a virus that is transmitted by the bite of a mosquito, and infection in horses precedes human infection. Common forms include Western equine encephalitis, Eastern equine encephalitis, St. Louis encephalitis, Venezuelan equine encephalitis and California encephalitis. Encephalitis may also be caused by other viruses that aren't transmitted by the mosquito. These include measles and mumps viruses, and prevention of encephalitis is one of the reasons for immunization against these diseases.

How is encephalitis diagnosed?   During an epidemic, the onset of fever, meningeal irritation and loss of consciousness occurring in someone with a history of mosquito bites is quite typical. The diagnosis is confirmed by a spinal tap and blood tests.

How dangerous is encephalitis?   As many as half of children with Eastern equine encephalitis may die, and many of those who recover have brain damage or seizures. The prognosis in adults is somewhat better, and the average mortality rate in other forms of encephalitis is 10 to 25 percent.

What's the treatment for encephalitis?   A specific antibiotic is not available, but the person should be admitted to the hospital for supportive therapy. Fever and convulsions can be controlled, and the person can be fed intravenously during the illness. Death may occur during the first week or the person may recover slowly over a period of several weeks.

Can encephalitis be prevented?   Widespread vaccination of horses has helped to control the epidemic infection, but the vaccine is not safe enough for use in humans. The main preventive measure during an epidemic is to avoid mosquito bites. Since the infection may be passed to the fetus, pregnant persons must be especially careful. Babies should be protected by having the crib covered with mosquito netting. Insect repellents and insecticides may prove useful in protecting those who work outdoors.

INTESTINAL INFECTIONS AND HEPATITIS

What causes intestinal flu?   A virus causes the disease, which is passed from one person to another. In epidemic form, it is most frequent in the winter and affects children more often than adults.

What are the symptoms of intestinal flu?   Nausea and vomiting are followed by diarrhea. Abdominal pain may occur. The onset is abrupt, and the illness usually runs its course in one to four days.

What's the treatment for intestinal flu?   Bed rest and sips of fluids are indicated. Medicine to control vomiting and diarrhea can be prescribed by a doctor. Hospitalization is rarely necessary.

What causes food poisoning?   It is caused by harmful germs that are introduced into food by those preparing it, but the food must be incubated as well as contaminated. The usual scenario is for many people to become ill after dining at a public facility or eating at a large picnic where food was provided by many persons. Investigation reveals that one or more dishes were left standing in warm temperatures for several hours or overnight. Frequently tainted foods include mayonnaise, potato salad, casseroles, whole-egg preparations or custard. Staphylococcal food poisoning and salmonella food poisoning are the two most common types, and the features of each are quite distinct.

What are the features of staph (staphylococcus) food poisoning? Symptoms begin one to six hours after ingestion of the tainted food, and include cramping abdominal pain and violent vomiting and retching. Diarrhea is often noted, but fever does not occur. The symptoms, due to a toxin produced by the staph, are usually over within six to eight hours. Symptomatic therapy may be given by a physician, but specific therapy is not available. When two or more persons who ate the same food develop symptoms, public health officials should be notified so that the source of the poisoning can be identified.

What are the features of salmonella food poisoning? Nausea and vomiting begin eight to forty-eight hours after ingestion of the contaminated food. Abdominal pain and persistent diarrhea follow, and the person develops fever in the range of 102° to 103° F. (38.8° to 39.5° C.) The illness runs its course in two to five days, but considerable variation occurs. Some persons may have mild symptoms, while others who ate the same food become seriously ill and require hospitalization. Treatment consists of fluids, medicine to lower fever, and symptomatic measures taken for the intestinal upset. The source of the outbreak should be identified so that health officials can investigate.

What causes botulism? This is a rare but dread form of food poisoning caused by a toxin secreted by *Clostridium botulinum.* Spores of the bacterium may enter food that is to be canned or preserved in fruit jars. The spores are destroyed by heating the food to 250° F. (121° C.), but may persist in food subjected to a temperature of less than 212° F. (100° C.). Because of inadequate sterilization, home-preserved vegetables and fruits are the most common sources of infection, followed by preserved fish products, such as canned tuna.

What are the symptoms? Five to thirty-six hours after ingesting the toxin, the person may develop nausea, vomiting and abdominal pain. Dryness of the mouth and throat occur. Blurred vision, difficulty in speaking, difficulty in swallowing and muscular weakness appear half a day to three days later. Weakness of the chest muscles causes difficulty in breathing, and respiratory failure is the usual cause of death.

How is botulism diagnosed?　　The diagnosis is not difficult when several persons who ate the food develop symptoms. The suspicious food can be tested to confirm the diagnosis. The toxin may also be detected in the victim's blood or stool.

What is the treatment for botulism?　　The person should be placed in the hospital so that airway assistance (perhaps including tracheotomy) can be given. An antitoxin is used to treat the disease, but even with treatment, the mortality rate averages 50 percent. Those who recover don't usually have residual weakness or paralysis.

How can botulism be prevented?　　Food should be boiled for three hours in the preparation for preserving it. An added precaution is to boil preserved food for fifteen minutes before it is used. A can or jar showing any discoloration or swelling of the container or lid should not be used, and containers of the same food made at the same time should also be discarded. Botulism from commercial products occasionally occurs, and is reported in the newspapers. Such recalled items should be returned to the store or disposed of.

What causes travelers' diarrhea?　　This condition, known as "turista" or "Montezuma's revenge," affects a large percent of Americans traveling to Mexico or other underdeveloped countries. The cause is a toxic form of *Escherichia coli,* a normally innocuous inhabitant of the colon. It presumably reaches the intestine through contaminated food or drink. The symptoms are watery diarrhea, abdominal cramps and, sometimes, nausea and vomiting.

Can travelers' diarrhea be prevented?　　Encouraging results have been reported with the use of doxycycline in a dose of 100 milligrams daily with breakfast. A long-acting form of tetracycline, doxycycline prevented diarrhea in most of the study subjects who took it during their first three weeks in Kenya. The medicine's preventive effect persisted for a week after it was stopped. Side effects of doxycycline include an exaggerated sunburn reaction and intestinal upset. It shouldn't be taken by children because it may stain their teeth, and it shouldn't be used during pregnancy because it may harm the fetus. Other ways of preventing travelers' diarrhea are to avoid raw, unpeeled fruits or vegetables, unbottled or poorly bottled drinking water, dairy products and highly spiced foods.

Are there any conditions that may resemble travelers' diarrhea?　　Yes, and one that is being increasingly recognized is giardiasis, an infestation with the protozoan *Giardia lamblia.* This condition, which may cause diarrhea, nausea, loss of appetite and abdominal discomfort, is worldwide in distribution but is seen more frequently among those who have visited the Colorado Rockies for a ski trip ("Pike's pique") or cities in Russia ("the Trotskys"). It is contracted through the ingestion of water or food contaminated with *Giardia* cysts.

Treatment includes the use of quinacrine or metronidazole. Quinacrine may upset the stomach or cause a yellowish tint to the skin, and metronidazole may cause nausea and a peculiar metallic taste. These side effects are not usually troublesome during the ten days or so of therapy.

Another condition that may be mistaken for travelers' diarrhea is dysentery, discussed below.

What causes dysentery?   The word is used to describe any disease characterized by diarrhea lasting more than a day or two. Most of the time a virus is responsible, but three treatable forms of dysentery are amebic, bacillary and salmonella.

· *Amebic dysentery* causes diarrhea of progressively increasing severity: the stools may become so bloody that they resemble fresh hamburger meat. Fever, dehydration and generalized weakness may occur. Amebiasis is capable of infecting the liver and other organs.

· *Bacillary dysentery* is a serious and possibly fatal disease when it occurs in a child under two. Chills and fever are followed by diarrhea and abdominal cramps. Initially watery and foul-smelling, the stool soon contains mucus and blood (see p. 159). Rapid dehydration and shock may occur. In older children the condition may be mild and self-limited.

· *Salmonella dysentery* is also most severe in children under the age of two. The symptoms are diarrhea, fever and vomiting. Sometimes the stool contains blood. Salmonella outbreaks may occur in epidemics among nursery school children. The infection also occurs in adults.

How is dysentery diagnosed?   The diagnosis can be suspected on the basis of the history and physical examination. Studies of the stool are usually diagnostic, but blood tests may be needed. A quicker way to diagnose amebiasis is to perform a proctoscopic examination of the rectum and lower colon, since characteristic mucosal ulcerations appear there.

What's the treatment for dysentery?   Ampicillin is used to treat bacillary or salmonella dysentery, and metronidazole, tetracycline and other drugs are given to eradicate amebiasis.

What is infectious hepatitis?   It's a viral infection of the liver that may occur sporadically or in epidemics. It is sometimes known as "yellow jaundice," though other medical conditions may also cause jaundice. Two forms of the infection are recognized: hepatitis A and hepatitis B.

Hepatitis A is passed by the fecal-oral route upon ingestion of con-

178

taminated food or water spoiled by untreated sewage. Two to six weeks later the person develops nausea, loss of appetite, abdominal pain and mild fever. A smoker may lose his or her taste for cigarettes. Darkening of the urine and a yellow discoloration of the eyes signal jaundice, which occurs in less than half of persons with hepatitis. Easy fatigue and loss of energy are additional symptoms.

Hepatitis B was originally thought to be transmitted only through blood transfusions or contaminated needles. Now it is known that the infection may be passed by the fecal-oral route as well as by blood transfusion, a contaminated needle, dental or surgical instrument, a dirty tattoo needle or a shared razor or toothbrush. Venereal transmission has been reported. The incidence of transmission through blood transfusion is much lower since blood banks began to screen donors for HBAg (hepatitis B antigen). HBAg is found in 1 or 2 percent of paid donors and one or two out of a thousand volunteer donors. Its presence in the blood indicates that the person may carry the disease, and he or she is excluded from donating blood. The incubation period for hepatitis B is six weeks to six months, but the disease itself does not differ markedly from hepatitis A.

How is hepatitis diagnosed?　Blood tests show evidence of liver infection, and the hepatitis B antigen will appear in the blood if this disease is present.

What is the treatment for hepatitis?　Rest and a good diet produce healing within two or three weeks, but the return to full physical activity may not be possible for several months. Alcohol must be avoided during the illness and for some time afterward. Steroid hormones may hasten healing when jaundice is severe or unrelenting, and such persons should be admitted to the hospital for therapy.

What about those exposed to hepatitis?　A single dose of gamma globulin, based upon body weight, should be given (the maximum dose is 2.0 milliliters). It will protect against hepatitis or make it milder if it does occur. Gamma globulin will also protect someone traveling to an area where the risk of contracting hepatitis is high. A special form of immune globulin must be given to anyone who has been exposed to hepatitis B. The main side effect of gamma globulin is an allergic reaction to it, and due caution must be taken where there is a history of allergies.

What about a carrier of hepatitis B antigen?　The person should have a medical evaluation to see if he or she has a smoldering case of hepatitis. A carrier should not donate blood nor share personal items with others.

BLADDER AND KIDNEY INFECTIONS

What are the symptoms of bladder infection?   Burning on urination and frequent urination are the main ones. Some persons also have fever and abdominal or pelvic pain. Slight blood-tinging or cloudiness of the urine may occur. Infected urine tends to have a strong odor.

What causes bladder infection?   Women are susceptible to this infection because of the nearness of the urethra (bladder opening) to the vagina and anus. The female urethra is much shorter than a man's, making it possible for germs to reach the bladder easily. A man is unlikely to develop a bladder infection unless his prostate gland enlarges. Stricture of the urethra is another cause of infection in a man.

What is "honeymoon cystitis"?   It is a bladder infection occurring soon after a woman begins an active sexual life and is thought to be caused by germs spreading from the vaginal entrance to the urine opening as a result of sexual intercourse.

What is the treatment for cystitis?   A visit to a general physician, internist, gynecologist or urologist is indicated. The doctor will do a urinalysis and urine culture. The infection should be treated for ten days to two weeks with an antibiotic. If the infection clears, no further therapy is needed.

What is the treatment for recurring cystitis?   Sometimes what starts out as honeymoon cystitis turns into an ordeal of recurrent bladder infections that goes on for months. The problem is an unusual susceptibility to infection by germs normally found in the genital region that are forced into the urethra during the thrusting motions of intercourse. Continuous therapy with an antibacterial agent is indicated. The woman should empty her bladder after sexual relations; she may benefit from drinking two glasses of fluid just before retiring, because the fluid may make her get up in the night and pass urine to wash out germs that may be multiplying in the bladder. It is uncommon for this infection to last more than six months. In the case of recurring cystitis not associated with sexual activity, a culture should be taken to identify the infecting germs, and if the condition persists, it should be evaluated by a urologist to see if the bladder and urethra are functioning properly.

What causes kidney infection?   It usually begins the same way as bladder infection: by germs getting into the urethra. From the bladder the germs make their way up the ureters to the kidneys. The infection is more common in women than in men.

What are the symptoms of kidney infection? Chills and fever of 102° to 104° F. (38.8° to 40° C.) begin abruptly. Pain in the back, flank and abdomen, a burning sensation on urination, frequency of urination, and nausea and vomiting are other symptoms, though not all these occur in each instance. Fever and nausea may be the main symptoms. A kidney infection known as pyelonephritis may mimic pneumonia, appendicitis, hepatitis, gastroenteritis or the flu.

How is the diagnosis made? Physical examination shows fever, and tenderness is present on one or both sides of the back where the two lower ribs join the spinal column (this is the position of the kidneys). White blood cells appear in the urine, and the urine culture is positive for the infecting bacteria.

What's the treatment for kidney infection? Hospitalization is indicated to allow the administration of intravenous fluid and antibiotic therapy. Four-fifths of kidney infections in women are caused by *Escherichia coli,* a bowel inhabitant that has entered the urinary tract. Ampicillin is specific for this germ, but other antibiotics or sulfa drugs may also be effective. A form of penicillin, ampicillin is relatively safe. Some persons are allergic to it, as shown by rash or hives developing during therapy. Safe usage during pregnancy has not been established. Sulfa drugs may also cause a variety of side effects and reactions. Therapy should be continued for two or three weeks, though hospitalization is usually not necessary for more than four or five days.

OTHER INFECTIONS

What causes mononucleosis? The Epstein-Barr virus is responsible for this disease. Communicability is low, but transmission may occur through kissing or the sharing of eating utensils and drinking glasses. Mononucleosis is most common in teenagers and college students, and is rare beyond the age of thirty.

What are the symptoms of mononucleosis? The main ones are fatigue, mild fever and sore throat. Lymph glands, particularly in the back of the neck, may enlarge, and a faint, sandpaperlike rash may accompany the infection.

How is the diagnosis made? The mono spot test done on a sample of blood will be positive in most patients within a few weeks after the onset of the disease. Findings on the blood smear and physical examination help to confirm the diagnosis.

What is the treatment for mononucleosis?   Rest and good diet are the main treatment, and the disease will run its course in several weeks. Steroid hormone therapy (prednisone) may shorten the duration of illness and lessen the degree of fever, soreness of the throat and glandular swelling, though the benefits of steroids must be balanced against their side effects (see p. 350–52.) Up to a third of mono patients have superimposed strep throat, which can be diagnosed by throat culture and should be treated with penicillin.

What's the main complication of mononucleosis?   Three-fourths of persons with mononucleosis develop an enlarged spleen. Every so often the spleen will rupture. Death may occur unless surgery can be done in time to stop the bleeding. To prevent splenic rupture, stressful activity and contact sports must be avoided until this organ has returned to its normal size, usually within several weeks after the onset of the disease.

What is blood poisoning?   This occurs when a bacterial infection enters the bloodstream and has the potential of infecting organs throughout the body. The medical term for it is septicemia, or sepsis.

What causes blood poisoning?   The infection may begin on the skin or in the lungs, kidneys, throat or genital organs, then spread to the blood. Direct infection of the bloodstream is possible when an addict injects a drug intravenously.

What are the symptoms of blood poisoning?   Chills, fever and prostration occur rapidly. Ineffective circulation may lead to a precipitous drop in blood pressure—shock—that is reflected by coldness of the extremities, rapid breathing and loss of consciousness.

What's the treatment for septicemia?   Hospitalization and intensive antibiotic therapy are indicated. Fluids and drugs to support the blood pressure may be necessary.

How serious is septicemia?   The mortality rate is as high as 30 to 50 percent, depending on the nature of the infection, its duration, and the age and general health of the patient.

What causes lockjaw?   This disease, tetanus, is caused by a toxin released by *Clostridium tetani,* a germ that may contaminate a wound. Three factors that favor tetanus are lack of immunization, a dirty wound (particularly a puncture wound) and failure to keep a wound clean until it heals. A tragic and often fatal form of the disease, neonatal tetanus, may follow the cutting of a baby's cord with rusty or dirty scissors.

What are the symptoms of lockjaw?   Muscle spasms begin two to six weeks or longer after the wound. Difficulty in opening the mouth—lockjaw —soon appears, and is followed by difficulty in swallowing. In a mild or moderate case of lockjaw these symptoms may not progress to the convulsions, respiratory failure and extreme muscle spasms of severe tetanus.

What's the treatment for tetanus?   The person must be admitted to a hospital and placed in a quiet room. Muscle relaxants, human tetanus antiglobulin and penicillin are given. The wound itself must be cared for with cleansing and careful debridement, or surgical removal of contaminated tissue. Feeding and airway assistance are often necessary.

How is lockjaw prevented?   It can be prevented by the routine immunizations described on pp. 150–51. The dirtier the wound, the more likely it is to cause tetanus, so even the immunized person should receive surgical care for a severe wound. The need for a booster shot and a shot of tetanus immune globulin can be decided by the attending physician.

What is rabies?   It is an almost invariably fatal disease caused by a virus that is transmitted to man by the bite or licking of a rabid animal. The biting animal is usually a dog, cat, bat, skunk, fox or coyote. Any bite by a wild animal or an unprovoked bite by a domestic animal should be considered rabies-prone. Wounds on the head, face or neck are more likely to lead to rabies.

What do you do in case of a bite?   Identify the animal if it's a dog or cat, and report the incident to the health or animal control department as well as to the physician. The animal will be picked up and held for signs of rabies. If no symptoms appear within ten days, the animal can be assumed not to have rabies and no further precautions are necessary. An animal that dies or is killed should be taken to a public health facility and examined for the presence of rabies.

A wild animal inflicting a bite should be killed if possible and taken in for rabies examination. If the examination proves negative, it can be assumed that the animal was not rabid, and no further precautions are necessary. When the wild animal isn't killed and shown negative by examination, or when the bite is by a stray pet that can't be located, rabies immunization *must* be given. Immunization is also indicated, of course, when the bite came from a domestic animal later shown to be rabid.

What do the shots consist of?   A vaccine made from rabies virus grown in duck embryos has been in use for years. Twenty-one doses of the vaccine are given over a two-week period, with booster shots ten days, twenty days (and sometimes three months) after the series is completed. The shots are given beneath the skin of the abdomen according to a "map" worked out at the beginning so that no two shots will be injected in the same spot.

A human diploid cell vaccine has recently become available for use in rabies prevention. Because of its limited availability, the vaccine is used only for persons known to have been bitten by a rabid animal, those who are allergic to the duck-embryo vaccine, or those who fail to show an antibody response to the duck-embryo vaccine. Only five or six doses of human vaccine are needed to provide protection, and it is given in the arms rather than in the skin of the abdomen. The human vaccine is available from the Communicable Disease Center in Atlanta. Injection of human rabies immune globulin is also indicated for persons bitten by rabid animals or by animals presumed to be rabid.

How effective are the shots?   From 1957 to 1968 eight deaths from rabies occurred in 225,000 persons who had received the duck-embryo vaccine. It is thought that the human diploid cell vaccine should give even better results.

What are the symptoms of rabies?   The time from the bite to the onset of disease varies from ten days to a year, and the longer the incubation period, the greater the likelihood that the shots will be effective. The first symptom is numbness and tingling at the site of the bite. Apprehension, excitability and convulsions appear. Paralysis of the throat muscles leads to an aversion to water—hydrophobia. Death usually occurs five to seven days after the onset, but in 1972 doctors reported the case of a man who was given intensive therapy and survived rabies.

What is cat-scratch fever?   It's a viral disease transmitted by the scratch of a cat or a kitten. Dogs and monkeys may also transmit the infection. A sore appears at the site of the scratch, and fever and swelling of the lymph glands are noted one and a half to four weeks later. The tender glands may remain swollen for two months or longer.

What's the treatment for cat-scratch fever?   Since the disease is self-limiting, specific treatment is not necessary. A doctor should make the diagnosis, for other diseases may cause similar symptoms.

What is parrot fever?   This infection—ornithosis or psittacosis—is transmitted to humans from birds. Parrots or parakeets were once the main source of infection, but we now know that ducks, chickens, pheasants, turkeys and wild birds may transmit the disease to humans. Bird handlers and those who work in pet shops are most susceptible. Rarely, transmission from human to human may occur.

The symptoms are fever, cough and generalized discomfort. Shortness of breath, chest pain and delirium point to pneumonia, a complication that proves fatal in 5 to 40 percent of those who develop it.

How is parrot fever diagnosed?   The history of contact with birds in someone with the symptoms of the disease is very suggestive. Blood tests and X-rays will confirm the condition, which should be reported to public health officials so that others can take precautions to avoid it.

What's the treatment for parrot fever?   Tetracycline is specific for this infection, and the fever is usually gone two or three days after the onset of therapy.

What is spotted fever?   Also known as Rocky Mountain spotted fever, this disease is caused by a germ that is transmitted by the bite of a wood tick such as *Dermacentor andersoni.* It was originally described in the Rocky Mountain region of Montana, but is now much more common in the southwest, southeast and eastern sections of the United States. Campers and weekend vacationers are most likely to get it.

What are the symptoms of spotted fever?   Two to seven days after the tick bite, the person has chills, fever and aching suggestive of the flu. The rash begins on the ankles or wrists and spreads to cover both extremities and the trunk. The spots are small and red at first, but enlarge and turn darker. The rash may take on a bruised, hemorrhagic appearance. It typically spares the face.

What's the treatment for spotted fever?   Tetracycline is specific for the infection, but the person should be admitted to the hospital for treatment. The earlier therapy is started, the better the chance for recovery. The mortality rate without treatment is as high as 40 percent, but drops to 7 percent when appropriate treatment is given.

What can you do to prevent spotted fever?   Since tick bites cause it, the use of repellents and appropriate clothing is indicated when you go into tick-infested areas. Remember that a dog can pick up ticks and spread them to family members. A twice-a-day tick inspection may help when you're on a camp-out. As a tick must be attached for several hours before it becomes infectious, prompt removal is indicated. The tick will detach if touched by a lit cigarette or covered with gasoline or Vaseline. Pulling it out without letting it detach may leave the infective head in the skin. (A doctor can remove the head with a small cut in the skin.) A vaccine has

185

proven helpful in immunizing those who must spend considerable time in the woods.

What is trichinosis?   It's a parasitic disease caused by ingesting meat containing the larvae of *Trichinella spiralis*. The usual source is pork, but infection may occur after eating bear or walrus meat that has not been thoroughly cooked. The larvae turn into adults in the small intestine, where they mate and produce more larvae which pass by way of the bloodstream to muscles throughout the body.

What are the symptoms of trichinosis?   Fever, muscle ache and swelling of the eyes are early symptoms. With severe infection, the heart and breathing muscles are weakened to the point that death may occur.

What's the treatment for trichinosis?   Thiabendazole and corticosteroids help to relieve the muscle symptoms and fever, though a mild case may be self-limited. Trichinosis can be prevented by cooking pork at 325° F. (or about 163° C.) for thirty minutes for each pound of meat. Bear and other wild meat must be cooked to at least this same degree.

7

EMERGENCIES

What are the main types of emergencies? Those that threaten life and those that don't. Among the former are conditions that interfere with breathing, stop the heart, cause profuse bleeding, produce unconsciousness or penetrate, poison, burn or crush a vital part of the body.

Less urgent emergencies include cuts, bruises, broken bones, stings or a fall that isn't too serious. A fishhook in a finger is a minor emergency; so is a penis caught in a zipper. Both hurt and require immediate attention, but they don't threaten life.

Where do emergencies occur? They're most likely to occur in your home, your yard, or on the street that runs in front of your home. The next most likely place is on the highway.

Can someone without medical training handle an emergency? Yes, effective help can be given by someone with common sense and a knowledge of first aid. Twenty percent of persons dying in auto accidents could be saved by simple lifesaving maneuvers performed at the crash site. As many as 100,000 persons who die each year from heart attack could have been saved by cardiopulmonary resuscitation.

How commonly do accidents occur? They are the leading cause of death between the ages of one and forty-four. Overall, accidents rank fourth as a killer behind heart disease, cancer and stroke. Since most injured persons are under thirty-five, accidents account for a disproportionate loss of work years. More hospital days are spent in the care of accident victims than in the care of persons with cancer or heart disease.

What are the main home accidents?   In order of frequency: cuts, falls, swallowed substances (poisonings), burns, crushed fingers and a foreign body in the eye, nose or throat.

What is the most dangerous type of accident?   Car wreck. Auto accidents account for half of the accidental deaths in this country, killing 55,000 people a year and disabling another 2 million. The number of people who have been killed on our highways is double the number of battle deaths the United States has had in all the wars it has ever participated in.

What are the main medical emergencies?   Heart attack, stroke, convulsion, choking on food and a severe allergic reaction are the most serious ones, but not the most common. You're more likely to have to deal with a poisoning, a sting, a bite, a minor allergic reaction, or simple fainting from heat or an emotional shock.

GENERAL MEASURES

How fast do you need to work during an emergency?   You have enough time to do what needs to be done. Don't rush, but work deliberately and without delay.

What are the general measures to follow in caring for an emergency?
Spend a few seconds evaluating the problem and what needs to be done to solve it. If there are two or more victims, see who needs help the most. Assess the person's state of consciousness, check the airway and establish breathing, check the heart and establish circulation, and only then, turn to such matters as bleeding and broken bones. A list of priorities is given in the accompanying chart. They apply whether the victim has been shot, drowned, injured in a car wreck, choked on a piece of food, or has had some other misfortune.

PRIORITIES IN AN EMERGENCY

1. Evaluate the injured person or persons. See who needs help the most.
2. Establish if the person is conscious or unconscious, and whether he or she can respond to questions.

3. Check breathing. If it isn't present or if there is any difficulty in breathing, clear the mouth and throat, extend the neck and give mouth-to-mouth resuscitation.

4. Check for a heartbeat. Feel for the pulse in the neck beside the Adam's apple. If it is absent, give heart massage.

5. Place a dressing or use your hand to cover a sucking wound of the chest or neck.

6. Control bleeding by applying pressure.

7. If the back or neck is injured, don't move the person until spinal support is established.

8. Apply a splint to obviously fractured bones.

Why is it necessary to work in this order? The brain can live for only four to six minutes without oxygen, so clearing the airway and establishing breathing are the first steps. Heart function comes next, to move oxygen to the brain. Other injuries don't matter until or unless effective breathing and circulation can be established.

What are the priorities in caring for car-wreck victims? To avoid having another accident, pull off the road beyond the wreck if possible and leave your hazard lights blinking. Unless the wrecked automobile is on fire or in jeopardy for some other reason, do not haul the victims out until you've established what injuries they have. Attend to the unconscious persons first. Gently tilting the victim's head back may open the airway and allow better breathing. Cover a sucking chest wound (a hole in the chest through which air blows or bubbles with each breath). Apply pressure to stop bleeding. Look and feel for obvious fractures of the bones and spine. If these are present or if the car doors are crushed, wait till help arrives before attempting to move the victim.

What should you avoid doing in an emergency? Don't panic. Don't try to get an unconscious or injured person to sit up or stand up. Don't give the victim water, whiskey or anything else by mouth. Do not apply a tourniquet when bleeding can be controlled by direct pressure. Don't jab things into the mouth of someone having a convulsion. Do not hit the victim in an attempt to cause him or her to regain consciousness. Unless immediate movement is mandatory, do not reposition someone after an injury until you're sure fractures aren't present or until splints have been applied. If you have to move the victim, hold the head in a neutral position in case of neck or spine fracture.

At what point do you summon help? If you're the only one giving aid, call out loud for help as soon as possible. Wait until you've done what you can before stopping to phone. When two or more persons are giving aid, one can summon help immediately. In the case of a car wreck, wait till someone else stops and send that person for aid.

How do you summon help?   A universal emergency number, 911, is now in use in New York City, Philadelphia, Boston, Chicago, Jersey City, Denver, Omaha, Birmingham and many other cities across the country. This number will reach a dispatcher who can send help to the site of the emergency. In cities that don't have the 911 system, call the Fire Department or the Emergency Medical Service.

What is the Emergency Medical Service?   Like the police and fire departments, it is an arm of public service. Emergency medical technicians have been trained to give aid and resuscitation, and paramedics have the training to do these things as well as to give certain drugs under the guidance of a physician.

Are you legally liable if you try to help someone who later dies?   Most states have "good Samaritan" laws that protect you from blame unless you are willfully or wantonly negligent or unless your services are rendered for a fee.

How can you tell when someone is dead?   Signs pointing to irreversible death are coldness of the skin, stiffness of the body (rigor mortis) and lack of breathing or a heartbeat. The person who collapses in your presence may be revived by the use of cardiopulmonary resuscitation.

RESUSCITATION

What is CPR?   It is the abbreviation for cardiopulmonary resuscitation, the modern term for artificial respiration. It goes a step beyond artificial respiration by restoring the circulation as well as the respiration.

What's the purpose of CPR?   It is only indicated when the victim has suffered a loss of breathing and/or heartbeat. The purpose is to substitute mouth-to-mouth breathing and heart massage for these functions. The hope is that the victim's own breathing and heartbeat will return during the resuscitation, or that the person's brain can be kept alive until definitive therapy can be given by a doctor or paramedic.

In what instances is CPR indicated?   It is most likely to be effective when the person has a heart stoppage in the presence of others, provided the witnesses lose no time in recognizing what has happened and administering CPR. The instances in which CPR is indicated include:

· Sudden collapse of a person due to cessation of breathing, heartbeat or both. The cause may be a heart attack, stroke or allergic reaction to an injection or insect sting.

· Revival of a drowning victim

· Revival of someone overcome by carbon monoxide or other poisonous gas—such as persons removed from burning buildings

· Revival of someone struck by lightning

· Revival of someone after an injury, head wound, strangulation, or accidental or suicidal hanging

How do you determine that breathing and heartbeat have stopped?   Go to the victim and shout, "Are you okay?" Someone who can respond by saying "Yes" is not in need of CPR. The person who doesn't respond may only have fainted. Get down so that your ear is over the mouth and listen for breathing. Watch to see if the chest is expanding with respiration. Feel over the mouth and nose for air. When none of these signs is present, breathing has stopped.

Place two fingers in the groove beside the Adam's apple and feel for a pulse. This pulse, caused by the carotid arteries carrying blood to the brain, is normally felt on both sides of the neck. (Check your own neck to learn what the pulse feels like, but press gently.) When the neck pulse is absent, the person's heart is not beating. Begin CPR immediately.

How do you give CPR?   Place the victim on his or her back on a hard, flat surface, such as the ground or floor. This enables you to get to the person more easily and provides support for the chest massage. Think of what you're doing as providing the ABCs of Airway, Breathing and Circulation—in that order.

Place one hand under the victim's neck and lift, while pushing down on the forehead with your other hand. This tilts the head back. The purpose is to lift the tongue away from the throat and clear the air passage. Pinch the nostrils shut and cover the mouth with yours. Give four quick puffs of air. Blow about twice as hard as you normally would, and make sure that your breaths cause the person's chest to expand. For a child or baby you don't have to breathe nearly so hard.

Check the carotid pulse again, and if it's still absent, begin heart massage. Put the heel of one hand over the lower half of the victim's breastbone, and place the heel of the opposite hand on top of the first. Lock your elbows and rock forward from your knees, pressing inward to massage the heart between the breastbone and backbone. You have to apply eighty to a hundred and twenty pounds of pressure in an adult, and this should lower the breastbone about one and a half to two inches with each compression. For a child, use the heel of only one hand, and for a baby, use only the tips of the index and middle fingers; do not apply too much pressure.

191

How do you alternate breathing and heart massage?   When you're the only rescuer, give the heart compressions at a rate of eighty a minute. Stop every fifteenth compression to give two mouth-to-mouth breaths, then resume heart compression. Two rescuers make resuscitation easier. The heart massage is given at a rate of sixty compressions a minute, and every fifth beat a mouth-to-mouth breath is administered by the second rescuer. To avoid fatigue, the two rescuers should change places every five minutes.

What do you do if the victim vomits?   Turn the head to one side so that the material can drain from the mouth. Wipe out the remaining material with a handkerchief or your fingers. Resume CPR.

How can you tell if CPR is being effective?   Effective heart massage will produce a pulse that can be felt through the carotid arteries. The victim's pupils will not dilate and become fixed in that position as they would without CPR (or dilation will occur very slowly). Movements of the victim or spontaneous breathing efforts indicate improvement. If these occur, stop CPR momentarily and see if the heartbeat has resumed on its own.

How long should you continue CPR?   Until a paramedic or physician can take over or until complete recovery has occurred. If help hasn't arrived in half an hour, if the victim's pupils are widely dilated and fixed, and if no spontaneous breathing or heartbeat has been noted for this length of time, the decision to stop may be made.

Can CPR be harmful?   Yes, heart massage may break the ribs or breastbone, injure the lungs, damage the liver or spleen, or bruise the heart. It's less likely to have these effects when administered properly. In any case, the risks must be weighed against the choice between certain death and possible recovery. The chance of harm is greatest when CPR is given to someone who doesn't need it, such as the person who has fainted but not had a cardiac arrest.

How can you learn to do CPR?   It is taught by local chapters of the American Heart Association and the American National Red Cross. The training is free, and is recommended for every adult. CPR is also taught in many schools, and may eventually become a required part of the driver's education course. Many businesses offer this training to their employees, and police and fire departments give CPR courses to the public.

LOSS OF CONSCIOUSNESS

What causes sudden unconsciousness? Fainting is the most common event, but others include drug or alcohol intoxication, head injury and convulsion. The most serious causes include heart stoppage (cardiac arrest), stroke, asphyxia and electric shock.

How do you know if the problem is critical? Assess the person's airway, breathing and circulation as described on p. 191. Give resuscitation if it is indicated. When breathing and a strong neck pulse are present, the situation is not so urgent. Call for help or send someone while you watch the person. Evaluation by a physician is indicated to establish whether the problem is serious.

How do you tell between the different causes of unconsciousness? The distinction must be made by a physician, but here are some guidelines:
· *Fainting* usually occurs in someone previously in good health. A reaction to pain, fear or an emotional shock, it is caused by a precipitous drop in blood pressure. Rarely, fainting is the first symptom of a viral illness, such as the flu. Leave the person on the floor until consciousness returns.
· *Postural syncope* is a form of fainting that occurs when a person suddenly stands upright. Blood pools in the legs and abdomen, and the faint may be preceded by a "graying out" sensation. A person recovering from surgery or a medical illness, or who is taking blood pressure medication, or an older person is most susceptible. Keeping the head low will allow consciousness to return.
· *Convulsion* is signaled by rhythmic jerking of the arms and legs. Breathing may stop, but the heart continues beating. The main need is to protect the person from fire, water or a sharp object or machine. Mouth-to-mouth resuscitation is indicated if breathing doesn't return promptly, as when the convulsion lasts for more than a minute.
· *Low blood sugar* is most apt to occur in a diabetic on insulin. Drinking alcohol may cause an attack. Hunger and sweating precede the blackout. Medical help is needed, but the person who is conscious enough to swallow may benefit from drinking orange juice or a regular soft drink, or eating sugar or hard candy.
· *Head injury* as a cause of unconsciousness is always serious. The problem may be a concussion or brain hemorrhage. It's possible for the person to regain consciousness in a few minutes, feel fine, and then slowly lose consciousness over several hours as blood collects between the brain and the skull.
· *Drug or alcohol intoxication* may be suspected by the odor of alcohol or by the finding of drug containers in the vicinity of the victim. Medical evaluation is indicated. The drunk may have a head injury, and the user of

drugs may need stomach pumping, breathing assistance and other measures.

· *Cardiac arrest* is most likely to occur in a man in his forties, fifties or sixties, usually when heart disease is known or suspected to exist. Stroke may occur at any age and in either sex.

ASPHYXIA

What is asphyxia?   It is an emergency condition created by a lack of oxygen reaching the brain. Anything that prevents breathing or oxygen uptake may cause it. Early symptoms are dizziness, agitation and shortness of breath. Loss of consciousness and bluish discoloration of the skin and mucous membranes occur later.

Is recovery from asphyxia possible?   Yes, when the problem is corrected and CPR is given, recovery may occur after ten or fifteen minutes of asphyxia.

What are the general measures for treating asphyxia?   Remove the source —or the victim from the source—as quickly as possible. Lay the person on a flat surface such as the ground. Examine for airway, breathing and circulation. Give mouth-to-mouth resuscitation if the airway is open, and give heart massage if the heart is not beating.

How do you know when someone has choked?   In a child the signs are coughing, gagging, wheezing and distress. An adult will not be able to talk. The frantic person may thrash about and gesture toward his or her throat, and will soon collapse if the obstruction isn't relieved. When this happens during a meal, the cause of the problem is usually apparent.

What is the "café coronary"?   It's a term used to describe choking on food while eating at a restaurant. The victim, who may have had too much to drink, attempts to eat a large item of food, usually meat, that gets stuck in the throat. Others may not notice the person's distress until he or she collapses. In the past the death was sometimes attributed to a heart attack, hence the reference to "coronary."

What do you do for the person who has choked?   If you can see something in the throat, hook your finger around it and remove it, or give three or four sharp blows to the back. Unless you can see the foreign body in the throat, don't try to remove it—you might push it farther down. Here are the steps to take:

1. *Apply the Heimlich maneuver,* which uses the lungs as a bellows to blow out the obstruction. Stand behind the victim and make a fist with one hand.

Clasp this fist in your other hand so that your thumb is jammed into the victim's upper abdomen. Apply pressure with a quick upward thrust just below the breastbone. If the first attempt doesn't dislodge the foreign body, the maneuver may be repeated several times. The Heimlich maneuver may be performed with the rescuer sitting astride a victim who is lying face up. Here, the pressure is exerted downward with the body weight transmitted through the arms. The direction of the push should be toward the chest as described above.

2. *Give mouth-to-mouth aspiration* if the obstruction persists. This is the reverse of mouth-to-mouth resuscitation, as air is sucked from the throat in an attempt to dislodge the obstruction.

3. *A sharp blow to the back* may help dislodge a persistent obstruction. Swing a small child upside down in the air by holding the feet before delivering the blow. Position an adult with the torso hanging down from a bed or piece of furniture before striking the back between the shoulder blades.

4. *Give mouth-to-mouth breathing* as a last resort, and get the person medical help as quickly as possible. A doctor may insert a large-bore needle into the trachea below the site of obstruction. This will provide temporary relief, but the operation known as tracheotomy will probably be necessary. Afterward the obstruction can be removed with the help of a laryngoscope to peer into the throat.

Does the Heimlich maneuver cause any side effects?   It may damage the liver, spleen or stomach, which underscores the need to use it correctly and only when someone is choking from a foreign body lodged in the throat or windpipe. The Heimlich maneuver is not indicated when someone has choked on liquid, had a cardiac arrest or is having difficulty breathing because of an injury of the throat, face or head.

What should be done for the drowning victim?   Here are the steps:
1. *Remove the person from the water* as soon as possible.
2. *Place the victim on a firm surface* and let water drain out of the mouth and throat. Feel in the mouth to clear other material and to pull the tongue forward.
3. *Extend the person's neck,* pinch the nostrils closed, and begin mouth-to-mouth resuscitation.
4. *After four or five breaths, feel for the carotid pulse* to see if the victim has a heartbeat. If one is present, continue mouth-to-mouth resuscitation. If the heart is not beating, give chest compressions along with breathing assistance (see CPR, p. 191).
5. *Summon help as soon as possible,* and switch to mechanical ventilation with oxygen when it becomes available.

What should be done next? Every person who is resuscitated from drowning or who stands a chance of being resuscitated should be taken to an emergency room for therapy and subsequently admitted to the hospital. Pneumonia and an outpouring of body fluids into the lungs may cause complications. The treatment varies depending on whether the person was in fresh or salt water, but it usually includes a day or two of mechanical ventilation, oxygen therapy and the use of intravenous fluids and bronchodilators. If these measures and someone skilled in their use are not available at the first hospital, the resuscitated person should be moved as soon as feasible to a facility where lung specialists are available.

What determines survival from drowning? The critical factor is the period between the time the victim goes under and the time resuscitation is started. Resuscitation has a good chance of reviving someone who's been under for less than five or six minutes. The person who makes spontaneous attempts to breathe when brought up will probably recover. So will the individual who responds quickly to mouth-to-mouth resuscitation. Revival has occurred after the victim has been under for ten or fifteen minutes, but the longer the delay, the greater the chance that the revived person will have permanent brain damage.

How long should the resuscitation be continued if the victim doesn't respond? CPR may be stopped after thirty minutes if the victim shows no response at all (see p. 192).

Can a hanging victim be resuscitated? Yes, if the person's neck isn't broken. Judicial hanging involves a drop of five or six feet, and the upward jerk of the rope snaps the neck; this is instantly lethal and recovery is not possible. Hanging by suspension without a drop is more likely to kill by asphyxia, and recovery is possible. An example is suicidal hanging when the victim swings off a chair or footstool, or accidental hanging when a child playing near a window is found hanging from the pull cord of the Venetian blinds or drapes.

What is the emergency treatment? Remove the victim from the noose as quickly as possible; evaluate airway, breathing and circulation; and administer CPR (see p. 191).

What are the chances for recovery? Rescue is more apt to be successful if it can be established that the person was suspended for less than five or ten minutes. Recovery after longer periods of suspension is possible when the constricting effects of the noose are delayed by the efforts of the victim, when the victim is a child or is an adult of less-than-average body weight,

196

or when the noose is made of a nonconstricting material such as bed sheets or a chain. Revival is unlikely when the victim is cold, stiff or suffused with a bluish or mottled discoloration.

What should be done for a child who has been trapped in a refrigerator or other airless place?   Remove the victim as quickly as possible. Evaluate airway, breathing and circulation, and administer CPR (see p. 191) if necessary. Follow the same sequence when someone is overcome by a poisonous gas, such as carbon monoxide, or when an infant is found with its head trapped in a plastic bag.

What should be done for the victim of an overdose of drugs?   If the person has stopped breathing, give mouth-to-mouth resuscitation. Accompany it with heart massage if indicated. Summon help. Transport the person to a hospital as soon as possible.

ELECTRIC SHOCK

How does electric shock occur?   The most likely cause is touching a hot wire in the home. The back of a color TV and a garbage disposal unit that has a short circuit are two likely sources. Even though the voltage is relatively small, the amount of current may be sufficient to cause the heart to stop beating or the breathing to stop. Outdoor sources of electric shock are high-voltage lines and lightning; in both instances the victim suffers burns as well as stoppage of the heart and breathing.

What is the treatment for electric shock?   Remove the person from the source of electricity, but take a few moments to assess the safest way of doing this. Above all, do not touch the person who is still in contact with electricity. (Doing this just adds you to the circuit.) Instead, shut the power off if this can be done quickly. Or stand on a dry board or something made of rubber, and knock the wire away with a nonconducting substance, such as dry wood or dry paper. When the source can't be knocked away, stand on wood or rubber and grab the person's foot through a heavy insulation of paper or rubber; then pull the victim to safety. (The power must still be shut off to prevent someone else from being shocked.)

After the victim is removed from the electricity, evaluate airway, breathing and circulation, and give CPR (see p. 191).

What if lightning strikes someone?   Some persons recover spontaneously, but give CPR if respiration and heartbeat are absent. The chances of revival are very good if resuscitation is begun immediately, and in one instance a boy recovered completely even though effective CPR wasn't begun until twenty minutes after he was struck by lightning.

How do you avoid electric shock?   Make sure home appliances are properly wired. Don't touch a switch while standing in water or with wet hands. Cap electrical outlets so that small children can't jam things into them. Avoid downed high-voltage lines. People have died from touching them or even coming close, since electricity can jump from a high-power source to the human body. Persons in a car that is in contact with a downed line should not attempt to leave the vehicle until power in the line has been shut off.

Don't take refuge under a tree during a thunderstorm. Toss aside golf clubs, fishing rods or an umbrella. Get out of a swimming pool. If you are outdoors, lie flat on the ground away from trees and poles. Lie on top of a rubber raincoat if you have one. If you're indoors, don't stand between an open door and an open window, as lightning may strike horizontally between the two.

BLEEDING

What causes bleeding?   It occurs when blood vessels are cut, crushed, punctured or pulled apart by the force of injury. Hemorrhage is the medical term meaning blood has escaped from the vessels.

What are the important types of bleeding?   External bleeding occurs from the skin or nose, and is readily visible. Menstrual bleeding is also considered external. Internal bleeding occurs in a body cavity such as the abdomen or chest, or in an organ such as the kidney, liver or lung. Though the blood is not visible, this is by far the most dangerous type of hemorrhage.

How do you distinguish between arterial and venous bleeding?   Arterial blood is bright red. It's under high pressure and tends to spurt. Blood from the veins is darker and oozes out because of the lower venous pressure. Most injuries cause arterial and venous bleeding, and the way of controlling the bleeding is the same.

How do you control bleeding?   Apply pressure directly to the site of bleeding through a piece of gauze or cloth. Bleeding will usually stop after five to ten minutes of pressure, though it may recur if the wound is deep. A wound that continues to bleed or that seems big enough to require stitches should be managed by a physician. Other tips:
  · *For serious wounds,* apply a pressure dressing while the person is en route to the doctor. Use an Ace bandage or gauze strip to hold the dressing firmly on the wound.
  · *Nosebleed* can usually be controlled by applying pressure from the side of the bleeding nostril toward the midline. The pressure should be kept up

for five to ten minutes with the person sitting up quietly at rest. A clot may form in the back of the nose and later be cleared from the throat. Brisk bleeding that continues down the throat despite pressure on the nose calls for medical evaluation. The physician may need to insert a nasal pack.

· *Bleeding from a finger* is a special matter, since the use of a tourniquet can do more harm than good. Unless a part of the finger is completely severed, apply pressure to the cut with the thumb or another finger, and keep the hand elevated en route to the doctor.

When is a tourniquet indicated?   This constricting band, twisted around an arm or leg to stop bleeding, should be used when a hand, arm, foot or leg has been amputated, or when bleeding from an extremity is so profuse as to threaten life. It should never be used when pressure alone will control bleeding.

How do you apply a tourniquet?   Tie a piece of cord, light rope, belt or strips of cloth around the extremity, and use a stick to twist it tightly enough to just control bleeding. The tourniquet should be placed between the wound and the trunk, an inch or two above the site of bleeding. It is not a good idea to loosen a tourniquet once it's in place, but try not to leave it on for longer than twenty to thirty minutes. In most instances this is enough time to reach medical help.

What about internal bleeding?   Injury to the internal structures may cause profuse bleeding even when no external bleeding is present. Be alert to this form of bleeding when a child has been hit by a car, when a child or adult has been in a car wreck, or when someone has struck his chest or abdomen in a fall. The same blow that may fracture ribs in the lower right chest may also puncture the liver; a blow breaking ribs in the lower left chest may rupture the spleen. Either situation is a life-threatening emergency. Sometimes the victim of internal injuries may cough or vomit blood, or complain of severe chest or abdominal pain. The most likely event is that the person will develop the medical condition known as shock.

What is shock?   It is the body's way of reacting to a crisis created by excessive blood loss, hemorrhage of more than a pint in an adult. The brain, heart and lungs get top priority. Blood continues to reach these organs, but very little goes to the skin, muscles and abdominal organs. The inadequate circulation creates its own problems, and shock tends to worsen when the hemorrhage is not controlled promptly. Other causes of shock are heart attack, severe infection and a bad burn.

How do you recognize shock?   The victim becomes dizzy and cannot stand up. Lying down offers some relief, but thirst and a slight chill persist. Some persons in shock are extremely anxious, but others seem almost too calm. The skin is cool and moist, the hands and feet feel cold, and white persons will become pale. The heartbeat is fast, the blood pressure is low and the pulse is weak.

What should be done for the person in shock?   Realize that shock is not an entity in itself but the body's reaction to injury or disease. Supportive measures are aimed at keeping the person in the best possible shape until definitive treatment by a physician can be given. Here's what to do:

1. *Apply pressure to stop bleeding,* and use pressure dressings over the wounds.

2. *Splint broken bones.*

3. *Keep the person lying down,* and elevate the feet six to twelve inches higher than the head. This improves circulation by keeping blood from pooling in the legs.

4. *Cover the person with a light blanket* or one or two layers of clothing. Do not apply too much cover, because the heat will draw blood to the skin, where it is not needed.

5. *Do not give anything by mouth* if medical help is less than an hour away. Give sips of orange juice or water if there is to be a long delay in reaching help. Under no circumstances should you give whiskey, which, by dilating the blood vessels, will worsen the shock. Do not continue to give fluid by mouth if the victim vomits or has abdominal pain.

BROKEN BONES

How do you recognize a fractured limb?   Broken bones are painful, and the person may be unable to move that part of the body. Swelling or bleeding may mark the site of fracture. A severe break may distort the normal alignment of the arm or leg.

Which limb fractures are the most dangerous?   Breaks of the thighbone (femur) or leg bone (tibia) are more apt to cause serious problems than breaks of the upper arm (humerus) or lower arm (radius or ulna). The danger is that the sharp edge of a fractured bone may cut a vessel or nerve to cause bleeding or paralysis.

What are simple and compound fractures?   A simple fracture is a broken bone not accompanied by a break in the skin. With compound fracture the broken bone sticks out through the skin or the skin has been cut to leave an open gash above the fracture. Compound fractures are worse than simple fractures, but the latter may also be dangerous. It is possible for someone with a simple fracture of the thighbone to go into shock from bleeding into the tissues around the bone.

What's the treatment for a limb fracture?   The fracture should be treated by a doctor. Emergency treatment consists of immobilizing the bone above and below the break, and transporting the person to the emergency room. Bleeding from a compound fracture should be controlled by a pressure dressing. Occasionally it is necessary to use a tourniquet to control bleeding from a compound fracture. The injured person should be kept quiet and at rest. Treat for shock if it develops (see p. 200).

How is a splint applied?   A complete description of splinting is beyond the scope of this chapter, but here are some guidelines:
· *The splint should extend from one joint below the fracture to one joint above it.* For a fracture of the forearm, the splint should reach from the hand to several inches above the elbow. For a fracture of the lower leg, the splint should reach from the foot to several inches above the knee. For a fracture of the thighbone, the splint should reach from the foot to above the hip.
· *A splint may be made* from pieces of wood, pieces of chrome stripping, or folded newspapers or magazines.
· *Tie the splint on with strips of cloth* torn from bedding, jeans, shirts or the like. Take care not to tie so tightly that the ligatures interfere with blood circulation.
· *When moving the injured person,* one rescuer should lift nothing but the splinted extremity while the others lift the remaining body weight.
· *For a compound fracture,* apply a pressure dressing and then splint as for simple fracture.
· *Do not try to reduce a fracture* (that is, align the broken bones) before splinting it. You might create bleeding or nerve injury, so it's best to let an orthopedic specialist do the reduction. When the victim is conscious and has only an arm fracture that is not likely to be jostled en route to the doctor, splinting may not be necessary.

What about a spinal fracture?   A fracture of the back or neck may be made worse if the victim is not transported properly. The first step is to determine if the fracture is present or may be present. If the person is conscious, ask about pain in the neck or back. See if the person can move the arms, hands, legs and feet. Inability to move the arms or hands suggests a fractured neck. Inability to move the feet or legs suggests a fractured neck or a fractured back. When the victim is unconscious and has been involved in an auto accident, a diving accident or severe fall, it's best to assume that a spinal fracture may be present and to take appropriate precautions.

How should a person with a spinal fracture be transported to a hospital?
The spine must be immobilized so that no further injury occurs during

201

transport to a medical facility. If possible, do not move the victim until Emergency Medical Service people arrive. These trained individuals have splints that can be used to protect the person with a suspected spinal fracture. When professional help is not available, plan to move the victim on a long board or flat piece of metal that reaches from below the feet to above the head. Three persons are needed to lift the person onto the board: one at the legs, another at the trunk and another at the upper back and head. The idea is to avoid twisting the spine and to keep it as near as possible to its natural alignment. Gentle, coordinated efforts are essential.

The person with a broken neck should be transported on his or her back; the person with a broken back should be transported face down if this position can be achieved without having to turn the person over. If necessary, a stretcher made from a blanket or clothing may be used in the transport, but a flat board reinforced with other boards is preferable.

What should you not do when you suspect someone of having a spinal injury? The five things to avoid doing are given in the chart below.

FIVE DON'TS IN CARING FOR THE VICTIM OF SPINAL INJURY

1. Don't try to do everything yourself; call for help and wait till it arrives.
2. Don't grasp the person's head and move it from side to side to see if there is a neck fracture; if there is, the movement may kill or permanently paralyze the person.
3. Don't scoop up the victim in your arms so that the spine bends and the head falls back; this will worsen the injury.
4. Don't move the victim even a few feet until a correct support has been made.
5. Don't transport the person in an auto or in the back of a truck or stationwagon; wait for an ambulance.

What is the management of skull fracture? If the person is unconscious, check the airway, breathing and heartbeat; give CPR (see p. 191) if indicated. Apply pressure to stop bleeding from a head wound, and cover the wound with a dressing. Keep the victim lying down. When spinal fracture may also be present, transport on a board as described above. Do not give the person anything to drink even if he or she is conscious and asks for something.

BURNS

What are the types of burns?   Burns may be classified according to what caused the injury (grease burn, sunburn, chemical burn, fire burn, electrical burn, etc.), but the medical categories grade the severity of the burn. *A first-degree burn* is the least severe. Redness of the skin and pain on movement of the area are the main symptoms. *A second-degree burn* is slightly deeper: blisters appear in the burned area and pain is a prominent symptom. *A third-degree burn* goes through the skin to the fat beneath it. The burn may appear black, brown, white or red. Though this is the most serious of the categories, it may not be painful because the nerves in the skin have been destroyed. Pain may be present in the adjacent skin, which may have first- or second-degree burns.

How dangerous are burns?   They cause 10,000 deaths a year, and are especially dangerous in young children and persons over sixty. A third-degree burn of any extent is serious; when it involves more than 40 or 50 percent of the body, recovery is unusual. A second-degree burn of more than 10 or 15 percent of the body is serious. First-degree burns are usually minor, but can be uncomfortable for several days, as in the case of severe sunburn.

What's the treatment for first-degree burn?   Relief of pain may be obtained by immersing the area in cool water or by applying ice packs. An antibiotic ointment, such as Neosporin or Bacitracin, will make the area feel better and may prevent secondary infection. The various sunburn ointments may bring relief, but water-soluble preparations, as opposed to those with a petroleum base, are preferable. The burn will heal with flaking of the skin in several days.

What's the treatment for second-degree burns?   These usually occur in association with first-degree burns. For blisters that are small and few in number, the treatment is the same as for first-degree injury. When large or numerous blisters appear, apply a cold wet dressing and take the person to the doctor.

The physician may open the blisters or leave them intact. Healing is quicker when the blisters are broken, but the chance of an infection is greater. In either case, antibiotic ointment, an occlusive dressing and frequent dressing changes are necessary. Second-degree burns usually heal in a week to ten days.

What's the treatment for third-degree burns?   Remove the victim to safety, and check the airway, breathing and circulation. Give CPR (see p. 191) if indicated. Remove clothing and other debris from the burn.

Apply clean wet dressings, splint fractures and transport the person to a medical facility as quickly as possible. Keep the victim's feet elevated en route.

Treatment at the hospital will consist of the use of intravenous fluids and antibiotics, airway assistance if needed, and local treatment of the burn. Since the management of third-degree burns is a highly specialized field, the victim should be cared for by a plastic surgeon or transferred to a facility having the services of a plastic surgeon. The healing process may take months or years, and burn centers, such as those run by the Shriners, are excellent sources of help.

POISONING

How frequently does poisoning occur?   It is the fourth most common cause of death in children. The youngster is almost always under five, and "curious two" is the age of greatest susceptibility. Except in rare instances, childhood ingestion is accidental. It occurs when something is left within reach of the youngster. In adults, poisoning is more likely to be purposeful. Suicide is the ninth leading cause of death in the United States, and self-induced poisonings account for over half of such deaths.

What are the common causes of poisoning in children?   The use of safety caps has reduced the incidence of drug ingestion. Poisoning with aspirin, acetaminophen, tranquilizers or sleeping pills may still occur, but house-hold items such as bleach, perfume or cologne are more likely to cause problems. Petroleum products, such as charcoal lighter and paint thinner, and insecticides, such as benzene hexachloride, constitute a continuing source of severe poisoning in children.

What are the symptoms of poisoning in children?   The symptoms depend on the substance and the amount of it that is ingested.
 · *Aspirin poisoning* produces rapid breathing, though the onset may be delayed for several hours after the child has taken the aspirin. An early symptom is ringing in the ears. Nausea and loss of appetite may occur as the breathing becomes deeper and more rapid. Loss of consciousness is a late symptom.
 · *Acetaminophen poisoning* (the drug is sold under the name of Tylenol and other brands) is unique in that there are no immediate symptoms. Even so, the overdose may cause fatal liver damage. By the time symptoms appear it may be too late to reverse them, but the antidote, acetylcysteine, is effective when given within ten hours after the ingestion.
 · *Iron poisoning* (from taking iron tablets) damages the stomach and intestines. The symptoms are vomiting and bloody diarrhea, and the child rapidly goes into shock from blood loss.

· *Petroleum products* may produce coughing, gagging and vomiting soon after ingestion. The child may appear agitated or lethargic, and the poisoning can be recognized by the smell of the substance on the breath and clothing and by the container lying nearby.

· *Cleaning agents and detergents* irritate the mouth and esophagus. The child may complain of burning in the throat and chest, and may refuse to take liquid or food. Vomiting may occur. Difficulty in breathing points to injury of the upper airway by the caustic agent.

What are the common causes of poisoning in adults?　Self-induced poisoning is most likely to be done with sleeping pills or tranquilizers (often on top of alcohol), but adults sometimes ingest insecticides, rodenticides, cyanide or strychnine for suicidal purposes. Poisoning from an illicit drug is most apt to occur from an overdose of sleeping pills (downers), hallucinogenic drugs ("acid" and similar agents), amphetamines (speed) or narcotics (heroin). Poisoning may also result from the inhalation of the vapors of certain chemicals—glue-sniffing.

What are the symptoms of poisoning in adults?　As the agent is most likely to be one affecting the central nervous system, the person may appear drunk. Confusion, garbled speech and a staggering gait are early symptoms of an overdose of sleeping pills, narcotics or alcohol. Loss of consciousness and labored breathing are late signs. Unusual or bizarre behavior, agitation, confusion and increasing excitement characterize a "bad trip" from an overdose of a hallucinogen. Symptoms of an overdose of amphetamines include insomnia, agitation, hyperactivity, mania and delirium; convulsions may occur.

What should be done in a case of poisoning?　When you suspect that a child or adult has ingested a harmful quantity of any substance, here are the five steps to take:

1. Evaluate airway, breathing and circulation. Give CPR (see p. 191) if indicated. The victim who is conscious or has good vital signs should be watched closely.

2. Determine what happened. Look for evidence of poisonous substances that may have been ingested, such as empty vials, pills or spilled chemicals on the floor. Look for stains on the clothing or burns about the mouth. Smell the breath for signs of the substance. In an adult, look for other signs of self-injury, such as slash marks on the wrist or neck.

3. Notify your physician or the Poison Control Center for further instructions. Give treatment, such as an emetic or antidote, only under the direction of the physician or someone from the Poison Control Center.

4. When the seriousness of the poisoning dictates, call the Emergency Medical Service for rapid transportation of the victim to the hospital. Do

not do this until you have talked to the Poison Control Center, as steps you take at home could prove lifesaving.

5. Take the container, label and any of the remaining ingested material with you to the doctor's office or hospital. Save any material the person might vomit. A sample of the vomitus in a plastic bag is sufficient.

How do you get in touch with the Poison Control Center?   There are 650 Poison Control Centers nationwide. Each is in or near a large hospital, is open twenty-four hours a day, and will dispense free information on the poisonous effects of the thousands of substances that may be ingested by a child or adult. The best way to locate the one closest to you is to call the nearest emergency room and ask for the number. Include this number in your list of emergency telephone numbers.

Under what circumstances do you induce vomiting at home?   Attempt it when:
  · The ingestion occurred within the last thirty or forty minutes (in some cases even longer).
  · The substance ingested was a drug.
  · The person is fully conscious and not liable to aspirate during vomiting.

How do you induce vomiting?   The older methods of tickling the throat or having the person drink warm water or dishwater are not as effective as using syrup of ipecac. If your child is prone to swallowing whatever is at hand, keep a bottle of this substance at home. *Do not get tincture of ipecac or fluid extract of ipecac, either of which is so toxic that it might cause fatal poisoning.* The dose of syrup of ipecac for a child above the age of one is fifteen milliliters (one tablespoon, or three teaspoons). The child must drink at least a cup of water or juice—the more the better—after taking the ipecac. Vomiting will usually occur within fifteen minutes. The dosage may be repeated once if vomiting doesn't occur in twenty to thirty minutes. For a large child or adult, the dose of syrup of ipecac is thirty milliliters—two tablespoons, or one ounce—with ample fluid; the dose may be repeated in twenty to thirty minutes. Tickling the back of the throat may be necessary to induce vomiting when the ipecac fails.

Under what circumstances do you not induce vomiting?   Vomiting may be harmful when the child has ingested kerosene, gasoline, charcoal lighter or other petroleum products. The danger is that some of the substance may be aspirated into the lungs and cause pneumonia. A caustic substance, such as lye, bleach or acid, should not be removed by vomiting, for to do so would expose the esophagus and throat to it once more. It is dangerous to induce vomiting in someone stuporous, unconscious or uncooperative, as the vomitus might be aspirated.

What is a universal antidote?   The traditional universal antidote was made of two parts powdered charcoal, one part tannic acid and one part magnesium oxide. It is no longer in use because of the discovery that the ingredients are mutually inactivating.

Activated charcoal *is* useful in absorbing poisons. The dose is ten to fifteen grams of charcoal for each gram of poison. The usual dose is thirty grams mixed with distilled water. Cherry syrup can be added as flavoring. Charcoal should be given after vomiting has occurred, for if given before ipecac, it may prevent vomiting. (Sometimes the charcoal itself will cause vomiting.) Another use of charcoal is as a marker; once it appears in the stool, it can be assumed that the poison has also passed through the intestine.

What other antidotes are available?   Doctors and persons trained in pharmacology know or can look up the antidotes to most poisons. Often the effects of the poison are neutralized by giving a drug that has an opposite effect: a stimulant to combat a depressant, a sedative to counteract a stimulant. The effects of an acid may be neutralized by giving milk of magnesia or sodium bicarbonate, and the effects of an alkali by giving vinegar or lemon juice. The effects of an irritating poison may be reduced by giving olive oil, vegetable oil, egg white or milk. These foods help to coat the stomach and intestine and to slow the absorption of substances such as kerosene.

How can child poisoning be prevented?   Some of the ways to prevent this unnecessary cause of death and disability are given in the accompanying chart.

TEN WAYS TO PREVENT CHILD POISONING

1. Don't leave medicines within reach of children.
2. Don't let a child watch you take medicine.
3. Don't compare taking medicine to eating candy.
4. Don't store medicines, chemicals or poisons in food containers or near food.
5. Don't leave gasoline, charcoal lighter, paint thinner or similar products in a cup, glass or soft-drink container.
6. Do go through the house and identify all substances that might be poisonous to a child.
7. Do use the "Officer Ugg," "Mister Yuk," or another labeling method to indicate unsafe substances. Information about "Officer Ugg" is available from the Rocky Mountain Poison Foundation, 1722 Prudential Plaza, Denver, Colo. 80202. Information about "Mister Yuk" is

available from the Pittsburgh Poison Control Center, Children's Hospital, 125 Desoto Street, Pittsburgh, Pa. 15213.
8. Do store medicine in a high, locked cabinet.
9. Do keep aspirin and acetaminophen in safety-capped bottles.
10. Do keep chemicals, petroleum products, cleaning agents and insecticides on a high shelf out of sight and reach of children.

SNAKEBITE

How dangerous is snakebite?   Each year, about 7,000 people in the United States are bitten by a poisonous snake. Fewer than a dozen of these persons die, but many are left with disability of a limb and scarring at the site of the bite.

Which snake is the most dangerous?   The rattlesnake accounts for 80 or 90 percent of fatal bites. It is irascible, occurs in most parts of the country, and turns up near towns as well as in the rough. The eastern and western diamondbacks may grow to lengths of seven or eight feet.

Other poisonous U.S. snakes are the water moccasin (cottonmouth), the copperhead moccasin and the coral snake. All but the coral snake are pit vipers: they inject venom via fangs, and the venom acts mainly on tissues and the blood. The coral snake is responsible for only 1 or 2 percent of bites in this country. It has a small mouth, and its venom flows passively into the wound after the bite. Coral-snake venom acts mainly on the nerves, and is fifteen to twenty times as deadly as venom from a rattlesnake.

Who is most likely to be bitten?   Persons at greatest risk are those who handle snakes for purposes of entertainment, religion or science. Outside the high-risk group, hunters, farmers and fishermen are the most susceptible. In the eastern United States, most bites occur in persons between the ages of five and nineteen who are near home at the time of the poisoning.

Which bites are most likely to be fatal?   Snakebite in a child under five is most dangerous, because the child's body is not big enough to readily dilute the poison. Bites on the face, neck or trunk are more severe than those on the extremities, because a ligature cannot be used to slow the absorption of the poison.

One reassuring point is that in about a third of bites by pit vipers, no venom is injected. And even when the snake injects venom, it's rare for the animal to put all its venom into one bite.

Can a snake strike the same victim more than once?   Yes, especially a child who stands and cries instead of moving away from the animal.

208

What are the symptoms of poisonous snakebite?   The bite of a pit viper (rattlesnake, cottonmouth or copperhead) causes severe pain and swelling. Blood blisters may form at the site of the bite and obscure the puncture marks. A rapidly spreading bruise is common. Additional symptoms, generally indicating a severe bite, are nausea, vomiting, dizziness and generalized weakness. The mean time of death following poisonous snakebite is eighteen hours.

Rattlesnake bites tend to be the most severe and to cause most fatalities. The bite of a coral snake doesn't cause much pain or swelling. Symptoms may not develop for one to ten hours, and include weakness and difficulty in swallowing or speaking. Muscle paralysis, convulsions and death may occur within twenty-four hours after the bite.

How do you tell between a poisonous and nonpoisonous bite?   The best way is to identify the snake. A nonpoisonous bite doesn't usually cause much pain or swelling, though the wound may bleed freely. Only one puncture mark or more than two marks may be seen in nonpoisonous as well as poisonous bites. When there is any doubt as to whether the snake is venomous or when the bite occurs at night and the snake isn't seen, presume that the bite was poisonous and take the precautions given below.

What first-aid measures are indicated for poisonous snakebite?   The following method is based on recommendations by several leading authorities:
1. Get to medical help as quickly and safely as possible. Do not waste time on home remedies, and do not hesitate to walk to help if you are alone.
2. Identify the snake if you can do so without danger. Do not waste time looking for the snake, however.
3. Do not make cuts at the site of the wound or attempt to suck the poison out. Even those authorities who still recommend the "cut and suck" first-aid measure admit that it is of no use unless done immediately, and that the cut itself may harm a vital structure.
4. Place a ligature two inches above and below the bite to impede the absorption of venom. A rubber tubing is preferable, but shoelaces, cord or a strip of clothing may be used. The ligature should be applied firmly but carefully so as not to cut off the circulation, and should not be so tight that you cannot slip a finger under it. Leave it in place until you reach medical help, or for up to an hour en route, but you may have to reposition it to keep it ahead of the swelling.
5. Apply a chemical cold pack or ice in a plastic bag to the site of the bite as soon as possible. It will slow the absorption of venom and can be left on for up to an hour or two if necessary without causing skin damage.
6. When bitten by a snake with red, yellow and black markings, gently wash the bite area with water to remove venom that may have been left on the

209

skin. The venom of a coral snake is not injected; it runs into the wound made by the snake's teeth.

7. If possible, splint the arm or leg while the person is en route to the doctor. Have the victim lie down, and take a positive, reassuring attitude to allay the person's fear.

What is the definitive treatment for poisonous snakebite?　Treatment is best given by a surgeon or someone skilled in snakebite therapy. Antivenin therapy is the specific antidote, but because of the possibility of an allergic reaction from its administration, the decision to give it should be based on an evaluation of the type of snakebite, its severity and other considerations. It is important to note that these preparations are *specific* for the various kinds of bites, and that the patient will not respond unless the correct antivenin is used. Various surgical measures are sometimes used as adjuncts to antivenin therapy. After emergency treatment, including prophylaxis against tetanus, hospitalization and observation are indicated. Tetanus immunization and wound care are indicated even if the snake was nonpoisonous.

What should be done about a nonpoisonous bite?　Evaluation by a physician is recommended. The wound should be cleaned and dressed, and an antibiotic ointment may help to prevent an infection. Depending on when the last tetanus shot was given, a booster may be desirable.

ANIMAL BITES (see pp. 183–84)

SPIDER BITES AND SCORPION STINGS

What are the most dangerous spider bites?　The bite of the black widow may be fatal in up to 5 percent of victims, with most fatalities occurring in small children. The black widow is responsible for more bites than the next most dangerous spider, the brown recluse. Tarantula bites resemble those of the black widow, but occur much less commonly.

What are the symptoms of black-widow bite?　Not infrequently the bite is on the buttocks or genitals, because of the black widow's tendency to frequent outhouses. Two tiny red spots may occur, or a bruise and swelling may be noted. The pain may be severe or minimal. Beginning fifteen minutes to several hours later, symptoms of generalized toxicity occur. These include nausea, vomiting, abdominal pain and boardlike rigidity of the belly muscles. Sometimes an erroneous diagnosis of perforated ulcer is made. In severe bites, labored breathing, convulsions, shock and coma may occur.

What's the treatment for black-widow bite?   Incising and sucking the bite are not useful. It's better to clean the skin thoroughly and rush the person to medical help. An antivenin is available and could be lifesaving for a young child. Injections of calcium gluconate may relieve muscle spasm, and steroids or other drugs may control some of the symptoms.

What are the symptoms of brown-recluse bite?   The bite may occur on the genitals or buttocks, but is more likely to be on the hand or leg when the spider is encountered in a woodpile, cave, cellar or closet (where it may get into infrequently used clothing).

A mild stinging sensation or very little pain may accompany the bite. Six to eight hours later, severe pain begins and progresses. A blood blister or a clear blister may form, and the skin around the bite turns a white, red or purplish color. Within a day the bite and the area around it become exquisitely tender. The person may have chills, fever, nausea and vomiting. The skin around the bite turns progressively darker, becomes leathery, and will eventually die and slough off.

What's the treatment for brown-recluse bite?   Since the symptoms come from the persistence of the toxin in the skin around the bite, many doctors now favor an excision of the most severely involved area. This skin would die anyway, and removing it relieves the person's symptoms. Skin grafting can be done later. Short of excision, the treatment is symptomatic. An antivenin has not yet been developed.

What about tarantula bite?   Abdominal pain and pain at the bite may occur, and the skin around the bite may slough off. There is no antivenin, and the treatment is supportive or similar to that for a brown-recluse bite.

How dangerous is scorpion sting?   In most parts of the United States scorpion sting is not serious. A few species in the Southwest may produce severe symptoms, and in Mexico ten times more deaths occur from scorpion sting than from snakebite. Most fatalities occur in young children or in the very old.

What are the symptoms of scorpion sting?   The least serious stings cause pain and swelling similar to those of a beesting. Poisonous species in the Southwest, including *Centruroides sculpturatus* or *C. gertschi,* have a toxin that affects the nerves. Numbness near the site of the bite may spread to involve the entire arm and leg. Within an hour or two the tongue may feel numb. In severe cases, excessive salivation, runny nose, chills, fever, agitation, nausea, vomiting and convulsions occur. Death from respiratory paralysis is a possibility.

What is the treatment for scorpion sting?   Tie a tourniquet above the bite, apply ice to slow the absorption of the poison, and take the victim to the doctor. Loosen the tourniquet and remove the ice every twenty to thirty minutes; reapply these measures a few minutes later if still en route to the hospital. Specific antiserum is available in places where dangerous scorpions are endemic, and use of the serum will reduce the mortality rate.

INSECT STINGS

How dangerous are insect stings?   They kill more people than snakebite! Drop for drop, the poison of a honeybee is as potent as rattlesnake venom, but that isn't what kills. The forty persons who die each year following insect sting do so because of a catastrophic allergic reaction to the insect venom.

Which insect stings may cause the allergic reaction?   Honeybees cause most fatalities, but the sting of a hornet, wasp or yellow jacket may be just as dangerous.

How do you know if you are allergic?   You may not know until you develop symptoms following a sting. The reaction of a nonallergic person is to develop pain and swelling at the site. Itching and reddish discoloration are common. Nausea, vomiting, headache and fainting may occur when many stings have been sustained or when the victim is a small child.

An allergic reaction may consist of hives near the sting and on other body parts. The lips and fingers, as well as the site of the sting, may swell. Wheezing and difficulty in breathing are danger signs. In a severe reaction, shock, collapse and an obstruction of the airway (laryngeal edema) may prove fatal within a few minutes. A blood test known as the RAST, or radioallergosorbent test, can be used by an internist or immunologist to document that the allergy exists.

What is the treatment for an allergic reaction to an insect sting?   The reaction is an emergency, though not every reaction will be catastrophic. If the victim has collapsed, evaluate airway, breathing and circulation. Give CPR (see p. 191) if indicated. Summon help and make plans to take the person to an emergency room as soon as possible.

Meanwhile, tie a piece of rubber tubing or similar ligature above the sting to slow the absorption of venom. A honeybee may leave its barbed stinger in the skin. Remove it by gentle scraping with a knife or fingernail. Do not grasp the stinger with fingers or tweezers, as this might inject more venom from the sac that is still attached to the stinger.

If it is available, epinephrine (adrenaline) should be given. It counteracts the severe allergic reaction and opens the victim's airway. The allergic victim may be carrying a kit containing it (see below).

What precautions should the allergic individual take? Persons who survive an allergic reaction are at risk of having another one. They should avoid insects, carry a kit in the event of a reaction, see an immunologist for desensitization therapy, and wear an appropriate identification bracelet telling of the allergy.

· *Avoiding insects* requires the use of "knockdown" *insecticide spray.* The person should wear protective clothing outdoors and should not use perfume or cologne before going outside to play tennis or to jog. Car windows should be left rolled up.

· *Kits* containing epinephrine and instructions are available from various manufacturers, including Center Laboratories, Port Washington, N.Y. 11050, and Hollister-Stier Laboratories, Box 3145, Term. Annex, Spokane, Wash. 99220.

· *Desensitization therapy* can be offered by an immunologist. Pure venom extract is becoming available, and should prove more effective than whole body extract.

· *An identification bracelet* will tell others of the allergy in the event the person is unconscious or unable to speak.

AQUATIC STINGS

What should be done for jellyfish stings? Most jellyfish stings are not serious, but those caused by a Portuguese man-of-war (*Physalia* species) may cause severe pain and a generalized reaction consisting of shock and cessation of breathing. The first priority is to get the person out of the water. Use gloves or other protection to remove adhering tentacles. Pour alcohol on the sting and rinse the skin with sea water. Transport the person to the nearest emergency room for further therapy.

What about the stingray? This fish doesn't usually sting unless it is stepped on. Severe pain and swelling occur at the puncture wound, and the first aid is similar to that for snakebite. Apply a tourniquet, then wash the wound with sea water. Remove any visible part of the stinger. Suck the poison out of the wound, and transport the person to an emergency room for further therapy. A cold pack may be applied to the site of the sting.

ALLERGIC DRUG REACTIONS

Which drugs are most likely to cause allergies? Penicillin heads the list, and according to one estimate, 5 to 10 percent of Americans are now allergic to this antibiotic. Aspirin (alone or in combination with cold or pain remedies), sulfa drugs and insulin are frequent sources of allergic reactions. Other high-risk drugs are antibiotics other than penicillin or sulfa. Tranquilizers and iodide-containing drugs, such as the dye used for gall-bladder and kidney X-rays, sometimes cause allergies as do many kinds of preparations applied to the skin.

What types of reactions occur?   Skin rash such as hives is the most frequent symptom signifying a strong allergy. Many rashes are measles-like, and some do not occur unless the skin is exposed to the sun. Depending on the drug, other symptoms include fever, nausea, diarrhea, mouth sores, small skin hemorrhages (petechiae) and secondary infection due to a reduction in the white blood cell count.

What is the most dangerous type of reaction?   Anaphylactic shock, which begins as a sudden collapse within minutes after an injection of the drug. Breathing may cease or become difficult because of laryngeal obstruction. Wheezing and hives appear. Death may occur from stoppage of the heart or respiration. This reaction is identical with a severe allergic reaction to insect sting, and the same body mechanisms are involved in both situations.

What is the treatment for allergic drug reaction?   CPR (see p. 191) may be indicated for a severe reaction, but the definitive therapy consists of injecting epinephrine, corticosteroids and other medications as necessary. Obviously, the person should be rushed to the nearest medical facility if a physician is not in attendance. In less severe reactions the first step is to stop the offending drug or all drugs that the person is taking. Check with the prescribing physician about further therapy.

What are some general rules about drug reactions?   These are more likely to appear when a drug is injected than when it is taken by mouth, so don't insist on a shot of penicillin if you can get by with oral therapy. The more drugs you take, the more likely you are to develop an allergy, and people who have other allergic diseases such as asthma or severe eczema are more prone to drug allergy. Use drugs only when definitely indicated. If you develop a rash after taking a drug, you may have a more serious reaction, even anaphylaxis, if you take it again. An allergy should be pinpointed so that you can avoid the offending drug for life.

What precaution should the allergic individual take?   Since you may be involved in a serious auto accident or become too ill to give your medical history, you should wear a Medic Alert bracelet or necklace telling of the drug allergy. It can be obtained from the Medic Alert Foundation, P.O. Box 1009, Turlock, Cal. 95380. The bracelet will say something like "Allergic to Penicillin," and will give a telephone number that will be answered by someone who can give the caller the person's medical background. Medic Alert is a nonprofit organization that was founded by a doctor and has been in operation since 1956.

HEAT COLLAPSE

What are the causes of heat collapse?   Exposure to high temperatures may cause heatstroke, heat exhaustion or heat syncope.

What is heatstroke?   It is the most severe of the conditions and occurs when someone is exposed to the sun without relief, when a workman is confined to a very hot environment, such as the boiler room of a ship, or when a child is left in a hot car with the windows rolled up. It is especially severe in the very young and the very old, where the mortality rate is 50 percent. As few as two hours of exposure may lead to heatstroke in a baby, but several hours of exposure are necessary before the condition develops in an adult.

What are the symptoms of heatstroke?   Headache, nausea and dizziness are followed by confusion, fainting, coma and convulsions. The temperature is 104°–108° F. (40°–42° C.), the skin is hot and dry, and the person is no longer capable of sweating.

What is the treatment for heatstroke?   The treatment is aimed at reducing body temperature as quickly as possible. Remove the person's clothing and place him or her in a tub of cold water. Another way to lower the temperature is to put ice bags over the groin, in the armpits, at the front of the neck and over the trunk. Wet towels or sheets may be placed on the skin and kept moist while a fan blows on them. If facilities are available, it's best to lower the temperature quickly and then take the person to an emergency room for further treatment and observation.

What is heat exhaustion?   It takes longer to develop this condition than heatstroke, and it results from sweating profusely and not replacing the fluid by mouth, or replacing it with plain water containing no salt. Susceptible individuals include a football player during training, a jogger running in the heat, and a visitor to a hot climate before acclimatization has occurred.

The symptoms are weakness, dizziness and muscle cramps. The skin has a wet, clammy feel in comparison to the hot, dry feel of sunstroke. The body temperature is only slightly elevated. In a severe case of heat exhaustion, the person may collapse from shock and circulatory failure.

What's the treatment for heat exhaustion?   Take the person to a cool place and give cold water and electrolyte-containing drinks, such as Gatorade.

215

Intravenous fluids are indicated when the person can't take nourishment by mouth. Prevention of heat exhaustion requires the intake of enough liquid and salt to make up for the losses caused by working and training. This may require six to eight quarts a day, and twenty or twenty-five grams of salt, preferably in the form of salty foods and liquids rather than salt tablets. It's now recognized that athletes training in the heat should be allowed to stop and replenish body fluids as often as necessary.

What is heat syncope?   A fainting episode following exposure to the heat. It may occur in band students or soldiers required to stand for half an hour or more in formation on a hot day, or in a jogger or competitive athlete at the end of a taxing run. The blood pressure drops, causing dizziness and fainting. Recovery occurs quickly once the person lies down and is removed from the heat. Moving the knees slightly and pumping the calves while standing in formation may prevent it. The athlete who is prone to dizziness or fainting at the end of a run should train more slowly.

FROSTBITE

What is frostbite?   A skin reaction to severe cold. The low temperature, often twenty or thirty below, frosts the outer layer of skin. The nose, ears, hands and feet are most commonly affected. Unchecked, frostbite may progress to freezing injury or deep frostbite.

What are the symptoms of frostbite?   The normal reaction to cold is pain. Sudden cessation of pain, perhaps accompanied by a tingling sensation, is a sign of early frostbite. The facial muscles stop working when this is the area of exposure. Frostbitten skin is crisp, nontender, and cold. Loss of feeling in the hands and feet signals that they are becoming frostbitten.

What is the treatment of frostbite?   The purpose of treatment is to restore blood flow to the skin by warming the frostbitten part. *Under no circumstances should the skin be "thawed" by rubbing it with snow!* Placing a warm hand over the affected ear or nose may help, and frostbitten fingers may be warmed by placing them in the opposite armpit. A frostbitten foot may be warmed on the skin of a companion's belly.
    When warm water is available, the affected part should be immersed in it, preferably under the supervision of a physician. Dry heat in the form of a heating pad or electric blanket is not desirable, for it may burn the skin.

How is frostbite prevented?   Prevention entails wearing proper clothing when exposed to cold weather, avoiding alcoholic beverages during exposure, and resting and warming at the first signs of excessive coldness.

MINOR EMERGENCIES

How do you know when a cut needs suturing?   To minimize scar formation, even a small cut on the face may need sutures. A cut up to an inch long on another body part may heal well without sutures, providing the bleeding stops quickly and the wound is kept clean. Any cut involving a tendon or nerve, or in someone with inadequate tetanus immunization, should be evaluated by a doctor.

What are butterfly sutures?   They are thin strips of Band-Aid or Steri-Strip placed across a cut to keep the edges closed so that suturing isn't necessary. For best results, the wound edges should be painted with tincture of benzoin prior to applying the strips. Because it is sticky, the benzoin holds the strips in place. After five or six days the butterfly sutures may be removed.

Which wounds should not be sutured?   Very dirty wounds may become infected if sutured. The dirtiest of wounds is that due to human bite; usually it is left to heal without stitches. Small cuts on the fingers and toes may do better without stitches, as sutures don't hold well in these areas. Stitches also don't hold well inside the mouth.

What do you do for a penis caught in a zipper?   Try to free the penis with a steady downward motion of the zipper. When this isn't possible or a child is screaming with pain, cut the zipper out of the trousers with scissors, dress the young man in pajamas or a robe, and take him to your pediatrician or to the emergency room. Local anesthetic can be injected to relieve pain, and the zipper can be cut apart with wire cutters to free the penis.

How do you get a fishhook out of the skin?   If the fishhook is embedded in the finger, arm or leg, the easiest way to remove it is to force it the rest of the way through its arc until the barb has cleared the skin. Cut the barb off and draw the hook back out the way it entered. A hook in the face or ear should be removed by a physician. Two methods have been developed that allow removal without forcing the barb the rest of the way through its arc, but these methods should be employed only by those skilled in their use.

What will remove the pain of a beesting or insect bite?   Add a drop or two of water to a dash of meat tenderizer and rub this into the skin after the stinger has been removed. Massage gently for several minutes. If pain persists, apply an ice cube or cold pack, or soak with Epsom salt to relieve pain and reduce swelling.

What will stop hiccups?   A method that works for many is to swallow a teaspoonful of white sugar. It should be swallowed without water or other fluid and will give immediate relief in most persons. Another teaspoonful of sugar can be taken if the hiccups persist.

8

SKIN CARE

How frequently do skin conditions occur? Skin problems are said to be the most frequent of all medical problems and account for a fourth of visits to doctors.

What functions does the skin perform? The largest organ in the body, the skin is also the most visible and it bears the brunt of protecting the rest of the body from the environment. It helps to cool the body by sweating, and the fat beneath the skin is an insulation against the cold. Activated by the sun, the skin makes vitamin D. It helps us display emotion, and has a role in sexual attraction.

Special sweat glands, the apocrine glands, are situated in the armpits, around the nipples and in the cleavage between the buttocks. At puberty, the apocrine glands are stimulated by the sex hormones to release a cheesy substance and certain chemicals. The scent of these chemicals has an aphrodisiac effect on members of the opposite sex and forms a part of one's sexuality.

What causes oily skin? Inheritance plays a part, and persons with darker skin and hair tend to have more oil than those who are blond and fair-skinned. Boys are oilier than girls. Factors that increase oiliness are use of birth-control pills or other hormones, eating a high-fat diet, and using creams and heavy cosmetics that add to the body's own oils.

Where does skin oil come from?   Most of the body is covered by hair, and each hair is attached to a tiny smooth muscle in the skin's deep layer. Contraction of this muscle causes the hair to move into a more vertical position—goose bumps occur when many of these muscles tense—and each time the muscle tightens it expresses a small amount of oil from the sebaceous gland near the root of the hair. These oil glands are the source of skin oil.

What can be done for oily skin?   Washing the face or other oily area two to four times a day is usually effective. Once a day apply a nonprescription drying lotion. Products containing 5 to 10 percent benzoyl peroxide are best. Stay away from face creams and fatty foods.

What causes dry skin?   The skin dries with aging; other factors include too frequent bathing, frequent exposure to the sun and sleeping under an electric blanket. Dry skin is more likely to occur in the winter than in the summer. Too little fat in the diet may contribute to the dryness.

What can be done for dry skin?   Moisturizing products can be applied to the bath or directly to dry skin, and bathing less frequently is also helpful. Some soaps are more creamy and less likely to cause dryness. Instant oatmeal can be used to add oil to the skin: Add a cup of hot water to an envelope of the cereal, then tie up the congealed oatmeal in a large handkerchief. Use this as a large soap pad having both cleansing and emollient properties.

What causes itching?   It can be a symptom of rash or dry skin, or it can occur in its own right for poorly understood reasons. In some instances, itching produces scratching, which irritates the skin and causes more itching. To be successful, treatment must interrupt this "itch-scratch" cycle.

What's the treatment for itching?   General measures include the use of a bland soap, adding lubricating or moisturizing creams to the bath, and applying such creams or lotions to the itching areas. Itching skin should be babied: don't rub it with a washcloth or towel. Wash it gently with the fingers and let it air-dry.

What causes wrinkles?   After the age of thirty the skin begins to lose its elasticity. The supporting fibers stiffen and wrinkles are the result. Cigarette smoking and excessive exposure to the sun are two factors that increase the rate of wrinkling. The obese person who suddenly loses weight in middle age is more wrinkle-prone because of the loss of supporting fat beneath the skin.

What can be done for wrinkles?   Repeated sunburn speeds skin break-down and hastens the onset of wrinkling, so prevention by avoiding the sun is the best treatment. When you're in the sun, wear headgear and use a sunscreen containing para-aminobenzoic acid (PABA). The sunscreen will protect the skin from the harmful rays of the sun. Dry skin wrinkles more quickly than oily skin, so the use of a mild moisturizer containing urea may slow wrinkling. Since such a product doesn't clog pores, even the person with oily skin may use it.

What is involved in cosmetic surgery?   Face-lifts are becoming increas-ingly frequent among those who can afford them (average cost: $1,500 and up). The operation is performed by a plastic surgeon under local or general anesthesia. It takes three to four hours, and depending on the person's age, weight and general health, will last four to eight years. Cosmetic surgery is also performed to treat wrinkles on the eyelids, neck and breasts.

How do I find a dermatologist?   Family practitioners and internists have been trained in the treatment of skin problems and can handle most skin conditions. See one of these first, and ask for a referral if the condition persists or you're not satisfied with the treatment. A qualified dermatologist will have completed three or four years of training in this specialty and will be certified by the American Board of Dermatology. Because most diag-noses are made simply by looking at the skin and since confirmatory lab tests aren't usually necessary, it is not unusual for the skin specialist to see many patients in an hour. Find a doctor who will take the time to explain your condition and its treatment.

COMMON SKIN CONDITIONS

What are some general measures for treating skin problems?   The main consideration is that it is the type of problem more than the cause that dictates treatment. For a wet rash, use soaks or lotions until the skin is dry. For a dry rash, use ointment or cream. Use only one preparation at a time, and keep track of what you use.

What are some soaking solutions to use on inflamed skin?   You can add half a cup of plain white vinegar or a tablespoon of 2 percent boric acid crystals to a quart of water, or add one Domeboro tablet or one packet of Domeboro powder to a pint of water. Dip a piece of clean cotton sheet into the solution and lay it on the rash. Keep it in place and wet for twenty or thirty minutes. Use the soaks three or four times a day; as the water in the dressing evaporates, it dries up the skin. Soaking solution that isn't used at one treatment may be kept in the refrigerator until the next application.

221

What are some lotions to use?   Calamine lotion is a good all-purpose product to relieve itching from poison ivy and similar rashes. Shake it well before using it three times a day. Be sure to gently wash the old lotion off before applying a new coat. Plain calamine lotion is preferable to products that contain antihistamines that could cause an allergic reaction in the skin.

What is the difference between creams and ointments?   Creams disappear into the skin when rubbed, whereas ointments do not. Plain cold cream, known to the pharmacist as "ointment of aqua rose," is useful on a dry rash as are ointments based on white petrolatum or zinc oxide. Many of these can be purchased without prescription. In general, water-washable creams have a drying effect, and should not be used on dry rash. Cortisone creams are useful in treating many rashes, but this medicine must be prescribed by a doctor.

What causes acne?   Acne, or pimples, is due to excessive oiliness of the skin and an inability of the skin to resist this problem. The oil is secreted in such copious amounts that it may cause a plug, or blackhead, to form in the oil gland opening. A pimple may form beneath the blackhead. The pimple is like a small boil caused by staph bacteria which are normally present on the skin.

Can acne occur in adults?   Yes, about one out of ten adults continues to have problem acne, often on the neck, back and chest. An acne-like condition known as rosacea occurs in middle-aged men. Characterized by redness, it affects the nose, cheeks and lips, and is associated with excessive drinking, high-fat diet and a lifelong condition of oily skin.

Why is acne worse at times?   The disease tends to flare up during highly emotional times or periods of stress. It is not associated with masturbation, as the folk myth has it, but it may get worse just before the menstrual period or just afterwards. Because sunlight tends to improve acne, the summer months are best and the condition is often worse in the fall and winter.

What is the treatment for acne?   The purpose of treatment is to keep the face clean and reduce oiliness. Here are the steps:
1. Wash the face three or four times a day using soap or an acne preparation or lotion. Your fingers are sufficient to work in the lather, or you may use a washcloth. You should wash before breakfast, at noon, before supper and at bedtime.
2. Apply a drying agent once or twice a day after the skin has been washed. Agents containing 5 to 10 percent benzoyl peroxide are best. The drying

agent may cause slight chapping; if the face becomes tender, reduce the use of the agent to once a day or every other day.

3. Squeeze blackheads and pimples only after a doctor has shown you how. Too much face-picking may produce scarring.

4. Limit your intake of greasy foods, milk products, chocolate, nuts and other foods that promote oiliness of the face, if your own experience shows that these contribute to your acne.

5. Don't use face cream or oil-based cosmetics or lotions (lipstick, dry rouge and face powder are okay). Boys with acne shouldn't use hair oil.

6. Visit a physician if these measures don't relieve the acne.

What is the medical treatment for acne?   Tetracycline, an antibiotic, can be prescribed to reduce the problem with pimples, but it is not prescribed for children under twelve. Exposure to sunlight should be reduced when tetracycline is used. The drug can be taken at a low dosage for extended periods, and though it may cause rash, upset stomach or diarrhea, the overall incidence of side effects is low. Vitamin A can be taken orally or as a topical preparation to relieve acne. Too much vitamin A may cause loss of appetite, hair loss and other problems, so the prescribed dosage should not exceed 50,000 to 100,000 units a day, and the vitamin should not be taken continuously for more than two or three months. These medicines are to be used in conjunction with the steps given above.

What will reduce acne-scarring?   By a technique known as dermabrasion, a skin specialist or plastic surgeon can plane down the rough skin of acne scars. A scab forms over the new skin, and after healing, the face is much smoother in appearance.

What is hidradenitis suppurativa?   It is a chronic infection of the apocrine sweat glands. Large, acne-like lesions appear in the armpits, groin and anal areas. Antibiotics and local therapy give some relief, but the condition tends to persist.

What causes a boil?   It is an infection of the hair follicle caused by staphylococci. The body's natural resistance usually controls the infection, as evidenced by the formation of pus.

What's the treatment for a boil?   Apply moist heat twice a day, but otherwise keep the area clean and dry. When the boil is "ripe," its tip should be punctured with a sterile needle and the pus gently expressed. For a large boil, this procedure should be done by a physician. Penicillin therapy is helpful when fever or a sick feeling accompanies the boil. Tender or swollen glands in the area of the boil may indicate spread of the infection and the need to seek medical attention.

Why do boils recur? Oily skin, profuse sweating and irregular bathing favor persistence of harmful staph bacteria on the skin. Probably a decreased resistance to infection is the primary cause, though this factor is not really understood. To prevent recurrence, keep the skin clean and dry. Be especially careful to cleanse the surrounding skin after pus is expressed from a boil. Penicillin or tetracycline may have to be given for several weeks to prevent the boils from coming back.

What is a carbuncle? This once dread condition, which commonly occurs on the back of the neck, is like several boils bunched together. It is a serious infection and should be treated medically with penicillin and incision and drainage of pus.

What is erysipelas? An acute streptococcal skin infection, erysipelas was once as dreaded as scarlet fever or carbuncle. It may erupt on the face, arms or legs, and is distinguished in Caucasians by its bright red color. Penicillin is curative, though some persons have recurrences.

What about "barber's itch"? It is a skin infection of the beard area that is spread by shaving. A man notes a pimple or two on the face one morning, shaves, and finds that several more soon appear. Within several days the beard area may be covered by small boils in various stages of healing.

What is the treatment for barber's itch? Stop shaving for several days until the infection is under control. Wash the face four times a day with Phisohex or plain soap and water. After each washing, apply a light coat of an antibiotic ointment, such as Mycitracin or Neo-Polycin. If several of the boils have pus, oral penicillin therapy will hasten healing. Ingrown hairs must be removed with tweezers. An uncommon form of barber's itch is caused by a fungus and must be treated by a physician.

Change blades each day when you return to shaving, or clean the head of the electric razor thoroughly with alcohol (be sure to unplug it first). Wash the face after shaving, and apply a light coating of antibiotic ointment. Continue doing this for two weeks after the infection has cleared. Twice-a-day face washings and the daily use of a drying agent such as benzoyl peroxide may prevent recurrence.

Can you get barber's itch of the legs? Yes, a similar condition may occur after shaving the legs. The treatment is generally the same as for barber's itch of the face.

What causes athlete's foot? Any of several funguses that have a predilection for warm, moist areas such as between the toes. The infection may be spread through shower rooms or among family members using the same bathtub. Boys are more susceptible than girls, and adults who use public swimming or exercising facilities are apt to contract the infection.

What are the symptoms of athlete's foot?   It usually begins with itching between the toes. As the infection progresses, flaking of the skin is noted and a dry, scaly rash may spread across the sole or to the top of the foot. Small blisters may appear but usually go unnoticed.

What is the treatment for athlete's foot?   Tolnaftate, a drug available without prescription, is excellent for treating athlete's foot. It is available in cream, liquid or powder form, and should be applied to the affected areas twice a day for two or three weeks. When the skin between the toes is severely inflamed and weeping, the liquid medicine is preferable. The drops may also be used on dry athlete's foot, as may the cream or powder. Several drops are enough to treat one foot and should be rubbed in gently. The medicine should not be applied when the foot is still wet from showering.

How do you keep athlete's foot from recurring?   Some authorities claim it's impossible to completely eradicate the infection, so recurrence is likely. It may help to sprinkle a small amount of tolnaftate powder into the shoes and socks each day. Keeping the feet clean and dry is probably the best preventive. So that the fungus is not spread to the groin and other body areas, the feet should be toweled *last* after a bath.

What causes fever blisters?   *Herpes simplex,* a virus, causes fever blisters. The agent is classified as Type 1 Herpes to distinguish it from the Type 2 infection that causes herpes venereal disease.

What are the symptoms of fever blisters?   A group of painful blisters form at the angle of the mouth or elsewhere on the lips. These crust over, become more tender, and gradually heal in a week to ten days (the first time they may last two to four weeks). Some people have them once and never again, but others are prone to recurrent fever blisters. As the name indicates, recurrences may accompany fever, a common cold, exposure to sunlight or injury to the mouth.

What is the treatment?   There is no specific treatment, but antibiotic ointment applied to the sores once or twice a day may help to relieve symptoms.

What causes mouth ulcers?   The cause is unknown, but recurring attacks of these sores afflict one out of five adults and bring untold misery to the sufferers. Theories as to the cause include infection by a virus or bacteria and a self-destructive body process. Anxiety plays a role. Biting the lip or jaw, using a hard toothbrush, or eating nuts or other sharp-pointed foods may bring on an attack. The ulcers are misnamed canker sores ("canker" is derived from the Latin word *cancer*), and doctors prefer the term "recurrent aphthous stomatitis."

What's the treatment for mouth ulcers? A dermatologist or general physician may be able to help by giving symptomatic therapy. A steroid cream may reduce pain when the sores first appear, and 2 percent viscous zylocaine is a local anesthetic that can be applied directly to the ulcers or held in the mouth for a minute to relieve the pain before eating. Both medications require a prescription.

What causes warts? A virus, *Verruca vulgaris,* causes warts. Most persons develop a resistance to this virus by the age of puberty.

Where do warts occur? They may occur anywhere on the body. The most common sites are the feet and hands, but warts on the soles of the feet tend to be the most resistant to therapy.

What's the treatment for warts? Magic is involved, for children may suddenly develop antibodies that destroy warts following the rubbing of them with saliva from an elderly individual possessed of the power to heal warts. Even a modern physician may get results by rubbing each wart with a bright new penny, wrapping it carefully, and giving it to the child with instructions to bury it in a certain place at a certain time while reciting, "Wart, go away, wart, go away, and do not come again my way!"

Medical treatment consists of removing the wart with liquid nitrogen, solid carbon dioxide or electrosurgery. It may help to use a daily application of 10 percent salicylic acid in flexible collodion, made up by the pharmacist. Another method that gets the child involved in the therapy is to apply a drop or two of castor oil to each wart and cover it with adhesive tape. The tape is left on for a day, then removed, and the process is repeated. After six to eight weeks, the wart may come off. Warts on the face, lips, palms or soles should be treated by a physician.

What causes moles? A mole is a normal skin growth consisting of nevus, or pigmented, cells. ("Nevus" comes from the Latin word for birthmark.) Babies either have no moles or very few, but the cells that will eventually form moles are present in the skin at the time of birth. Some moles appear during childhood, but most become apparent in the years right after puberty. Still others become evident during adulthood.

How many moles is it normal to have?   No normal limit has been set, and the chance that a mole will become malignant is not related to the total number of moles that are present.

What are the danger signs of a mole?   Most moles grow slowly and change gradually over the course of years, but a sudden change in growth or appearance is abnormal. A mole that takes on an irregular dark color, or that begins to have pigment growing outward into the skin from its base, should be examined by a physician to make sure it has not changed into a malignant melanoma. Bleeding from a mole or the formation of a sore or irritation over it are other danger signals.

What is the treatment for moles?   Treatment isn't necessary unless the mole bothers you, changes in appearance, or occurs in a high-risk area. Any mole that is of concern to you should be evaluated by a physician and removed if indicated. Certain other moles should probably be removed: those that occur on a frequently injured area, those found on the lips, genitals or anus and those occurring next to a fingernail or toenail.

Self-examination of all moles should be performed every three or four months. The examination is especially important in individuals who have a fair complexion or who have a family history of melanoma, since these persons have a higher risk of developing this form of cancer.

What causes spots on the skin?   Depigmented spots may appear on light-skinned or dark-skinned persons. Among the causes are skin infection, skin allergy, chronic skin disease, drug reaction or internal disease. When the spots appear for no known cause, the condition is called vitiligo. Common sites for vitiligo are the face, neck and hands.

Spots of increased pigmentation are more common. These may appear during pregnancy, after exposure to the sun, or after taking birth-control pills. The so-called liver spots of brown pigmentation that appear most commonly in older persons bear no relationship to liver disease. Medical conditions such as Addison's disease or cirrhosis of the liver may, however, produce brown spots. In a rare instance the spots reflect an internal malignancy of the chest or abdomen.

What is the treatment?   The person should visit a physician to find out if a treatable condition caused the spots. Pigment due to pregnancy usually disappears within a few months after delivery. Light spots from an infection or rash may persist for several weeks. The light spots of vitiligo may be covered with makeup. A medication is now available which will repigment these spots, but it must be used under medical supervision. Brown spots may be minimized by avoiding the sun and using a sunscreen.

227

What causes dishpan hands?   Also known as housewives' dermatitis, this condition is due to irritation of the hands by soap or detergent. It is worsened by frequent wetting of the hands.

What are the symptoms of this condition?   An itchy, irritating rash appears on the fingers and hands. Small blisters form and the rash is worse on the undersides of the fingers. It may get better for a day or two or leave completely, then recur.

What is the treatment for housewives' dermatitis?   The use of a dishwasher is recommended. When you must do the washing by hand, you should wear cotton gloves inside of rubber gloves to protect your hands. Soaks and steroid cream will relieve a severe rash.

SKIN DISEASES IN CHILDHOOD

What causes cradle cap?   It's due to a temporary shedding of dead skin and oily secretions from a baby's scalp. The flaking, crusty material is most prominent at the front and sides of the head. Contributing factors are failure to keep the baby's scalp clean and the use of baby oils either on the scalp or elsewhere on the body.

What is the treatment for cradle cap?   Shampooing two or three times a week with a mild agent such as baby shampoo is usually all that's necessary. The looser crusts may be removed gently after the hair is dry. Persistent cradle cap should be treated by a physician.

What are the symptoms of prickly heat?   Also called heat rash, this is an eruption of tiny bumps on the face, neck and trunk of a baby. In an older child or adult, it is most common where two areas of skin rub together, such as in the folds of the arms or beneath the breasts of a woman. The rash burns and itches, and in a white person, may have a pink to red color.

What causes prickly heat?   Sweating gets it started. The sweat may become mixed with dust or dirt to plug the gland openings, and bacteria on the skin then invade the sweat ducts to create the rash.

What's the treatment?   A cool bath or shower is needed to wash material from the sweat glands. After the skin is dry, a light coating of antibiotic ointment should be applied. Calamine lotion may be used to reduce itching. Light, loose-fitting clothing should be worn. Prickly heat won't occur if the individual is kept cool by air conditioning; even several hours of cooling a day will usually prevent it.

How should diaper rash be treated?   The treatment depends on whether it is caused by primary irritation, candidiasis (thrush) or ammoniacal products in the baby's urine:

· *Primary irritation* from the urine and feces is treated by keeping the baby's bottom clean and dry. A sprinkling of talcum powder is useful in taking up some of the irritants after a diaper change. Disposable diapers are more likely to cause rash than cloth diapers, and if the rash continues, permanent diapers should be used.

· *Thrush* is an infection with the fungus *Candida albicans.* The rash is fiery red with clear borders. It may cover the genitals and also be found in the mouth as white plaques. Diabetics and very obese persons may get thrush in the skin folds. The treatment is nystatin by mouth and as a cream applied to the rash.

· *Ammoniacal diaper rash* may occur in babies wearing washable diapers. Blisters break out in the cleft of the buttocks and form red sores. The sores become confluent in a severe case. The odor of ammonia is very strong when the diapers are removed. What happens is that a germ capable of breaking urine into ammonia gets into the diapers and resists removal by laundering. As soon as the baby urinates, the urine is turned into ammonia, which irritates the skin. The treatment is to switch to disposable diapers and put Diaparene cream on the baby's bottom. Before the cloth diapers are used again, they must be thoroughly disinfected by applying an antiseptic to the final rinse water. Commercial antiseptics are available, and certain wash powders are specific for correcting this problem. The diapers must continue to be laundered in this way to prevent the rash from recurring.

What is impetigo?   It is an infection of the skin caused by streptococci. The infection may accompany a strep throat or occur on its own. Commonly known as "infantigo," it is not usually a serious infection.

What are the symptoms of impetigo?   Rash appears on the face or trunk. In mild cases, it is a raised, dry area that looks as if an extra piece of skin had been stuck on with glue. In more severe infections, blisters break out and fill with honey-colored serum, which may form into pus. Crusts and new areas appear as the fluid is discharged. The infection may progress rapidly to other body parts.

What's the treatment?   Mild impetigo can be treated by washing the area three or four times a day with soap, and applying an antibiotic ointment. When the child has fever or when the impetigo is extensive, penicillin therapy is indicated. Rarely, impetigo may occur in an adult and the treatment is the same as when it appears in a child.

What causes scabies?   A mite, *Sarcoptes scabiei,* is responsible. The infection, which in times past was known as the "seven-year itch," is spread by close body contact and is most common in conditions of wartime, famine and poverty. Recent years have brought an increase of this infection throughout the world to persons of all socioeconomic groups and even to individuals who maintain good body hygiene.

What are the symptoms of scabies?   Severe itching and rash are the main symptoms. In a baby, the rash may appear on the buttocks and resemble diaper rash, but the lesions also occur on other parts of the body. In older children and adults, the rash is usually on the trunk, neck and extremities, usually at the belt line, the front of the armpits and between the fingers. A characteristic of the rash is the appearance of many tiny scabs that look like someone had poked a pencil lead into the skin. Secondary infection of the sores is frequent.

What is the treatment for scabies?   In adults and children over the age of two, a single application of gamma benzene hexachloride is usually curative. It should be left on the skin for four hours and washed off. Eurax cream (crotamiton) is used in children under two. Both medicines require a prescription and should be used under the direction of a physician. Recent reports have indicated that enough gamma benzene hexachloride may be absorbed from the skin to cause brain damage if it is left on for longer than four hours. The drug's potential for harming the developing brain is why it shouldn't be used in young children or during pregnancy.

What causes ringworm?   It is a fungal infection of the skin that is most common in children. The fungus may be transmitted to the child from a dog or cat, from another child, or from the soil. Less commonly the source of infection is athlete's foot of an adult or older child in the family.

What are the symptoms of ringworm?   As the name suggests, there is a ring of inflammation, which may vary in size from less than a dime to as big as a softball. Characteristically, the outer edge of the ring is the most severely infected, and the central area may be clear. The child may have several dime- or penny-sized scaly patches on the face or chest. Itching may occur, but is not severe.

Where on the body is ringworm most likely to occur?   On the face, neck or chest of a child, and on the hands, arms, trunk or groin of an adult. The toenails are infected much more commonly than the fingernails.

What is the treatment for ringworm?   Tolnaftate cream or powder will give relief when the ringworm is on the face, trunk or extremities. The medicine should be applied to the involved areas two or three times a day until at least a week after the rash has disappeared. Ringworm of the scalp, fingernails or toenails calls for griseofulvin therapy under the direction of a dermatologist or pediatrician. Resistant ringworm of the smooth skin must be treated with griseofulvin. This drug should not be used during pregnancy or by a person with liver disease or porphyria (see p. 409). Side effects of griseofulvin include allergic rash or hives, stomach upset, dizziness, headache, insomnia and a depression of the white blood cells.

ALLERGIC CONDITIONS

What is eczema?　　The term is from a Greek word meaning "to boil over," which refers to the weeping inflammation of classic eczema. In modern usage, eczema refers to an allergic skin reaction that is most common in children.

What causes eczema?　　The cause is not known, but inherited allergies to food and other substances are thought to be important factors. A third of children with eczema develop asthma, and almost three-fourths of them will have hay fever. Eczema, asthma and hay fever are often grouped as differing manifestations of similar underlying allergies.

What are the symptoms of eczema?　　Eczema may begin on the cheeks and scalp of an infant two or three months old. Irritated by wool and lanolin, the rash is worse during the winter, and is more severe after the ingestion of certain foods. Blisters may form, break and ooze. More often the rash is dry and scaly: bright red in a white child, and irregular and light-colored in a black or brown child. Spread to the back, abdomen and extremities is common. The rash itches and the baby is irritable. Even without treatment the eczema usually disappears by the age of one and a half or two.

In older children and adults, eczema is more likely to occur in the creases between the arm and forearm or the thigh and leg. It is characterized by intense itching, dryness and a raised, crusty or scaling rash.

What is the treatment for eczema?　　Skin irritants such as wool should be avoided, and the skin should be kept as moist as possible with drip-dry baths and the use of moisturizers afterward. A topical steroid will relieve itching. Elimination of foods that provoke the rash is indicated. Therapy is similar in an adult, with the most attention given to treating the rash and reducing itching.

What is contact dermatitis?　　It is a rash created when the skin touches a substance that irritates it or incites an allergic reaction. The most common

231

form of contact dermatitis results from touching poison ivy. It isn't that the resin from the plant is poisonous; it's that everyone has an allergy to it to some degree.

What are the symptoms of contact dermatitis?   Rash and itching occur at the site of contact. In severe instances, blisters form, break and ooze, and gradually heal if no further exposure occurs. Continued exposure may produce an itching, scaly rash with few or very small blisters.

The site of the rash may identify its cause. Housewives' dermatitis occurs on the fingers and hands, which suggests that water and soap are the primary irritants. A rash developing beneath a new watch and watchband points to a reaction to the new material. Rash on the face may indicate an allergy to cosmetics, on the ear to earrings, on the feet to shoes or socks, and in the anal area to colored toilet paper.

What are some common causes of contact dermatitis?   The rash may follow contact with almost anything, but frequent sources are the resin from poison ivy, poison oak or poison sumac; nickel, nylon, rayon, lipstick or other makeup; soap, rubber, insect spray, detergent, shampoo, perfume, deodorant or cologne.

What is the treatment for contact dermatitis?   The first priority is to determine and eliminate the cause. A weeping rash should be treated with soaks, and a dry one with a topical steroid cream. It is advisable to avoid future exposure to the substance that caused the rash.

What about hypoallergenic cosmetics?   Thanks to an FDA ruling, manufacturers must now subject a product to testing before claiming that it is "allergy-tested," "safe for sensitive skin," or "hypoallergenic." You may still react to one of these substances, and if the problem persists you may have to do without it.

What's the treatment for poison ivy?   For a weeping rash, make up soaks as described on p. 221 and apply them four times a day to relieve itching and to dry the skin. Domeboro soaks are best. When the lesions have dried, use calamine lotion or a topical steroid for itching.

Won't steroid injections or pills shorten the course of poison ivy?   Not really, though the medicine may give symptomatic relief. Steroid side effects may also occur, including increased risk of infection, menstrual irregularities and puffiness of the ankles, wrists and face.

Can you be immunized against poison ivy rash?   Yes, but it takes a long course of taking the allergen orally. Injections do not produce immunity, and if given during an acute case of poison ivy the injections could be harmful.

What's the best way to prevent poison ivy?   Learn to recognize the plant, as well as poison oak and poison sumac, which produce a similar reaction. Wear protective clothing when going into the woods. Be aware that you can get the rash by changing a tire that has recently been driven through poison ivy, that smoke from burning the plant may cause the rash, and that you can get it from a dog, clothing or shoes that have been in contact with oil from the plant's leaves or fruit. Thorough washing of the skin after exposure may help to prevent the rash, but washing that is delayed for thirty minutes or an hour is of no use. Ordinary laundering of clothing will remove the causative plant oil.

What drugs are most likely to cause skin rashes?   Penicillin, ampicillin, sulfa drugs and tetracyclines are often responsible, but a skin rash may result from taking any drug to which you are allergic.

What agents may cause a rash only when the skin is exposed to the sun?
The most common drug offenders are tetracycline, sulfa drugs and thiazide diuretics (used to control high blood pressure). Halogenated salicylanilides in certain soaps may cause itching when the skin is exposed to the sun. Other causes are perfumes and plant products containing psoralens. The giveaway for this type of reaction is the line of sharp demarcation between the normal skin that wasn't exposed to the sun and the inflamed skin that was.

HAIR PROBLEMS

What causes baldness?   In an adult man baldness is usually due to heredity. The trait is passed in an autosomal dominant fashion from father to son or in a sex-linked manner from mother to son. The hair loss becomes pronounced in the twenties or thirties. Loss of hair at the sides of the forehead (temporal recession) is a universal male trait due to the action of testosterone. Complete baldness in a woman may be hereditary, but this occurs infrequently and usually not till after age fifty. A more frequent problem is thinning of the hair. The cause is not always understood, but the problem tends to correct itself.

Can an illness cause hair loss?   Yes, baldness may follow high fever, nutritional deficiency (including severe dieting), systemic lupus erythematosus, endocrine disease, syphilis or cancer. Drugs such as Cytoxan, Imuran and vincristine that are used to treat cancer or to prevent rejection of a transplant may cause baldness. Taking the Pill sometimes causes the hair to fall out.

Does wearing a hat cause baldness?   No. Most bald men wear hats for protection and appearance, and that's probably how this mistaken notion got started.

What causes patchy hair loss?   In a child the most common cause is ringworm of the scalp. An overlooked cause is trichotillomania—the nervous plucking of one's own hair. In adults, alopecia areata may cause patchy hair loss.

What is alopecia areata?   Hair loss appears in certain areas of the scalp. The bald spot slowly enlarges, and the characteristic feature is the appearance, at its outer rim, of hairs that have broken off just above the surface of the scalp. Because these hairs are thin at their base and thicker at the broken end, they are known as "exclamation-point hairs." Several hairless patches may appear, and hair of the eyebrows, eyelashes and beard may be lost. Fortunately, alopecia areata is self-limiting. In almost every instance the hair grows back within six to twelve months. The cause of the condition is unknown.

What is the treatment for baldness?   There is no known treatment for hereditary baldness. Griseofulvin is the treatment for ringworm of the scalp. Steroid cream is sometimes used to treat alopecia areata, and steroid injections have helped when a young woman loses most of her hair for an unknown reason. A wig can be worn to cover the bald scalp, and hair transplants have been successful in many persons.

What causes hair to turn gray?   The pigment responsible for its color is replaced by air spaces in the shaft of the hair, and the process usually begins in middle age and progresses slowly. Hair does not turn gray overnight, nor does gray hair occur more frequently in those who worry a lot than in those who don't. The most important determinant of when graying begins is heredity; if either or both parents had early onset of grayness, so may the children. Hair that grows into a certain type of bald spot may be white or gray even when the rest of the hair remains its usual color.

What can be done for gray hair?   No drug or other remedy will reverse the graying process, but the hair can be dyed if a change in color is desirable. Many dyeing agents are available, but these should be used with caution (see p. 240).

What causes dandruff?   The cause is unknown, but dandruff occurs in at least a third of people and varies from mild flaking of the scalp to a rash extending to the forehead and eyebrows, behind the ears and to other body parts such as around the bellybutton. An oily skin contributes to it.

Is dandruff infectious?   No, it can't be spread by a comb or any other means.

Can dandruff be cured?   No, but it can be controlled.

What is the treatment?   Frequent shampooing with any agent (even plain soap) will remove the flakes of dandruff. The shampooing may have to be done every two or three days, and the scalp, not just the hair, should be washed thoroughly. The use of a specific agent, such as selenium sulfide, will prolong the effects of each shampooing and work better for severe dandruff. Certain of these products can be bought over the counter. Changing shampoos every six months to a year may also help. Topical steroids are indicated to relieve the itching of the rash (known as seborrheic dermatitis) when it is the main problem on the head or other body part.

Does it hurt to shampoo the hair every day?   There's no medical evidence that frequent shampooing will harm normal hair, though it might dry or irritate the scalp of some persons. Choosing an appropriate shampoo or using an oil treatment afterward should prevent most problems.

What causes head lice?   The head louse, a bloodsucking parasite known as *Pediculus humanus capitis.* Other forms of pediculosis may affect the genital area ("crabs") or trunk (body lice). Head lice are spread from person to person as well as via combs, brushes and headwear. Lack of body hygiene is a contributing factor, and children are infested much more frequently than adults.

What are the symptoms of head lice?   Itching may be so intense that the scalp becomes raw and secondarily infected through scratching. The lice remain hidden, but the eggs (nits) appear as tiny white particles attached to the hairs. Two things help to differentiate these particles from the flakes of dandruff. Flakiness from the latter is adjacent to the scalp, while the nits may be found near the ends of the hairs. Dandruff flakes come off easily, but nits stick tightly to the hairs.

What's the treatment for head lice?   Shampooing with gamma benzene hexachloride is usually curative, though the treatment may have to be repeated in a week. It shouldn't be used on infants or pregnant women. The lotion is used to treat body lice and the shampoo is used for pubic lice. Nits must be removed from the hair with a brush or comb after the sham-

235

poo, and the bedding and clothing should be laundered in hot water to kill lice and nits. When more than one member of a family is infested, all should be treated simultaneously.

What causes unwanted hair?   Racial characteristics determine hair growth. Caucasians have more hair than blacks, who have more hair than Orientals or American Indians. Caucasians of Mediterranean origin are more hairy than those of Anglo-Saxon or Nordic stocks. Dark hair growing on the face of a woman is most often an inherited trait and not the result of disease. Another consideration is age. A woman tends to grow more hair on her lips and chin after the menopause.

What diseases can cause excessive hairiness?   Hormonal imbalance due to a tumor or disordered metabolism of the adrenal gland or ovary may cause menstrual irregularities, deepening of the voice and growth of hair not only on the face but also on the chest, abdomen and extremities. Medical evaluation is indicated when these symptoms occur. It's safe to assume that a tumor isn't present if the unwanted hair is limited to the face, the menstrual periods are regular, and similar hair growth occurred in the person's mother, aunts or sister.

What drugs may contribute to growth of body hair?   Steroid hormones such as prednisone may cause excessive hair growth, but a return to the normal pattern will occur after the steroids are stopped. Birth-control pills containing a relatively large dose of progesterone may stimulate growth of facial hair.

What's the treatment for unwanted hair?   When the cause appears reversible, as when the Pill is responsible, switching to a different Pill or to an alternate method of birth control may help. Four possible remedies for nonreversible hair growth are to dye the hair, pluck it, use a depilatory agent, or have it removed by electrolysis.
  · *Bleaching the hair* will make it less noticeable. Prepare a soft paste out of baking soda and bleach containing 6 percent hydrogen peroxide; add a few drops of household ammonia to the mixture and apply it to the unwanted hair. After several minutes remove the bleach and wash the skin. If the skin becomes irritated, use less bleach and more baking soda next time.
  · *Plucking them* is a satisfactory way of dealing with only a few unwanted hairs. The hairs will grow back, but not at a faster rate. For that matter, shaving the lip or chin doesn't make the hair grow any faster.
  · *Depilatory agents* contain chemicals that break the hairs off even with the skin. Newer agents smell better and act more quickly than those in use a few years ago. Some people are sensitive to these chemicals, so you should

try them first on a small spot on your leg before using them extensively.

· *Electrolysis* gets rid of hair by destroying the hair root. The hair doesn't grow back if the treatment is effective, but the treatment takes a long time, is expensive, and may produce scarring if done incorrectly. If you opt for this method, it's best to have facial hair removed by a professional. A dermatologist can refer you to one.

MISCELLANEOUS SKIN CONDITIONS

What are some causes of rash in an adult?   Three fairly common causes are neurodermatitis, tinea versicolor and pityriasis rosea.

What causes neurodermatitis?   The key feature of this entity, which apparently has no physiologic cause, is that nervous itching and scratching produce rawness of the skin that lead to additional itching. Soon the itch-scratch cycle is born.

How do you recognize neurodermatitis?   The most likely sites are the back of the neck, the wrists or the ankles, but neurodermatitis may occur on the anus, scrotum, labia, back or abdomen. The rash is scaly and raised above the surrounding skin. Crisscrossing of the skin lines is more visible in the area of rash. The person will scratch the area frequently, sometimes without realizing it, and itching tends to be worse during stress and may also occur at night during sleep.

What is the treatment for neurodermatitis?   The itch-scratch cycle must be interrupted. This may be accomplished by applying a topical steroid to the rash, with or without a covering of plastic wrap, or by giving the person medicine to control itching. Neurodermatitis may persist for months or years. The earlier treatment is started, the more likely it is to be successful.

What causes tinea versicolor?   This mild skin infection is caused by the fungus *Malassezia furfur.* Certain persons are more susceptible than others, and the individual who develops tinea versicolor may expect to have recurrences even after treatment.

How do you recognize tinea versicolor?   It may cause light spots on the skin in both whites and blacks. In a person with very light complexion, the spots may be darker than the surrounding skin. A frequent complaint in white persons is that the skin doesn't tan evenly on exposure to the sun. The areas occur on the neck, upper back, chest and the front of the arms. The involved skin is scaly but doesn't itch. The rash is most prominent after a day of hard work and sweating.

What is the treatment for tinea versicolor?   Selsun shampoo (obtained by prescription) contains an ingredient that will kill the fungus. The yellow shampoo is applied to the rash, taking care to spare the face, before retiring. Next morning it is showered off. This is repeated after one week. Another way to use Selsun is to apply it for thirty minutes and wash it off, and to repeat this treatment weekly for a total of three treatments, then monthly for three months. Selsun will eradicate the infection, but the light areas of skin may persist for several weeks. Tolnaftate solution or cream may also be used in the topical treatment of tinea versicolor.

What causes pityriasis rosea?   The cause of this condition is unknown, but it is thought to be a viral infection with a low degree of contagiousness.

How do you recognize pityriasis rosea?   It occurs mainly in young adults, and may begin as a large spot on the chest or back that is mistaken for ringworm. This herald patch may be an inch or two in diameter. It is the same rose color in a white person as the smaller lesions that break out on the chest, abdomen and sometimes the extremities two to ten days later. In a black person the rash may have a light or slightly pink and scaly appearance. Because of its distribution, the rash produces a Christmas-tree effect on the back; the spots parallel one another and appear in rows that are slanted down on either side from the backbone. The skin may itch, but many persons have no symptoms other than the rash.

What is the treatment for pityriasis rosea?   The rash will regress spontaneously in about six weeks. Itching may be relieved with a body oil or calamine lotion. Recurrence is rare, and spread to a family member is uncommon.

What is psoriasis?   A chronic skin disease that causes scaling rash on the scalp, elbows, knees or other body part. The cause is unknown, but many persons with psoriasis have a family history of it.

How do you recognize it?   The rash is raised, white to reddish in appearance, and has a rough, dry texture. Discrete spots of psoriasis are the rule, but in a severe case the lesions may merge to produce large patches that cover the knees and elbows. Itching is a complaint in about a third of affected persons.

What's the treatment for psoriasis?   Topically applied coal-tar cream is a time-honored remedy. Selsun shampoo helps to control scalp involvement. Steroids may be used as a cream, or the hormone may be injected directly into involved areas. Strong drugs given by mouth are sometimes used to treat severe psoriasis, especially when a rare form of arthritis complicates the disease.

What causes shingles?   The same virus that causes chicken pox.

What are the symptoms?   Blisters and rash break out on the chest, back, neck or abdomen, and less commonly on the face or extremities. The rash always occurs along the distribution of a nerve that runs close to the skin's surface. The blisters form pustules and crusts just like the lesions of chicken pox. New crops may appear for several days, and healing occurs in two or three weeks.

Pain in the area may antedate the rash or, primarily in older people, may persist for weeks or months after the rash is healed. This neuralgia that follows shingles can be a disabling problem.

What is the treatment?   Shingles is most apt to occur in an older person who is chronically ill, and treatment should be given by a physician. Sometimes an underlying blood condition is discovered. Painkilling drugs and local anesthetics may be used to relieve the neuralgia. A short course of oral cortisone may decrease the likelihood that the pain will persist.

What are the skin changes of lupus erythematosus?   Lupus may be limited to the skin (discoid lupus) or it may cause rash, fever, arthritis and damage to the kidney and other organs (systemic lupus, or SLE). The skin changes are similar in both forms of the disease. The classic "butterfly rash" appears on the cheeks and across the bridge of the nose. It may persist for weeks or months, doesn't itch, and is aggravated by sunlight. More common are red to scaly splotches on the face, trunk or extremities. Scarring is more likely to occur after the rash of discoid lupus.

What causes lupus?   It's thought that one inherits a predisposition to develop the disease, given certain variables such as exposure to sunlight, infections and certain drugs. The precipitating drugs include Mesantoin (an anticonvulsant), Pronestyl (for heart irregularities) and Apresoline (for high blood pressure). Lupus is five to ten times more common in women than in men.

What is the treatment for lupus?   Avoidance of sunlight is indicated. Steroid hormones, topically or systemically, will usually control the symptoms. Good nutrition, vitamins and lots of rest are thought to help. Systemic lupus may be a severe disease and treatment should be sought immediately by an internal medicine specialist or a rheumatologist (see p. 316).

What is scleroderma?   Less common than lupus, scleroderma is a disease that may also cause skin changes or affect the internal organs.

Plaques or scar-shaped configurations may appear in the skin. Sometimes the skin swells and loses its elasticity, becoming tightly adherent to underlying bone. Typical changes occur in the fingertips. A frequent internal disorder is loss of function in the esophagus. Specific therapy is not available, though steroid hormones may be of benefit. Scleroderma may be a very serious illness, and treatment from an internal medicine specialist should be sought.

What is pemphigus? It is a rare disease characterized by the breaking out of large or small blisters on the skin. The disease may be inherited or may occur as an autoimmune process. The blisters appear in crops in the mouth or on the trunk or extremities, and each enlarges slowly before rupturing to leave a festered sore. Secondary infection is common. An attack may subside spontaneously after several weeks, but recurrence is the rule. Steroid hormones may help in the treatment, or the disease may run a progressive course causing death a year or two after onset.

SKIN CANCER

What is the incidence of skin cancer? It's one of the most frequent forms of cancer. Over 300,000 new cases are reported each year, and about 6,000 people a year die from it.

Who is most susceptible to skin cancer? A fair-skinned, blue-eyed individual who works outdoors or spends a lot of time in the sun.

Do hair dyes cause skin cancer? The Food and Drug Administration has issued a warning that many of the common hair dyes contain carcinogenic chemicals. This was determined by feeding the chemicals to rats and mice and observing an increased cancer rate. The question is not so much one of skin cancer but of an increased cancer risk to the bladder, liver and intestine. (A small amount of the dye may be absorbed into the bloodstream.) Much more research will be necessary before this issue is decided; in the meantime, avoidance of these chemicals seems advisable. Certain companies, Clairol, for example, have removed these chemicals from their products.

Is there more than one type of skin cancer? Yes, the three types are basal cell cancer, squamous cell cancer and malignant melanoma.

How do you tell them apart? They differ in symptoms, appearance and degree of malignancy:
· *Basal cell cancer* is the least malignant and most common form of skin cancer. It doesn't spread to other body organs. The slow-growing tumor

starts as a nodule on the face or neck, sometimes at the site of a scar. It has a waxy or pearly appearance and blood vessels are visible on its surface. As it grows, the central part of the nodule sinks and forms into a sore.

· *Squamous cell cancer* grows rapidly and does spread to organs. It begins as a scaly, ulcerated nodule with a rough red border. The outside of the tumor is not shiny and blood vessels are not visible in it. It may arise in a sun-damaged area of skin or at the site of previous radiation therapy.

· *Malignant melanoma* is the worst form of skin cancer. It arises in a mole and is most common on the face, head or legs. The earliest sign is a change in appearance of the mole. It may begin to grow, form a notch on one edge, or take on a different shade of blue, gray, pink, or brown. Pigment may spread into the surrounding skin from the base of the mole or appear as satellite spots of pigment around the mole. The mole may enlarge, bleed or form a sore, but these are not early symptoms.

What is the treatment for skin cancer?   A suspicious nodule or growth should be removed by a skin specialist. Removal is usually curative for basal cell cancer, but additional forms of therapy may be indicated for squamous cell cancer or malignant melanoma. Most of the time squamous cell tumors respond to treatment, but malignant melanoma is not likely to be curable unless it is caught early. It alone accounts for one and a half percent of cancer deaths each year in this country.

What's the best way to prevent skin cancer?   Avoid excessive exposure to sunlight and use a sunscreen when you do go outdoors. If your job or your outdoor activities keep you out in the sun a lot, you should examine your skin regularly and be periodically examined by a physician. Should a suspicious growth appear, or should a mole or other skin nodule change, have it examined by a doctor. Nine out of ten times the diagnosis won't be cancer, but it could be, and the sooner the diagnosis is made, the better your chances of survival.

241

9

EYES

How do the eyes work? Somewhat like a camera in that light enters the eye through an aperture (the pupil), is focused by the lens, and strikes the back of the eye (the retina) to create a visual image. The image is transformed into nerve impulses that travel from the optic nerves to the brain for interpretation. Since the eyes work in concert, it's impossible to focus on more than one thing at a time. The brain interprets the two visual fields to create a three-dimensional image, which is responsible for depth perception.

What exactly is the pupil? It is the round hole in the center of the iris, at the front of the eye, through which light enters. Due to the action of an involuntary muscle, it gets larger when the amount of light is reduced and smaller when you're in bright light. Excitement dilates the pupil, while relaxation causes it to remain relatively small. Many drugs also have an effect on pupillary size.

What is the iris? It is the round, pigmented part of the eye surrounding the pupil. If you have blue eyes, your iris lacks pigment and appears blue; if your eyes are brown, so is your iris. Muscle pull from the rim of the iris is what accounts for changes in the size of the pupil. The more dilated the pupil, the smaller the amount of iris that is visible; the smaller the pupil, the larger the visible iris.

What is the cornea?　It is the transparent, saucer-shaped part of the eyeball that is in front of the iris and pupil. You can't see it well unless you look at someone's eye from the side. A protective shield, the cornea is exquisitely sensitive to touch. An eyelash floating on it is incapacitating, and even the slightest irritation will produce blinking.

What other protective layers does the eye have?　The white of the eye, or sclera, is a tough coat of protective tissue. The conjunctiva is the inner lining of the eyelids. Attached to the upper and lower aspects of the eyeball, it forms a protective sac that keeps particles from reaching the area above or below the eye. A bony fortress, the orbit, consisting of the bridge of the nose, the lower forehead and the cheekbone, protects the eye from blunt trauma.

What is the lens?　It is a transparent, elliptical structure located behind the iris and serving to focus the image on the retina, much as a projector focuses the image on the screen. Involuntary muscles can change the shape of the lens to allow you to focus for near or far vision.

What is the retina?　It is a sensitive and complex structure composed of ten distinct cell layers. It covers most of the back side of the eyeball, and transmits the visual image to the optic nerve, to which it is attached.

What are the optic nerves?　An optic nerve is attached to the back of each eyeball. The nerves join at the base of the brain, where the fusion of visual images begins. The nerve tracts continue to the right and left sides of the brain at the back of the head. In this visual center, the left brain interprets what is seen by the outer part of the left eye and the inner part of the right eye; the right brain does the same for the images from the inner part of the left eye and the outer part of the right eye.

What are the eye muscles?　Each eye has six muscles that arise in the back of the eye socket and pass forward to attach to the sclera around the circumference of the eyeball. They permit movement of the eyes in all directions, with the brain coordinating the synchronization of eye movements.

EYE CARE

What can go wrong with the eyes?　The most common problem is a refractive error that can be corrected by wearing glasses or contact lenses. Other mild conditions include inflammation of the conjunctiva and irritation of the eyelids. Visual loss may follow injury, cataracts, glaucoma, infection, tumor or severe diabetes.

243

Can eye problems be prevented?   Eye injury is the most preventable condition. Wear safety goggles when pounding steel on steel or working around machinery. Keep chemicals, spray cans, acids and lye out of reach of children. Close your eyes when using an aerosol can, and make sure the nozzle is pointed away from you. Wear sunglasses on a clear day on the ski slopes, and protect the eyes when under bright sun, a sunlamp or treatment lamp. Wear seat belts to prevent head and eye injury in the event of an auto accident, and wear protective glasses when engaging in vigorous sports, such as squash or hockey, where eye injury is not uncommon.

Maintenance of good general health, with close supervision of such conditions as diabetes, is also important. Irritation or pain in the eye or any difficulty with vision calls for an eye examination.

Who should perform the exam?   The best eye exam is done by an ophthalmologist, a medical doctor specializing in the treatment of eye disease. This physician is trained to prescribe glasses or contacts, treat other visual problems, and examine the eyes for glaucoma, cataract or diabetes. Should surgery become necessary, the ophthalmologist is qualified to perform it.

An optometrist is not a medical doctor. Most optometrists are competent to fit you for glasses, but by law in many states they cannot use the eye drops necessary to give an accurate reading of what strength glasses you need. This may change in the future. An optician is trained to make glasses' lenses under a physician's prescription, and doesn't do eye examinations.

How do you find an ophthalmologist?   Your primary physician can refer you to one, or you can do the selecting yourself. A qualified ophthalmologist has completed a four-year postgraduate training program in an approved hospital, and has been certified by the American Board of Ophthalmology. He or she may also be a member of the American Academy of Ophthalmology. You can find the names of ophthalmologists in your area by looking in the *Directory of Medical Specialists* in the public library or by writing to the American Academy of Ophthalmology, 15 Second Street SW, Rochester, Minn. 55901. A referral by another physician or by a friend whose judgment you trust is the best method.

What questions should you ask the doctor?   Before the first visit you may want to call about the price of an examination, though fees in a given area tend to be standard and average about thirty dollars. Probably the most important factor in assessing the doctor is his or her medical reputation as well as how comfortable you feel with him or her. If you have a choice, find someone who can explain things, answer your questions clearly and give you a thorough, unhurried examination.

What does the examination consist of?   It begins with a history of your general and visual health. If you've had eye surgery or any problem, the doctor will want to review the past records and note what medicine you are currently taking. If you wear glasses, the physician will measure the thickness and type of lens to compare these with the findings of the present examination.

The doctor will test movements of the eye, pupillary reactions and your ability to focus. With an ophthalmoscope he or she will look at the inner eye. The retina is the only place in the body where one can see small arteries and veins to assess whether they show the effects of high blood pressure or diabetes. Next comes an exam with the slit lamp, a biomicroscope that magnifies images so that the doctor can see things inside the eye that wouldn't show up otherwise.

Eye drops to dilate the pupil and paralyze the focusing muscles are given next. These drops are uncomfortable. Their effects may take up to half an hour to develop fully, and depending on the type of drop that is used, the effects may last for several hours to a day after the exam, creating discomfort if you have to go into bright light and making it difficult for you to drive. In many instances, the shorter-acting dilating drops are all that's necessary and their effects are over fairly quickly. The drops are necessary to give a true reading of the need you have for glasses, and to find out what strength of lens will work best for you. This is determined by examining you with the phoroptor, the heavy black instrument through which you look while the doctor changes lenses to find the one that gives you the best vision. To check for glaucoma, the doctor will also use a tonometer to measure the fluid pressure in the eye.

What if I give the wrong answer about which lens gives me the best image?
The doctor can get a 95 percent accurate reading of your glasses' needs without asking any questions. This is accomplished by peering at the back of your eye through various lenses until a sharp image appears. Questions are used to confirm the findings. Should you respond the wrong way, the physician will repeat the question then or later to give you a second or a third chance to say which image is best. The chances of error are very small.

How often do you need to have a routine eye examination?   A child should have an eye exam at age three and again at age five or six before entering school. The individual who wears glasses should be seen every year and a half. Persons under age forty who do not have eye problems may get by without eye examinations, but the current recommendation is to have an exam about every three years. After age forty, all persons should have an examination every two years. Any difficulty with the eyes calls for an examination at once without waiting for the next appointment. Among the

245

problems indicating an eye emergency are the sudden onset of eye pain—especially one increased by light—a visual problem such as double vision, blurred vision, loss or reduction in vision or the appearance of visual aberrations, such as seeing halos around lights.

When do I need eye drops? Over-the-counter preparations may have a soothing effect when the eyes are irritated from dust, smog or smoke, but if the irritation continues, an ophthalmologist should be consulted. These products are probably overused, and the main need for eye drops is to treat a condition such as infection or glaucoma under prescription from a physician.

Can eye drops harm the eyes? One may have an allergic reaction to over-the-counter or prescription eye drops, and the symptoms of allergy include pain, swelling and excessive tearing in the eye. Eye drops may also become contaminated by bacteria after the container is opened. Probably the main harm from over-the-counter drops is that they can cause a delay in seeking expert help for a serious eye problem.

How do you use eye drops? Most drops come in plastic containers; you release the medicine by removing the cap, holding the container upside down and squeezing. The best position is lying down. Aim the drops for the corner of the eye, and don't squeeze the eye shut immediately, since this may force the drops out. Remain lying down for several minutes and the drops will diffuse across the eyeball. Wash the remaining medicine from the eyelids with water.

When would I need eye ointment? Usually only under the prescription of a physician. Because the effects last longer, ointment is the preferred treatment for eye infections in an infant. When there is a choice, most people prefer drops; they're easier to use and less likely to blur the vision.

How is ointment used? Pull the lower lid down and instill the amount of ointment prescribed. The medicine will diffuse slowly upward as blinking occurs.

Is it all right to use someone else's eye drops or ointment? Definitely not, since the medication might harm your eyes.

What is the optimum amount of light to read by? The light supplied by a 100-watt bulb placed no more than several feet from the printed page is optimal. The light should come from over the shoulder or at the side so that it won't glare back at you from the page or desk.

Will reading in poor light harm the eyes?   No, using less than adequate light might cause eyestrain, but it won't harm the eyes.

What is eyestrain?   A tired feeling in the eyes that occurs after a period of reading or using the eyes for close work. Headache may accompany the eye fatigue. Eyestrain may also be caused or aggravated by failing to use glasses when they are needed or by using glasses with the wrong prescription.

What do you do for eyestrain?   Rest the eyes by gazing off at a distance for several minutes. Do this every half-hour. Getting enough sleep will help, and glasses or a new prescription may be indicated.

VISION

How is vision tested?   The usual way is to have you stand twenty feet away from a chart containing rows of black letters that become smaller from top to bottom. For small children or persons who cannot read, charts with illustrations are available. A visual test can also be done through the phoroptor or an instrument with optics set up to simulate the twenty-foot distance. Near vision is tested by having the person read material in standard-size type held at a normal distance from the eye.

What is 20/20 vision?   It is normal vision, meaning that the individual can see at 20 feet what people with normal vision see at that distance. This does not take into account the fact that people who are farsighted may not be able to read material held at a normal reading distance (see p. 248).

How bad must vision be before you need glasses?   It depends on the visual needs of the person. For someone who reads or does close work, 20/20 is desirable. Vision of 20/40 or better is required to pass the driver's test in most states: the person's eyesight must be good enough to see from 20 feet what a person with normal vision can see from 40 feet away. 20/60 may be adequate vision for watching television, but the person whose vision is worse than this will generally request glasses. In many states, vision of 20/200 or poorer that cannot be corrected with glasses is considered to constitute blindness.

What causes blurred vision?   A refractive error creating less than average vision is the usual cause. The possibilities include nearsightedness, farsightedness, astigmatism and presbyopia. Sometimes the blurring develops so slowly that the person is hardly aware of it. One woman recalled that after getting her first glasses she discovered that grass was made up of individual blades instead of being a solid, carpetlike growth. Blurred vision developing suddenly is more likely to be due to an eye infection, cataract, glaucoma, eye injury or disease such as diabetes, and this symptom calls for an immediate eye examination.

What is nearsightedness?   This condition occurs when the eyeball is too long for the image to focus correctly on the retina. Because light rays come together in front of the retina, they diverge out of focus and create a blurred image. Concave lenses will focus the image correctly and allow normal vision.

Who is most apt to have trouble with nearsightedness?   It may occur in men or women, but tends to run in families. Blurring of vision usually becomes a problem between the ages of fourteen and twenty-one, and the condition may stabilize or it may worsen steadily, requiring stronger lenses as one grows older. Symptoms of nearsightedness are squinting, holding objects up close to the face while reading, and, in children, an inability to see the blackboard from any but the front row of the classroom. Nearsighted persons are often very sensitive to sunlight, and use protective hats and sunglasses out of necessity.

What is farsightedness?   Since the eyeball is a little too short in a farsighted person, the rays of light don't quite meet at the retina. The image is out of focus and perceived as blurred vision. Theoretically, the light rays would come together on the far side of the retina, and the purpose of corrective convex lenses is to pinpoint the image on the retina and allow normal vision.

Who is most apt to have trouble with farsightedness?   A farsighted person under the age of forty or fifty can get by without glasses by using the focusing power of the human lens. This is a normal body mechanism, but overuse of the focusing muscles may lead to eyestrain and headache. Since the focusing power of the lens diminishes during middle age, the older farsighted person is most apt to have trouble. Blurred vision for close and faraway objects becomes an increasing problem requiring corrective lenses. Sensitivity to sunlight is not usually a problem in farsighted persons.

Do eye exercises help either of these conditions?   No, eye exercises are only useful in some children with muscle imbalance. By the same token, wearing glasses to correct nearsightedness or farsightedness does not worsen the refractive error or harm the eyes so long as the glasses are properly fitted and worn.

What is astigmatism?   It is an optical error created by unevenness in the shape of the cornea. Instead of being completely symmetrical, the cornea is steeper or flatter on one side or at its top or bottom. Light rays are reflected unevenly, creating blurred vision. Glasses can correct for the problem.

Who is most likely to have astigmatism?   It may occur in either sex, and the symptoms usually begin between puberty and adulthood as blurred vision and eyestrain. The degree of astigmatism tends to stabilize after age twenty-one.

What is presbyopia?   This term refers to the loss of the focusing power of the lens that begins in the mid-forties and is complete about ten years later. It occurs in both sexes. The farsighted individual may find that corrective lenses are now a necessity. The person whose vision was previously normal may note blurring of close objects, such as newsprint or needlework. By supplying the focusing power of the lens, reading glasses will correct presbyopia.

Are these refractive errors the same as eye diseases?   No, they represent developmental variations, and presbyopia is a part of aging. The eyeball is not diseased, and glasses will correct the visual impairment.

What causes double vision?   Eyes that don't work in concert may see different images resulting in double vision. "Lazy eye" and crossed eyes are the common causes in a child, and both result from muscle imbalance. In an adult an infection, tumor or hemorrhage may paralyze an eye muscle, so that double vision occurs because one eyeball can't move normally. Double vision always calls for an eye examination to determine the cause.

What causes muscle imbalance?   Five percent of children are born with an inability to coordinate eye movements. Double vision occurs, and the child's brain will correct for this by shutting out vision in one eye, the so-called lazy eye. Unless the problem is corrected before age five, the child will never learn to see out of the neglected eye. Another cause for what appears to be muscle imbalance is a severe problem in only one eye. The brain may shut out the image from this weak eye, which tends to wander while the other eye is focusing on an object.

How do you recognize these conditions?   The eyes may be obviously out of balance, though crossed eyes may not be noticeable except during an eye exam. Muscle imbalance is usually noticed soon after birth or by the age of two or three.

What's the treatment?   Glasses may be prescribed and are sometimes accompanied by instructions to place a patch over the good eye to force the use of the weak one. Eye exercises may also be useful. Surgery to align the eyes may be necessary. Surgery after five years of age is more likely to be of cosmetic than of functional value.

GLASSES AND CONTACT LENSES

What conditions do glasses correct?   Lenses can correct for nearsightedness, farsightedness, astigmatism, presbyopia or a combination of these.

Do glasses cure the defect?   They correct the visual error and may relieve eyestrain. They do not affect the length of the eyeball, the shape of the cornea or the ability of the natural lens to focus.

Do glasses weaken the eyes?   No, but by correcting a refractive error they may improve vision so much that the person comes to depend on them. Were the same person to go without glasses, his or her eyes would be no stronger.

Which glasses are best?   The choices include single-lens glasses, bifocals, trifocals and tinted lens. The selection depends on the person's refractive error and individual preference. Light frames are the most comfortable when the glasses are worn constantly.

Are glasses with plastic lenses preferable?   They have the advantages of being lighter and unbreakable, and therefore much safer for children. The disadvantages are that they're more expensive and that for a given prescription, the plastic lenses will be slightly thicker than glass lenses. They also get scratched more easily.

What are bifocals?   They are glasses containing two types of lenses: one for near vision and one for far vision. Since most persons look down to read, the near-vision lenses are at the bottom of the glasses.

Who needs bifocals?   They're most often worn by people over forty-five who have developed presbyopia in addition to a previous refractive error, such as nearsightedness or astigmatism. The individual could use two types of glasses—one for reading and one for distant vision. Bifocals make the logistics easier by combining both types of lenses into one frame.

What are trifocals?   They have three sets of lenses: one for close vision, one for middle vision and one for far vision. The person most likely to require these is one whose work requires visual acuity at several distances, but the problem may also be solved by wearing a different pair of glasses for different needs.

What are half glasses?   They're a type of reading glasses containing only the bottom half of each lens. The person can look over the top for distant vision or peer through the lenses for reading. Anyone who must continually refer to a data sheet while speaking to others may find half glasses useful. An alternative to half glasses is to fill in the top half of each lens with plain glass. The glasses then become a form of bifocals.

Which sunglasses are best?   Prescription sunglasses are best if you wear your ordinary glasses most of the time. Otherwise, prescription sunglasses are not necessary. Select a color and degree of darkness that is most comfortable. Glasses that lighten indoors and darken outdoors usually prove disappointing. They never clear completely inside, may not get dark enough outside, and always take a while for the color to change. At present, there is some professional concern about their use.

How do contact lenses work?   Placed on the cornea but separated from it by a layer of tears, the contact lens works like a glasses prescription to correct an optical defect. Blinking renews the supply of fluid beneath the lens to keep it afloat and bring fresh oxygen to the cornea.

What are the advantages of contact lenses?   Because contacts rest closer to the center of the eye, better vision is possible. You don't see a glasses' rim and you can more easily look up, down or to the side. Contacts don't steam up like glasses, nor do they catch raindrops or snowflakes when you're out in the weather. The cosmetic advantage is, of course, that you look more natural.

What are the disadvantages of contact lenses?   They cost more and are more trouble than glasses. You have to put them in and take them out every day. You may lose one. If you're not careful, you may harm your eyes by inserting contacts improperly, failing to keep them clean or wearing them for extended periods, such as while you sleep. Dust particles may become trapped between the contact and the eye to cause irritation, tearing and pain. Such problems are most apt to occur when the person is exposed to high winds.

Who can be fitted for contact lenses?   Almost anyone, although, particularly with hard lenses, there is a period of adjustment which varies from person to person, depending on the individual's tolerance. Your ophthalmologist can advise you.

What are the main types of contact lenses? All contacts are now made of plastic, but hard and soft varieties are available. The newer and more expensive soft lenses can be bent and will return to their original shape. Made of water-absorbing plastic, they cause very little discomfort and can be worn for as short or as long a period as you like. Lenses of hard plastic do cause discomfort during the adjustment period and must be worn regularly so that another break-in period isn't necessary. However, vision through soft contacts is not as good as through hard contacts. Another disadvantage of soft lenses is their tendency to absorb eye secretions and mists from hair spray, room deodorant and the like.

Who is most likely to benefit from contact lenses? Someone who must wear glasses all the time, such as a nearsighted person. Contacts are also helpful after cataract surgery (see p. 258). Besides producing grotesque magnification of the person's eyes, cataract spectacles often don't provide adequate vision. Contacts do, and are particularly useful when cataract surgery has been done in only one eye. An eye disease known as keratoconus calls for contacts as part of the treatment. By pressing against the cornea, the hard lenses help to retard the corneal bulging that is typical of this condition.

How often should someone with contact lenses have an eye examination? After the initial adjustment period, the person should have an examination every six months or at least once a year. New prescriptions are not generally needed as often as with glasses, and the main purpose of the examinations is to check the cornea for any problems that may be developing.

EYE INFECTIONS

What causes a sty? Staph bacteria get into an oil gland in the eyelid. An ingrowing eyelash also may set up the infection.

What's the treatment? Dip a very clean, lint-free cloth in warm water and apply it to the closed eye for ten minutes four times a day. Rewarm the rag as necessary. Your physician may instruct you to instill a prescription antibiotic ophthalmic ointment under the lid three or four times a day. Lancing and drainage of pus may be necessary if the infection persists.

What causes itching of the eyes? Itching may reflect irritation in the eyes due to sand or other particles, or result from an infection such as a sty, conjunctivitis or blepharitis. The sufferer of hay fever or similar allergies may note itching of the eyes during the peak of the pollen season. The usual treatment is to correct the underlying problem, and persistent itching calls for an eye examination.

What is "pink eye" or conjunctivitis?   It is an infection of the lining of the eyelid (conjunctiva) caused by bacteria or viruses. It's the most frequent eye problem in a child and may accompany a cold or a sore throat. Sometimes allergy or repetitive rubbing of the eyes causes conjunctivitis. Epidemic conjunctivitis, a form of pink eye that may spread rapidly through a classroom or nursery school, is caused by a species of Hemophilus bacteria.

What are the symptoms of pink eye?   The eye turns red and the lids swell and become sticky; they may be stuck together in the morning. There may be a feeling of scratchiness or sand under the eye. As the infection worsens, pus may drip from the corner of the eye or crust there. The pus may be yellow or green.

What's the treatment for pink eye?   Treatment should be given by a doctor, and includes the instilling of antibiotic ointment or drops into the infected eye. The drops are used every couple of hours at first, the ointment three times a day alone or just at bedtime to supplement the drops. A culture is made so that if improvement doesn't occur, a more specific antibiotic can be given. Any infection of the ear or throat must also be treated. Eyelids that are stuck together can be opened gently after wetting them with warm water.

How can pink eye be prevented?   The child should be kept at home until the conjunctivitis is over. Spread of infection in the household can be prevented by the washing of hands and use of separate towels, face cloths and other personal items. Thorough laundering will remove the infecting bacteria from linens and clothing.

What about chronic conjunctivitis?   Those most apt to have this condition include nearsighted persons, those whose eyes are very sensitive to sunlight and individuals with Down's syndrome (mongolism). The symptoms are burning of the eyes and production of matter, which are most noticeable early in the morning or late in the evening. The cause is unknown, but allergy and irritation of the eyes are sometimes responsible.

Drops containing a steroid are useful if an allergy is present, but their use must be weighed against their potential side effects. In nonspecific conjunctivitis, drops containing methyl cellulose and a 10 or 15 percent solution of sodium sulfacetamide usually provide relief.

What is blepharitis?   It is an inflammation of the lid margins along and in between the eyelashes. Crusting and flaking occur, and the person may note redness and burning of the lids. The treatment is with an eye drop or ointment specifically for blepharitis. Dandruff is frequently associated with this condition and it should also be treated.

EYE INJURIES

What are some common eye injuries? The eye and surrounding area may be cut, bruised, burned or irritated by a chemical. Getting something in the eye is the most common problem. The foreign body may be as harmless as an eyelash or as serious as a piece of steel that has penetrated the eyeball.

What do you do for something in the eye? If it is a piece of metal, glass or other sharp object that is deeply embedded, see the discussion under the next question. If it is a relatively harmless object—an eyelash or a speck of dust—go to a mirror and look at the eye. You may have to use your fingers to open the lids. If you can see the object inside the lower lid or at the side of the eye, wipe it off with the moistened tip of a clean handkerchief. Wipe toward the corner of the eye. The cornea is so sensitive that you shouldn't attempt to touch it; blink until the object moves to the side or below the cornea. If you know how, you can turn over the upper lid to remove whatever is caught there. A simpler way is to pull the upper lid out and down so that the lower lashes wipe its undersurface. When these measures don't give relief, go to a doctor's office or to the emergency room of a hospital.

What foreign bodies cause the most serious injury? A small piece of steel may penetrate the eye while one is hammering a piece of metal or working around a machine that cuts, shapes or resurfaces metal. Traveling at high velocity, the particle may enter the eye with a minimum of external injury. Sometimes only mild pain and smarting of the eye occur. The danger is that the foreign body may cause a delayed reaction resulting in loss of vision weeks, months or years later. Prompt removal is indicated, and may be accomplished by the use of a magnet.

Metal, glass or any object stuck to the cornea could scar it or lead to infection. Pain, blinking and tearing are usually present and the object may be visible as a small dot or irregularity on the cornea. Cover the eye with a patch and seek the services of an ophthalmologist.

What do you do for a cut around the eye? Use pressure to stop the bleeding, and if the cut is anything but a mild injury, go for a medical examination. Sometimes the eye is bruised by the same blow that caused the cut. The injury may provoke bleeding into the front part of the eye behind the cornea. This serious condition requires hospitalization and the attention of an ophthalmologist.

What do you do for a bruise of the eye?   A blow serious enough to cause swelling or discoloration of the eyebrow or eyelids merits a medical examination. This is especially true if the person develops double vision, blurred vision or pain in the eye.

What do you do for a burn of the eye?   Hot grease, scalding water or a flash burn may injure the eye. Wash grease out immediately by splashing water into the open eye. Immersing the face in water with the eye held open will also help to relieve the pain of scalding water or a flash burn. After five or ten minutes of flushing the face and eye, go to the emergency room for an examination. Antibiotic ointment is usually prescribed to prevent an infection.

What is the treatment for an irritating chemical in the eye?   Flush it out by using the spray nozzle of the kitchen sink. Don't use too much water pressure, and aim the nozzle from the side of the face so that the chemical is washed out and down into the sink. Flush for at least five minutes, longer if pain persists, then go to the emergency room or an eye doctor's office. Various eye solutions or ointments may be prescribed to neutralize the chemical and prevent infection.

GLAUCOMA

What is glaucoma?   It is a disease resulting from an increase of pressure in the eye. The pressure elevation may destroy vision, and glaucoma is one of the most common causes of blindness in this country.

What causes glaucoma?   It may be present at birth or occur during the first two years of life because of abnormal development of the eye. Injury, a cataract or bleeding into the eye may produce it. The most frequent mechanism causing glaucoma in an adult is a defective system for letting fluid leave the eye. This trait is usually inherited when one or both parents are carriers. However, a family history for glaucoma does not mean that you will develop it, while absence of a family history does not guarantee that you won't.

What is the exact defect?   The front chamber of the eye gets its nourishment from fluid that continually enters from just behind the iris. Normally the fluid is absorbed at the angle where the iris joins the cornea, but in glaucoma the fluid drains away too slowly. The effects of poor drainage become apparent around age forty, and since fluid still enters the eye at the same rate, the pressure goes up. If the higher pressure continues untreated, the person can gradually lose vision over a period of years and eventually become blind.

How common is glaucoma?   One out of 25 persons over the age of forty has it, but half of these individuals are unaware of the disease.

What are the symptoms of glaucoma?   There may not be any symptoms until eye damage is extensive. Slowly the disease destroys the outer parts of the visual field, creating tunnel vision. The eyeball is firmer than normal. The person may see halos around lights, but not till the glaucoma is advanced.

What is involved in an attack of glaucoma?   A less common form of glaucoma may occur when the susceptible person receives preoperative drugs or eye drops to dilate the eyes before an examination. Severe eye pain develops suddenly, and the eye turns red, swells and may become cloudy. Headache, nausea and abdominal pain occur. The condition will progress to complete and permanent blindness in two to five days if corrective surgery isn't done. A narrow angle between the lens and cornea is responsible for this form of glaucoma. It's estimated that one out of a hundred persons over thirty-five has the narrow-angle defect, but most of them go through life without ever having an attack of glaucoma.

What is the treatment for glaucoma?   Eye drops are prescribed which constrict the pupil and help fluid drain out of the eye. A new type of drop, timolol maleate, accomplishes the same purpose through a different mechanism. Both kinds of drugs are used once or twice daily for life.

Some individuals require water pills, such as acetazolamide, to reduce the rate of fluid formation in the eye. The pills are used in conjunction with drops. Surgery is indicated when medicine fails to keep the eye pressure down, and surgery is the preferred treatment for acute glaucoma. The removal of a small part of the iris provides a drainage area to keep fluid from accumulating in the eye.

What precaution should the victim of glaucoma take?   Drugs used to treat an ulcer, nervous stomach, irritable colon, diarrhea and similar problems may have an action that interferes with the eye drops and causes eye pressure to go up. Agents to avoid are Donnatal, Pro-Banthine, Lomotil and Pamine, but there are others that may also cause problems. Some drugs used to treat Parkinson's disease, such as Artane and Cogentin, may worsen glaucoma.

As a precaution, make sure before any physician prescribes medication that he or she is aware that you have glaucoma and that you cannot take drugs that might increase eye pressure. It is also important that anyone taking the above drugs or others that may increase eye pressure be examined regularly for the onset of glaucoma.

CATARACTS

What is a cataract?   It is a clouding of the lens that distorts or blocks passage of light through the eye. The loss of transparency, caused by precipitation of lens protein, leads to progressive blurring of vision in that eye.

What causes cataract?   Most cataracts occur in persons over sixty as a natural part of aging, and the lens opacity never becomes severe enough to require treatment. Cataract may occur in a young person following injury from a BB pellet or a rock striking the eye. Overexposure to heat or X-ray treatments may create cataracts. Lens opacities may develop as a complication of diabetes and of certain other illnesses.

Does cataract occur in one or both eyes?   Usually both, though not to the same degree. Cataract following injury develops only in the damaged eye.

What are the symptoms of cataract?   Progressive blurring of vision is the only symptom. Cataract does not cause pain or redness in the eye.

How is cataract diagnosed?   An ophthalmologist can make the diagnosis with a slit lamp examination. The doctor can get an idea of whether cataracts exist by having the seated person stare straight ahead in a darkened room while he or she stands to one side and shines the beam of a penlight into the person's eyes. In a normal person a red spot is seen behind each pupil; blood vessels in the retina are responsible for it. The red spot is either not visible or only slightly visible when a cataract is present, because the cloudy lens blocks the pathway for light.

How do you know when a cataract needs treatment?   The decision depends on the degree of visual impairment: treatment is indicated if the impairment interferes with the person's ordinary activities. Another consideration is whether cataracts are present in both eyes. If so, the eye with the poorer sight is usually treated first so that the other eye can serve the person's needs during the treatment period. Even if one eye is good enough, the cataract should be removed from the other eye so that normal activity is not restricted.

What is the treatment for cataract?   An operation is done to remove the opacified lens through a small incision in the eye. The lens is first frozen or emulsified to keep it from breaking apart during removal. The person

257

must wear cataract spectacles or contact lenses after surgery to make up for the loss of focusing power from the removed lens.

Are both eyes operated on at the same time? No, because the eye that was not operated on has to serve the person's needs for the three months before glasses or a contact lens can be fitted to the operated eye. Adjusting to the contact lens or the spectacles may take an additional period of time. Six months or a year later the second cataract can be removed if this is desirable.

What category of patients is most likely to have successful cataract surgery?
This is impossible to predict, because things don't always go as anticipated. Postoperative infection may develop, though in most instances this can be successfully treated. Those with arthritis or Parkinson's disease may have trouble manipulating the spectacles or contacts, yet without these the operated eye is virtually sightless. The spectacles may seem too heavy and it may be difficult to adjust to contacts. All these relatively minor inconveniences are as nothing, of course, when compared to the total loss of sight when cataracts are not removed.

Which are best, a contact lens or spectacles? The main problem with cataract spectacles is that to achieve focusing they must magnify the image by 20 to 30 percent. The magnification is so much larger than the image from the opposite eye that the brain reacts by shutting out the larger image. A contact lens gets around this problem by enlarging the image only 8 to 10 percent. This is not too much disparity for the brain to accept, and it's why ophthalmologists strongly encourage use of a contact lens following surgery on the first eye. When the other cataract is removed, the person can get a second contact lens or use cataract glasses. Still another advantage of contacts is that they don't magnify the eyes as cataract spectacles do.

What are the advantages and disadvantages of a lens implant? This has been hailed as a breakthrough for the person needing cataract surgery. After the natural lens is removed, an artificial one made of polymethyl methacrylate is inserted. The advantage is that it produces an image enlargement of only 2 percent, which poses no problem in the brain's fusion with the image from the unoperated eye. Neither contacts nor spectacles are necessary.

Many persons who've had a lens implant are extremely happy with it, but a disadvantage is that since it's usually done at the time of initial surgery, a lens implant must be planned before the person has a chance to know how well he or she might do with contacts or spectacles. Lens implant is more likely to cause a complication such as infection or eye damage. A reaction with progressive loss of sight in the operated eye is another possibility.

OTHER EYE PROBLEMS

What is night blindness?　　True night blindness, a rare condition due to vitamin A deficiency, is much less often a cause of poor night vision than conditions such as cataract or glaucoma, which may interfere with vision in bright or dim light. Difficulty in seeing at night may be an early symptom of retinitis pigmentosa, an inherited degeneration of the retina.

What is color blindness?　　It is an inherited condition causing an inability to perceive certain colors or shades of colors. Eight percent of men are color-blind, but the trait affects only one out of 250 women. It is particularly troublesome when the individual cannot distinguish between red and green —the color of traffic signals.

What diseases may cause blindness?　　Conditions that may cause a loss of sight are optic neuritis, diabetes and retinal detachment.

· *Optic neuritis,* inflammation of the main nerve to the eye, may follow the flu, measles, mumps or meningitis. The person notes sudden blurring in one eye accompanied by tenderness in the eye and pain on moving it. Visual loss may be complete, or the condition may improve after six to twelve weeks. A fourth of persons with optic neuritis are later found to have multiple sclerosis. The treatment of optic neuritis depends on its cause and is best undertaken by an ophthalmologist.

· *Diabetes* may damage the retina, and one in six persons with acquired blindness has it because of diabetes. Blindness rarely occurs before fifteen or twenty years of the disease, and good control of diabetes will help to protect against this complication. Laser beams have been used successfully to treat the retinal vessels.

· *Retinal detachment* may follow an injury to the eye or occur spontaneously, usually in someone over the age of forty. Nearsightedness predisposes to it. Spots and/or light flashes appear before the eye. The earliest symptom may be painless blurring of vision or a distortion of the visual field. Sometimes the onset is described as being like a curtain was pulled down over the eye. Though the eye may not look different from the outside, an ophthalmologist can make the diagnosis by looking at the retina. Surgery to reattach the retina is usually successful in treating this condition. Treatment should be sought as soon as possible after the onset of symptoms.

What causes spots to appear before the eyes?　　The person with migraine may see spots, as may someone who has high blood pressure or who has been using drugs or alcohol to excess. A very common cause of seeing spots that actually represent something in the eye is a situation where particles break off from the inner lining of the eye and float through the liquid in front of the retina. The particles shift when the eye shifts, and the vision can never seem to quite catch up to them. These floaters are absorbed in a day or so and don't usually mean the person has eye disease. Persistence of spots before the eyes calls for an eye examination.

When is a corneal transplant indicated?   It may be done to restore sight when a cornea has become opacified because of injury or infection. Because the cornea has no blood supply and hence can't reject a transplant, the surgery is successful in a high percentage of those who have it.

What causes excessive tearing from one eye?   Excessive tearing reflects an obstruction of the tear duct at the corner of the eye. This may occur in a baby as a mild abnormality of development, or in an adult as the result of infection or excessive matter in the eye. An eye doctor can probe the tear duct to relieve it of the obstruction, but antibiotic eye drops may be sufficient to cure the problem when an infection is responsible.

What causes a growth at the corner of the eye?   Pinguecula is a yellow nodule that may form in the corner of the eye, usually in someone over thirty-five. Since it doesn't interfere with vision, treatment isn't usually necessary. A pterygium is a layer of fleshy material that grows from either side of the eye toward the cornea. Exposure to dust and wind contributes to its development. An eye doctor can remove it under local anesthesia if it interferes with vision.

What causes a growth in the eyelid?   Infection of an oil gland causes a sty, and low-grade infection after the sty is healed may obstruct the gland, leading to accumulation of an oily material. The growth may reach the size of a peanut. The cheesy material can be removed by a doctor through a small incision in the eyelid.

What causes a ring around the iris?   A white or grayish ring around the iris in the cornea may signal an elevated cholesterol or triglyceride level in the blood. The ring may appear as a normal accompaniment of aging in older persons. Wilson's disease, a rare defect of copper metabolism, causes a golden brown or greenish brown ring around the cornea. The disease begins during the teenage years and affects the nervous system and liver.

How does a tumor develop in the eye?   A melanoma may arise from a pigmented part of the eye or a cancer may invade the eye from the adjacent tissues. Retinoblastoma is a tumor occurring in children under three. It is signaled by a white spot appearing in the pupil, and when it is diagnosed, the affected eye is sometimes removed and sometimes treated with radiation. Since the tendency to have this type of tumor is inherited, persons who have survived retinoblastoma should visit a genetic counselor to determine the risks of passing it to a child.

Can oxygen therapy damage a baby's vision?   Yes, a premature baby exposed to a high oxygen concentration during the first two weeks of life may, as a result of this treatment to sustain life, develop retinal damage. Such children may be blind for life. Babies at greatest risk are those who weigh less than three pounds at birth and who suffer from a lung problem requiring oxygen as treatment. This occurs less frequently than in the past now that the risk is understood.

How can oxygen damage be prevented?   An oxygen concentration of 40 percent or less is apparently safe, but the baby's blood level of oxygen must be followed while therapy is given.

10

EARS, NOSE
and THROAT

How does the ear work?   Noise produces vibrations that are caught by the outer ear and reflected into the ear canal causing the eardrum to vibrate. Three small bones behind the drum convey the vibrations through the middle ear to the inner ear, where fluid movement is transformed into nerve impulses. The impulses pass to the brain through the auditory nerve and are interpreted as sound.

What is the ear canal?   It is an opening in the bone that is lined with skin. Because it angles forward and slightly upward in the direction of the opposite eye, it is protected from wind, rain and foreign objects.

Where does earwax come from?   The ear canal contains specialized glands that secrete cerumen, or earwax. The wax lubricates the ear canal and the eardrum.

What is the eardrum?   It is a thin, tensed membrane measuring about a fifth of an inch in diameter. It resembles a snare drum, although it is slightly cone-shaped from the pressure of a small bone protruding into its middle.

How is the ear structured?   The outer ear is the part you can see, and the ear canal leads into the drum. Behind the drum are three small bones, the malleus, incus and stapes, that lie in the middle ear. The middle ear is a chamber connected to the throat by the eustachian tubes, which open a thousand times a day—each time you swallow or yawn—and serve to keep the pressure in the middle ears equal to the atmospheric pressure. The stapes transmits vibrations to the cochlea, a sensory organ in the inner ear. Containing fluid and specialized hairs, the cochlea can convert sound waves into nerve impulses. Another part of the inner ear, the semicircular canals, helps to maintain body position and equilibrium.

What's the best way to clean the ears?   The best course is not to clean the ears. Cerumen is secreted constantly, dries and falls out of the ear carrying with it hair, bits of lint and other particles that enter the canal. It is the natural cleaner, and should not be removed unless it is causing a problem. Try softening surplus dry wax with a few drops of baby oil or glycerine or a product created especially for this purpose. A little peroxide will also help rinse the ear. Instill the softener twice a day for several days, and the wax may leave on its own. Removal of problem wax should be done by a nurse or physician.

What physician should treat ear problems?   A general physician or pediatrician is competent to handle most ear problems. Seek help from an ear specialist when a problem recurs or is accompanied by a complication such as perforated eardrum or hearing loss. The otologist practices nothing but medical and surgical treatment of ear diseases, and the otolaryngologist (short for otorhinolaryngologist) treats ear disease as well as problems of the nose and throat. These specialists must complete four years of postdoctoral surgical training to obtain Board certification. The best way to find a good one is to follow the recommendation of your primary physician. If you're unhappy with the specialist, ask for referral to another one.

How often should your ears be examined?   They should be examined at each routine physical checkup. Hearing should be tested in a preschool child—earlier if hearing loss or speech delay is suspected—and regularly in an adult who has a loss, suspects a loss, or is around loud noises at work or play.

HEARING LOSS

How can hearing be tested?   A trained individual can use a tuning fork and the whispered voice to screen for hearing loss, but the two best tests are the audiogram and tympanometry. Both are available through an ear specialist or a speech and hearing department associated with a school district, college or university.

In the audiogram examination the person being tested indicates when he or she can hear sounds at various wave frequencies and decibels of intensity, and the responses are evaluated. Tympanometry is a simpler test by which sound waves are passed into the ear through a small device that picks up the waves as they are reflected by the eardrum. The test can be used with small children and retarded persons.

How common is hearing loss?   An estimated 5 to 10 percent of Americans have impaired hearing.

What are the main types of hearing loss?   A conductive or nerve defect may occur, and some persons suffer from both types of hearing impairment. A conductive defect results from anything that interferes with the transmission of sound waves to the inner ear. The causes include plugging of the ear canal by earwax or a foreign body, ear infection, fluid in the ear, perforated eardrum and otosclerosis (see pp. 266, 268 and 269).

A nerve defect results from damage to the auditory nerve by a birth injury, encephalitis, Meniere's disease or a brain tumor. The eardrum and middle ear may be normal, but the nerve or the brain's hearing center is unable to perceive sound. The condition known as presbyacusis is a type of nerve deafness occurring in many older individuals. Exposure to loud noise or, rarely, to certain drugs can also damage hearing.

What frequency of vibrations can the ear normally perceive?   The normal range is 30 to 20,000 cycles a second. Best hearing occurs at frequencies of 600 to 6,000 cycles a second, and, up to a point, the louder the sound in decibels the easier it is to hear. The voice emits a frequency of 1,000 to 2,000 cycles a second at an intensity of 45 to 55 decibels.

What is a decibel?   It is a unit of measurement for sound intensity. The level at which a normal person can perceive sound is set at 0 decibels. Changes in intensity of even one decibel can be perceived by the human ear, and noise greater than 55 or 60 decibels is uncomfortable.

How harmful is an excessive noise level?   A sound level of more than 90 decibels is capable of damaging the hearing if the exposure is repeated often enough. Since noise-induced hearing loss is greatest for frequencies above those of normal speech, it may go undetected until it is quite advanced.

What are the common sources of harmful noise?   At work, these include airplane engines, farm machinery, industrial machinery, a tractor or loud truck engine, a jackhammer and detonations from mining operations or explosives used in the building industry. Potentially harmful noises are those produced by a rock 'n' roll band, subway trains, gunfire or the firing of heavy ordnance during military maneuvers or wartime.

How loud must the noise be to damage hearing?   Levels above 90 decibels are potentially damaging, but the length of exposure must also be considered. Eight hours of exposure to 90 decibels day after day will certainly damage hearing, but exposure for a much shorter time may not. Even very limited exposure to noises above 150 decibels might damage hearing.

What are the early symptoms of noise-induced hearing damage?   Ringing in the ears and hearing loss are most pronounced at the end of the period of exposure. The person may not hear others well above the background of a radio or TV. High-pitched sounds, such as those made by a violin or oboe, may become hard to hear, especially for people over forty.

What is the treatment for noise-induced hearing loss?   Some of the loss is temporary and correctable if the person is removed from the source of the noise. This may require a change of job or leisure activity. Occupational safety standards require that the person wear ear protection in the form of earplugs or earmuffs during exposure to a noise level of 90 decibels or greater.

What drugs may cause hearing loss?   Drugs that may damage hearing include streptomycin, kanamycin, neomycin and certain other antibiotics. Aspirin, quinine and Lasix may also damage hearing. Ringing in the ears is an early sign of an overdose of aspirin or quinine.

What can be done to avoid a harmful drug?   One may have to make a trade-off, as when streptomycin therapy is necessary to treat life-threatening tuberculosis. In every instance, ask the doctor about the side effects of a drug and ask if a safer agent could be used. Consider getting by without drug therapy if possible. Certain new drugs, which haven't stood the test of time, may have side effects that no one is yet aware of.

How often is hearing loss inherited?   One in four deaf persons inherit the defect, and inherited deafness usually begins during childhood.

When is a hearing aid of use in treating deafness?   It may help when surgery or medical therapy cannot improve hearing. An aid should be purchased on the prescription of an ear specialist. The wearer must be trained in its use and should get regular checkups to make sure the aid is functioning properly. It is very important to obtain your aid from a reputable supplier. Ask your ear specialist to recommend a good, honest dealer.

In what other ways can the hearing-impaired individual be helped?   Lip reading is a very useful skill that most persons can learn, and it should

265

include training in the interpretation of facial expressions, body movement and gestures. Sign language is a way of communicating with the totally deaf individual.

In the classroom a child with poor hearing in only one ear should sit where the bad ear is on the side of the wall or windows and the good ear is turned to the teacher and classmates. A hearing-impaired person can understand you better if you look at him or her when speaking. Talk clearly and a little louder than normal, but don't shout. Turn off the radio and TV while speaking, and don't try to talk over the conversation of others.

OTOSCLEROSIS

What is otosclerosis?   A slowly progressive cause of conductive deafness beginning during early adulthood. Bony overgrowth limits the movement of the stapes so that sound waves can't be transmitted to the inner ear. An inherited condition, otosclerosis is passed from an affected parent to about 40 percent of his or her children. Because the condition is aggravated by pregnancy, otosclerosis is more likely to occur earlier and be more severe in a woman than in a man.

What's the treatment for otosclerosis?   Surgery to mobilize or replace the deformed stapes with an artificial one may be employed. Nine out of ten persons get good results from this operation, which is done on one ear at a time.

EAR INFECTIONS

What causes earache?   Infection is the most frequent cause, but earache may result from fluid in the ear (p. 267) or the presence of a wax plug or foreign body (pp. 263, 270). Perforated eardrum (p. 268) and stopped-up ear (p. 270) are additional causes of ear pain.

What are the main types of ear infections?   Infection of the middle ear is most common, but an infection may occur in the outer ear, the ear canal or the inner ear. A serious inflammation of the middle ear may penetrate through the adjacent bone to cause mastoiditis.

What are the symptoms of an infection of the outer ear?   Swelling, redness and pain occur in the ear, and pus formation may accompany a severe infection.

What are the causes of this infection?   A cut or blow to the ear may be followed by infection. Ear-piercing is a fairly frequent cause if the needle wasn't sterile or the post left in the hole was contaminated by bacteria.

What is the treatment?   Local application of heat may hasten healing of a mild infection, but antibiotics are indicated to treat a more severe infection of the outer ear. When the problem occurs after ear-piercing, the earring must be removed to allow healing.

What are the symptoms of an infected ear canal?   The ear hurts, and the pain is worse if you tug on the earlobe or apply pressure to the ear, as, for example, when you sleep on it. Itching is noted at the ear opening, and discharge of clear to pus-like material indicates that the infection is serious.

What causes the infection?   Getting water in the ear from showering or swimming is a frequent cause. Water may also collect in the ear from sweating or wearing earplugs on a hot day. Because the ear canal of a child is shorter and less well protected than an adult's, these infections are most common in children.

The person who scratches the ear canal with a matchstick or similar object may create the infection. Allergy to hair spray, soap, perfume, cologne or the constituents of an earplug or earmuff may set off an infection. Seborrheic dermatitis, the scaly scalp and facial condition that causes dandruff, may cause itching, swelling and discharge in the ear canal.

What is the treatment for an infected ear canal?   The discharge should be removed by a physician or nurse. Ear drops are instilled four times a day until several days after the infection has subsided. Prevention of another infection may require that the person wear plugs while swimming and use acidified alcohol drops (made by mixing equal parts of plain white vinegar and 70 percent ethyl alcohol) before and after swimming. The drops help to keep the ear canal dry. When allergy is suspected, the inciting agent must be avoided.

What are the symptoms of middle-ear infection?   Earache and fever occur, and fussiness may be observed in a small child.

What is the cause of middle-ear infection?   Very often the child or adult has had a cold or strep throat a week or two before the ear infection, and germs reach the middle ear by passing up the eustachian tube. Another common cause is changes in altitude, particularly in flying and especially when you have a cold. Avoid flying while you have a cold, or use a decongestant if you must fly.

What is the treatment for middle-ear infection?   Antibiotics are prescribed according to the tolerance and age of the patient. Ampicillin is often used to treat ear infection in a small child.

Is an injection better than pills?   The adage physicians learn is that you should never give a drug intravenously when it can be given intramuscularly, and that you should never give an injection if the person can be treated by pills. A shot produces a higher blood level of penicillin and a quicker relief of symptoms, but it is much more likely to cause a serious reaction in the event of an allergy.

What are the complications of a middle-ear infection?   An infection may perforate the eardrum, damage the middle ear or penetrate into the mastoid bone to cause mastoiditis. Hearing loss may accompany any of these complications.

What are the symptoms of a perforated eardrum?   The person may have hearing loss in that ear. Chronic drainage from the ear may occur, or there may be frequent bouts of infection in the ear. An older child or adult with a perforated eardrum may note at times that air entering through the eustachian tube escapes from the ear. Earache may occur.

What causes a perforated eardrum?   An infection of the eardrum is the most common cause, but poking a matchstick or hairpin into the canal could rupture the drum. Less common causes include a blow to the ear, lightning strike or injury from a firecracker or other explosive.

What is the treatment for a perforated eardrum?   It usually heals on its own in a couple of weeks. Should the hole in the drum persist, the child or adult may need surgery to close it. An operation is not indicated until any infection that may be present has been controlled. In the case of children, surgeons may prefer to wait until the child is nine or ten years old before repairing the drum. Intensive antibiotic therapy may bring about a slow healing without surgery.

What are the symptoms of mastoiditis?   Pain and swelling occur in the bony hood behind the ear. Pressure or tapping on this area will cause pain. The person's eardrum is perforated and the ear drains a pus-like material.

What causes mastoiditis?   It results from a continued middle-ear infection in the presence of a perforated eardrum. The disease is most common in children, but it is much less prevalent since antibiotics became available for ear infections.

What's the treatment for mastoiditis?   The patient should be admitted to the hospital and placed under the care of an otologist. Intensive antibiotic therapy is indicated, and if this fails to eradicate the infection, surgery must be done to remove infected bone and repair the damage to the middle ear. An element of urgency is indicated to prevent the formation of a cholesteatoma.

What is a cholesteatoma?   A tissue-filled cyst in the mastoid bone that forms as the result of a middle-ear infection and mastoiditis. Cells from the ear canal grow inward to contribute to the growth, which tends to enlarge, gradually destroying more bone and preventing the middle ear from healing. Though not a cancer, cholesteatoma may behave like a tumor in that it wears away bone and resists ordinary therapy.

What's the treatment for cholesteatoma?   The cyst and the surrounding mastoid bone must be removed.

What do you do for recurring ear infections?   After three or more middle-ear infections within six months, a child is a candidate for taking preventive doses of penicillin; the medicine must be taken by mouth each day or by injection once a month and the child should be watched closely for side effects and for the possible development of an allergy to the drug.

What are the symptoms of eustachian-tube obstruction?   An older child or adult will complain of hearing loss in the ear. The person's own voice sounds louder in that ear, and is heard with an echo quality, as though he or she were speaking into a barrel. A young child typically has few complaints other than frequent colds and hearing loss; pain doesn't usually occur unless the obstruction is accompanied by infection.

What causes eustachian-tube obstruction?   It may follow frequent colds or sore throats when swelling in the throat shuts off one or both tubes and creates a vacuum in the middle-ear cavity. The vacuum occurs because air is constantly being absorbed from the middle ear and the eustachian tubes can no longer bring in more air from the throat. The negative pressure generates a discharge of fluid into the cavity.

What's the treatment for eustachian-tube obstruction?   The tubes may open after treatment of the child's cold or sore throat. Air may be forced through the eustachian tubes by having the child blow up a balloon while holding his or her nose. Or the physician may use an inflator to increase pressure in the throat while the child swallows. To be successful, the inflations must be done six times a day until the eustachian tubes remain open. Surgically implanted ear tubes are needed when the obstruction persists.

What are ear tubes?   They are small, flanged polyethylene tubes that are inserted into the lower half of the eardrums by an ear specialist or physician trained in their use. The surgery may be done under local or general anesthesia.

What's the purpose of the tubes?   They serve to decompress the middle-ear cavity and take over the function of blocked eustachian tubes. The fluid in the middle ear will run out through the tubes.

How long are the tubes left in?   Long enough to give the eustachian tubes time to rest and heal, or several months to a year or more. The child should be examined every three or four months. Most children show a spontaneous improvement in eustachian-tube function at the age of seven or eight. Treatment of enlarged adenoids or nasal allergies, such as hay fever, may be necessary to prevent a recurrence of the eustachian-tube obstruction.

Can a child with ear tubes still go swimming?   One type of ear tubes is designed to make swimming possible; the tubes swell shut when in contact with water in the ear canal. The child who wants to continue swimming should ask for these before the ear-tube operation. Others should wear ear plugs.

OTHER EAR PROBLEMS

What are some common objects that may get into the ear?   Foreign bodies that may find their way into the ear of a child include a bead or small plastic item, a pebble, a piece of twig or an insect. Other items that may get into the ear are gum, food, string or a piece of cotton or crayon.

What's the treatment?   Instilling several drops of ethyl alcohol (or gin) into the ear may kill an insect, but it and the other items mentioned above will probably have to be removed by a physician or nurse.

What causes "stopped-up" ear?   This occurs when a eustachian tube stops functioning temporarily and the pressure in the middle ear doesn't stay the same as atmospheric pressure. It may occur when you're driving in the mountains, diving in deep water or descending in an airplane. Pilots often speak of it as "ear block."

What are the symptoms?   The ear feels stopped up and uncomfortable. You can't hear normally through it, though when only one ear is stopped up, you hear your own voice loudest in that ear.

What's the treatment? If you can yawn, the eustachian tube may open with a click announcing the sudden equalization of pressure in the ear. Try chewing some gum, drinking a glass of water or eating a meal, since swallowing may open the tube. Blowing against a closed nose may help, but do not blow too vigorously. Decongestants found in cold preparations may open the tube. Prescription drugs such as Dimetapp or Actifed may be useful. Aspirin and moist heat will relieve pain. The condition is self-limited and the tube will open in a day or so on its own. See a physician if symptoms are severe or persist for more than a day.

What causes vertigo? There are many causes of a light-headed feeling or a sensation of faintness, but vertigo is the true dizziness that accompanies ear disease. The person with vertigo feels as though he or she were revolving in space or that objects in the environment are moving about. The sensation often begins abruptly and is accompanied by incapacitating nausea, vomiting and an inability to stand up or walk. It is aggravated by any change in body position.

Vertigo reflects an inner-ear problem. The semicircular canals are filled with fluid, and when you bend your head to one side the fluid in the canals tilts with you so that the brain is aware of the change in position. Any disturbance of the fluid in these canals will garble the messages going to the brain and create vertigo.

What conditions are usually responsible? The causes of vertigo include Meniere's disease, viral infection of the inner ear, head injury, brain tumor, migraine and therapy with streptomycin, aspirin, quinine and other drugs. Benign positional vertigo is a frequent condition. It occurs only on sudden change of position, such as when one rolls over in bed. A momentary spinning or revolving sensation occurs, but everything soon returns to normal.

What's the treatment for vertigo? Hospitalization is indicated when a person develops severe vertigo. X-rays and other studies are done to determine the cause, and the acute symptoms are relieved with intravenous fluids and symptomatic drugs. Mild vertigo may improve when the person stops using coffee, alcohol and tobacco and goes on a low-salt diet. Dramamine may be used for symptomatic relief. Benign positional vertigo may return every few months or years, but it requires no treatment.

What is Meniere's disease? This inner-ear disease occurs most commonly in men forty to sixty years old and is characterized by attacks of vertigo, nausea, vomiting and hearing loss. The attacks last up to several hours, then leave as mysteriously as they appeared. Ringing or a roaring sound such as

271

that heard when a seashell is held against the ear occurs in the involved ear during an attack, and hearing loss may progress in this ear in between attacks. It's not unusual for the involved ear to become totally deaf after several years of Meniere's disease.

What causes Meniere's disease?   The cause is unknown, but excess production of fluid in the inner ear may contribute to the condition.

What's the treatment?   Intravenous infusion of Valium has been found to control the symptoms of Meniere's disease; the person must be hospitalized and observed during the treatment. Ear surgery may help when there is no response to medical therapy.

What causes motion sickness?   It's due to stimulation of the inner ear by repetitive motion as may occur during travel by air, auto, train or boat. Adolescents are the most susceptible, and psychic factors play a role.

What's the treatment for motion sickness?   Taken thirty minutes or an hour before a trip, Dramamine or Marezine may prevent motion sickness. It may be possible to avert an attack by leaning back, closing the eyes, drawing the shoulders together and breathing deeply. Fresh cool air is helpful. It's advantageous to sit in the front seat next to the window of an auto or toward the front of an airplane or train.

What causes ringing in the ears?   Though it's often a ringing sensation, noise in the ears may sound more like a buzzing, humming or roaring. It tends to be worse at night when there are no daytime noises to drown it out. Aspirin and other salicylates may cause it, especially if taken in high doses; ringing in the ears may be the first sign calling for a reduction in dosage. Ringing in the ears may accompany otosclerosis, Meniere's disease, hearing loss from excessive noise and almost any other ear problem. Vibrations from diseased blood vessels are sometimes responsible, especially when the person has anemia or hardening of the arteries—conditions favoring turbulent blood flow.

What's the treatment for ringing in the ears?   The underlying problem should be pinpointed and corrected if possible. Sometimes, it's possible to divert yourself from the anxiety the noise causes by going to sleep to the sound of a radio station or tape deck. In persistent cases, you might consider getting a pillow speaker.

FACE AND NOSE

What is the function of the sinuses?   The sinuses, which are connected to the nose by small openings, warm and clean the air that is breathed and give resonance to the voice.

What are the symptoms of sinusitis?   An attack generally begins with a cold and is accompanied by nasal discharge, nasal stuffiness and postnasal drip. Pain localizes in the face or forehead and is worse when the person leans forward. The painful areas are tender to the touch. Sometimes the teeth ache during an attack, and the person may have fever, generalized aching and severe headache. Smoldering sinusitis may cause few symptoms other than occasional stuffy nose and postnasal drip.

What causes sinusitis?   Because the sinuses open into the nose, forceful blowing of the nose, as, for example, when you have a cold, may propel secretions into them. Diving into the water or jumping in feet first may produce sinus contamination in a similar manner. Nasal allergies, nasal polyps, dental infections and facial injury are other causes of sinusitis.

What's the treatment for sinusitis?   Antibiotics and decongestants may relieve severe symptoms, or a physician can use a large needle to wash pus and fluid out of the sinuses. Repeat washings may be needed every week for several months. An operation to remove inflammatory material and promote better sinus drainage may become necessary, but should not be done until the person has had vigorous treatment for nasal allergies and has had all nasal polyps removed.

What are nasal polyps?   The polyps, which may be caused by hay fever or cystic fibrosis, are soft pink or grayish growths inside the nose. They're overgrowths of the lining of the nose that obstruct the flow of air and secretions.

What are the symptoms of nasal polyps?   A child with nasal polyps may constantly breathe through the mouth. An adult may note progressive nasal stuffiness and discomfort in the nose.

What is the treatment for nasal polyps?   They may have to be removed surgically, though small ones may regress when the person's allergies are brought under control.

What is hay fever?   Specifically, an allergic reaction to pollen, but other nasal allergies to dust, animal dander, industrial smog or other airborne particles produce the same symptoms.

What are the symptoms of hay fever and other nasal allergies?   Attacks of sneezing, runny nose and itching of the nose and eyes appear each spring and at other times when the causative allergens are most prevalent. Even between attacks, nasal stuffiness and postnasal drip are a problem.

When do symptoms usually begin?   Often during childhood but not usually till after age two or three (see p. 156). A fourth of afflicted boys improve spontaneously at puberty, while some girls have more difficulty after the onset of menstruation. The condition may persist for life and one out of ten people suffers from it.

What's the treatment for a nasal allergy attack?   Symptomatic relief can be obtained by using antihistamines. It is not a good idea to use nose drops because of a rebound worsening of nasal congestion after the effects of the drops wear off. Nose drops also may tend to be habit-forming.

What is allergy therapy?   It is the only definitive treatment for hay fever, and consists of desensitization against the offending allergens. An allergist, who has been trained in pediatrics or internal medicine and has had an additional year or two of training in the treatment of allergic diseases, should manage the desensitization program. Once the allergens are identified by skin testing, these substances are injected in progressively larger doses until the person is no longer allergic to them. Precautions against an allergic reaction must be observed each time the shots are given, and the injections have to be continued every few weeks at regular intervals even after the allergies have been brought under control. The treatment program lasts two to four years, and three-fourths of those who take it note a definite improvement in symptoms.

What else can be done for nasal allergy?   Avoiding the allergen is helpful:
· Keep animals outside the house or, if necessary, give up the pet.
· Remove feathers, felt, kapok and items containing them from the house. Substitute Dacron-filled pillows.
· Keep the house as dust-free as possible. Use dustproof coverings over the mattress and box springs. If you have air conditioning or forced-air heating, change the air filter on the blower very often. Keep books and furniture free of dust.
· Clean the showers and tub with a chlorine disinfectant twice a year to check formation of molds, and paint the woodwork and walls with special paint that will inhibit the growth of molds.
· Give up gardening or houseplants if you are very allergic to the pollen of flowers or vegetables or to leaf mold.

Will moving to another climate help?　　Obviously, if you have severe allergies to pollutants of various kinds, it would be better to live in an area where these aren't prevalent, if you can find it. Moving almost always brings a temporary relief from allergies. The problem is that since it's impossible to find an area having no pollen, dust, mold and other airborne particles, new allergies soon develop.

What causes nosebleed?　　The most common cause is irritation of the nose from frequent blowing. In a child the usual cause is a blow to the nose or a mild injury from picking or rubbing it. In an adult, high blood pressure is sometimes responsible. Ineffective blood clotting may cause nosebleed. The possibilities include leukemia, hemophilia, platelet disorders and the use of certain drugs, even aspirin. Severe sinusitis or a cold is occasionally a cause of nosebleed.

How do you know when nosebleed is serious?　　It's serious when it persists despite pressure on the front of the nose as described on pp. 198–99. It's also a sign of serious bleeding when enough blood is swallowed to cause vomiting, when the bleeding is accompanied by dizziness or loss of consciousness or when the bleeding interferes with breathing.

What's the treatment?　　A doctor may have to insert a pack into the nose to stop the bleeding. Sometimes a wedge of salt pork, which won't stick to the nasal lining, is used instead. Platelet transfusions or infusion of a specific clotting factor may be indicated when the person has a clotting disorder.

How can recurrent nosebleed be prevented?　　Daily application of petrolatum to the inside of the nostril may prevent a recurrence. The person should not take aspirin or blow the nose forcefully. Cauterization of bleeding vessels, a minor procedure that may be performed by a nose specialist, is sometimes helpful for recurrent bleeding.

What are the symptoms of a foreign body in the nose?　　The nose is stopped up on that side and a discharge begins if the item is not removed promptly. Such things as small plastic toys, gum, seeds, nuts or beans, are most likely to get into the nose of a child or a very old person. Because a bean swells as it absorbs fluid, it may be a particularly serious foreign body.

What's the treatment?　　The object should be removed by a physician.

What are the symptoms of a tumor of the nose?　　A tumor may cause nosebleed, obstruction of the nose, nasal discharge or pain and swelling.

With continued growth, the tumor may create facial enlargement and press upward on the eye to cause double vision.

What kinds of tumors may occur in the nose?   A benign tumor known as juvenile angiofibroma occurs in teenage boys. It grows slowly, erodes the surrounding tissue, and causes nosebleed and nasal obstruction. A malignant tumor may arise in the nose or spread to the nose from one of the sinuses.

What is the treatment for a tumor of the nose?   It should be removed by an ear, nose and throat specialist.

What may cause a deformity of the nose?   The nose may have been broken and healed imperfectly, or its natural structure may be uneven because of a beak or hump in the bony structure or a bulbous or drooping tip. The nasal septum may distort the face by curving to one side during the rapid-growth phase of adolescence. This is commonly called a deviated septum. Less common causes of deformity are loss of part of a nostril from an infection or injury, such as a human bite, and overgrowth of the tip of the nose due to the condition known as rhinophyma. The latter occurs most often in middle-aged men of oily complexion who drink heavily.

Can a nose deformity be corrected?   Yes, nasal surgery (rhinoplasty) is the most commonly performed cosmetic operation. It can be done by a plastic surgeon or by an ear, nose and throat specialist. Rhinoplasty is not usually done until after the nose has reached adult size, which usually occurs between the ages of fifteen and seventeen.

MOUTH

What causes bad breath?   Poor dental hygiene is the most common cause; food particles trapped between the teeth and gums putrefy and create an odor. Halitosis is especially apt to occur in someone who has periodontitis, a chronic inflammation of the gum margins. Other causes are sinus infection, lung infection, dental abscess, throat or nose infection, stomach or intestinal disorders and stagnation of saliva. The last is responsible for the fairly universal "morning odor" that is relieved by washing the mouth and teeth. Eating onions or garlic or drinking alcoholic beverages will obviously taint the breath temporarily. A child's body may absorb an offensive odor, as from dirty feet, and excrete it through the lungs to produce halitosis. Due to the lung's role in excreting an excess of metabolic by-products, a person with kidney or liver failure may have bad breath.

What can be done for bad breath?   The teeth should be brushed after each meal or at least three times a day, and the tongue should be brushed, too. The toothbrush should be firm enough to remove food particles. Many dentists advise dental flossing once a day: floss after brushing and you may be surprised at the number of food particles left between the teeth. Other dentists may advise the use of a Water Pik. Visit a physician if malodor persists, for it could be caused by a medical condition.

Does a mouthwash help?   It may, but it should not take the place of good oral hygiene.

What causes coated ("furred") tongue?   A coated tongue is not necessarily a sign of illness. Food stains may build up on the tongue of an adult unless these are brushed away. Coffee causes a yellow or brown coating, milk a white coating, and other foods may create shades of yellow or gray. Smoking contributes to furry tongue. Black tongue ("hairy tongue") may follow a course of antibiotic therapy or a febrile illness; it represents excessive growth of the papillae of the tongue and pigment formation by bacteria in the mouth.

What is the treatment?   Regular brushing of the tongue will remove the coating in many instances and prevent its recurrence. In the case of hairy tongue, brushing may suffice, or one may need topical medication as prescribed by a doctor or dentist.

What causes the tongue to turn red and painful?   Deficiency of iron, vitamin A, the B vitamins or niacin may irritate the tongue. A person with a condition called geographic tongue develops irregular red patches that are most pronounced during or right after an illness. The cause of this condition is not known. Infection of the tongue may follow injury from biting it, contact with very hot food or chewing sharp or pointed foods. Initially red, the tongue may swell and turn dark as the infection progresses.

What's the treatment?   A red or painful tongue should be evaluated by a physician. Correction of a vitamin or iron deficiency may be necessary, and symptomatic relief from geographic tongue can be obtained by using a dental paste containing a steroid hormone.

What causes white patches on the tongue?   In a baby or a diabetic, the likely cause is thrush, an infection due to *Candida albicans.* It can be cured by treatment with nystatin, available by prescription.

In an older person, especially one who smokes, uses a pipe or has bad teeth, a leathery patch on the tongue or anywhere inside the mouth may be a forerunner of cancer. The plaque may be yellow or white and tends to occur at a spot that is injured frequently by chewing or is repeatedly exposed to the hot stem of the pipe.

What's the treatment?   A firm white or yellowish patch that persists for more than two weeks should be evaluated by a physician, preferably an oral surgeon, dermatologist or ear, nose and throat specialist. Biopsy will show if the plaque is cancerous. If it is, its removal followed by X-ray therapy is usually curative. The person with a noncancerous plaque should be seen by the doctor twice a year and should give up smoking and have bad teeth pulled. Since teeth that are badly aligned may cause persistent injury to the tongue, these should be aligned.

How common is cancer of the mouth?   It accounts for 7 or 8 percent of all malignancies. Of the 24,000 persons who are discovered each year to have it, most have neglected the disease to the point that the cancer has already spread to nearby lymph glands when the diagnosis is made. Cancer of the throat is included in the statistics for mouth cancer, and accounts for 25 percent of these cancers.

Who is most likely to develop cancer of the mouth?   It's most likely to occur in older men, especially those who smoke.

What are the most common sites for mouth cancer?   In order of frequency, the tongue, lips, floor of the mouth, gums, palate and inner lining of the cheek. Throat cancer is most likely to occur at the back of the throat.

What are the symptoms of mouth or throat cancer?   A painless growth may begin as a white or yellowish plaque, a sore that won't heal, or a lump or enlargement in the tongue or other part of the mouth. Pain is not a prominent symptom for mouth cancer, but pain and difficulty in swallowing accompany throat cancer. Bleeding doesn't occur unless the cancer erodes the lining of the mouth or throat. Enlargement of glands beneath the jaw or at the top of the neck is a late finding indicating spread of cancer to these areas. Cancer-containing glands are firmer than the surrounding flesh and are not tender.

What's the treatment for mouth cancer?   When the cancer is caught early, surgery followed by radiation therapy is the usual treatment. Radiation therapy is the first choice when the cancer is too advanced to permit removal.

What are the chances of a cure?   The five-year survival rate is generally better than 60 to 70 percent. A cancer of the back of the tongue, the throat or the floor of the mouth carries a poor prognosis if spread has occurred at the time that treatment is started.

What is trench mouth?   An ulcerative infection of the gums, inner cheeks, floor of the mouth and throat. The symptoms are pain, bleeding from the mouth, fever and foul breath. Common in the trenches of World War I, trench mouth is also known as Vincent's angina after the French physician who first described it. It may accompany infectious mononucleosis or occur in a diabetic, alcoholic or one receiving cell-killing drugs for cancer or immunosuppression after an organ transplant. Leukemia and other blood problems also predispose to it.

What's the treatment for trench mouth?   Rest, good diet and mouth rinses with 3 percent hydrogen peroxide may be all that's necessary to clear up a mild case of trench mouth, and penicillin or erythromycin therapy will usually cure a severe infection within a week. A program of good oral hygiene must be maintained to prevent a recurrence.

How do you recognize cleft lip and cleft palate in a newborn?   A cleft lip is visible in a newborn, and a cleft palate can be diagnosed by feeling inside the baby's mouth for the defect. A palatal defect may involve only the membrane of the roof of the mouth, or both the membrane and the bone. Cleft lip (harelip) and cleft palate are the most common birth defects of the head and neck.

What causes these defects?   They are thought to be genetically determined, though the mode of inheritance is complex (see p. 148). Cleft lip and cleft palate may occur in children with chromosomal disorders, who tend to have other deformities as well.

Are these defects always in the midline?   No, and use of the term "harelip" is misleading. A rabbit's lip is creased in the midline, but cleft lip occurs on one side or the other, usually the left. Cleft palate may occur in the midline or to one side of center.

What problems does cleft palate cause?   Other than the obvious one of appearance, the baby may not be able to breast-feed. Feeding through a cup or rubber tubing is usually successful, and the baby must be kept upright to minimize the chance of milk getting into the nose where it could be aspirated into the lungs. Children with cleft palate have a higher incidence of middle-ear infections.

What's the treatment for cleft lip and palate?   A cleft lip can be repaired surgically when the child weighs twelve pounds or more, usually after the third or fourth month of life. So that the child can learn to talk at the usual age, cleft palate should be repaired at about eighteen months to two years of age. Before and after repair, the treatment requires cooperation between the oral or plastic surgeon (or ear, nose and throat specialist), the orthodontist, prosthodontist, pediatrician, and speech and hearing specialist. The initial surgery gives good results in three-fourths of afflicted children, but additional operations are sometimes necessary. Covering of the defect with a dental retainer may be successful when an older child or adult is discovered to have an unrepaired cleft palate.

What causes a bony protuberance in the mouth?   An overgrowth of the bones that join to form the roof of the mouth may create a hard midline bump that is easily felt with the tongue or seen during a mouth examination. Known as *torus palatinus,* it need not be removed unless it interferes with eating or the fitting of an upper dental plate. A *torus mandibularis* is a similar bony overgrowth occurring on the inside or outside of the jawbone below the teeth (generally two such knots are noted, one on either side of the mouth). In contrast to cancer, which appears as a new growth, both these conditions are present throughout life.

THROAT

What causes sore throat?   Most throat infections are due to the common cold. Beta-hemolytic streptococci (see strep throat, p. 167) is a less common cause of the infection. Other sources are viral infections other than a cold, infectious mononucleosis and, uncommonly, thrush, gonorrhea, diphtheria and trench mouth.

How do you tell the difference between strep throat and a sore throat due to a cold?   Strep throat begins suddenly. Fever rises to 101° F. (38° C.) or more, and pain on swallowing may be accompanied by tenderness below the angle of the jaw from enlarged glands. White patches of inflammatory material appear on the tonsils or in the throat. Runny nose and a productive cough are not usually present.

A cold may begin with scratchiness in the throat progressing to pain on swallowing. Runny nose, stuffy nose, sneezing, coughing, and other symptoms accompany the throat pain. The temperature rarely goes above 100° or 101° F., and white patches of exudate do not form in the throat. The glands below the jaw swell minimally, if at all. Since the symptoms of a cold depend on which of the hundred or more causative viruses is responsible, not every cold is accompanied by sore throat.

The only reliable way to distinguish between the two conditions is to take a culture from the throat and see if streptococci are present. This should be done promptly if strep throat is suspected, so that treatment can be started. If one member of the family has a strep throat, the others should be tested too.

What's the treatment for strep throat?   Penicillin by mouth or injection under the careful supervision of a physician will usually cure the infection. A fairly high dosage of oral penicillin will be prescribed for a full ten days, and it is important to stay faithfully with this treatment if complications are to be avoided. If an injection is administered, you should wait in the doctor's office for about fifteen minutes, the usual time it takes to see if a serious adverse reaction will occur.

The penicillin-allergic individual can be treated with alternative antibiotics. Tetracycline and sulfa drugs are not recommended to treat strep throat. Relapse or treatment failure occurs in about one out of ten or twenty persons treated for strep throat. If this happens, you simply have to start over with another course of treatment, usually given for a full two weeks the second time.

Why does strep throat recur?   One cause of recurrence is for the infection to "ping-pong" through a family. By the time it's passed among the children and adults, the first to have it may get it again. Fatigue, poor diet and emotional upset are factors that favor recurrent infection. The role of the tonsils and adenoids in allowing a recurrence is controversial.

What are the complications of strep throat?   A streptococcal infection of the throat or skin may give rise to a hypersensitivity reaction leading to rheumatic fever (see p. 157) or glomerulonephritis (see p. 425).

What are the tonsils and adenoids?   They are mounds of lymphoid, or antibody-forming, tissue in the throat. The tonsils are visible as fleshy domes behind the teeth and below the soft palate. Because the adenoids are up in the back of the throat behind the nose, they can't be seen without a special viewing mirror.

What purpose do the tonsils and adenoids serve?   By releasing germ-fighting white blood cells, they help to protect the body from an infection such as strep throat. They probably have other functions as well. The work of Dr. Robert A. Good at New York's Sloan-Kettering Institute for Cancer Research and of many others has shown that the tonsils and adenoids are like watchdogs that monitor food and air particles entering the body.

What is tonsillitis?   It's an infection of the tonsils usually caused by streptococci.

Won't a child have sore throat less often after tonsillectomy?   No, the frequency of strep throat is the same in those who have tonsils as it is in those who don't. The interesting point is that some children seem to go through a period of frequently having sore throat before building up a natural resistance. When this resistance occurs, the recurring sore throat stops. If a tonsillectomy has been done in the meantime, it gets the credit.

Does tonsillectomy have any risks?   One child dies for each 15,000 who have the operation, and one in twenty children have bleeding after the operation and require further surgery or emergency transfusions. Speech problems are noted in some children after tonsillectomy.

When is tonsillectomy definitely indicated?   The operation is indicated when a child's tonsils are so large that they interfere with breathing or eating. The adenoids should be removed if they're large enough to obstruct the nasal passages and cause troubled breathing, loud snoring or nasal speech. In an occasional instance chronically infected tonsils may have to be removed.

What causes hoarseness?   The most common cause is laryngitis, when the larynx (voice box) is inflamed or irritated. A growth or a paralysis of one of its nerves may also be responsible. Among the causes are laryngitis, singer's nodules and tumor. Persistent hoarseness following neck surgery usually indicates that the surgeon has inadvertently cut or bruised one of the recurrent laryngeal nerves and that one of the vocal cords is temporarily weakened or paralyzed.

What causes laryngitis?   A cold or flu virus may infect the larynx causing hoarseness and loss of voice. Throat pain and cough productive of phlegm may also be present if there is an accompanying cold or flu. Treatment consists of voice rest, moisturization of the air and symptomatic medicines for several days or a week. A bacterial laryngitis may be accompanied by fever and difficulty in breathing; this infection calls for antibiotic therapy by a physician.

What is spasmodic laryngitis?   Following a chest cold one may develop a nagging cough accompanied by a spasm of the vocal cords. A temporary difficulty in breathing may occur. Relief can be obtained by using a cough suppressant and taking a muscle relaxant. Addition of moisture to the air by a bedside vaporizer or other means may help. Once the cycle of cough and spasm is broken, recovery occurs.

What causes chronic laryngitis?   Smoking and other forms of irritation such as voice abuse are the usual causes of chronic laryngitis. Postnasal drip may contribute to the inflammation, and an allergy or alcohol consumption is sometimes responsible. Syphilis and tuberculosis are rare causes of chronic laryngitis. The treatment starts with a medical exam to rule out an underlying problem, and consists of resting the voice and avoiding irritants.

What are singer's nodules?   These tiny growths may appear along the edges of the vocal cords in one who strains the voice by singing or shouting. The nodules may go away with voice rest or they may have to be removed under local anesthesia.

Who is most susceptible to cancer of the larynx?   It is ten times more frequent in men than in women, and the most susceptible individual is one who has smoked heavily for many years. About 10,000 persons develop laryngeal cancer each year.

What are the symptoms of this cancer?   Hoarseness is the earliest symptom. Anyone who has hoarseness lasting for more than two or three weeks should have an examination to rule out cancer of the vocal cords. Other symptoms include discomfort and the sensation of a lump in the throat, difficulty in swallowing, cough, and trouble with breathing.

How is the diagnosis made?   By looking into the throat with a laryngeal mirror, a physician can see the vocal cords and tell if a tumor is present. A biopsy will show if the tumor is cancerous.

What's the treatment for laryngeal cancer?   An early cancer may be removed and the voice preserved. More advanced cases are treated by a combination of surgery and irradiation. The radiation therapy is usually given before the surgery.

What are the chances for a cure?   For an early cancer, the chances of a cure are excellent. The overall five-year survival rate is better than 50 percent, and half of those who are forty-five or younger at the time of the initial treatment are still alive ten years later.

Is speech possible without vocal cords?   Yes, esophageal speech can be accomplished by swallowing air and then belching it in a controlled manner to form words. The technique can be taught by a speech therapist. An artificial larynx is a battery-operated device which the person holds to the neck to transform words formed by the mouth into speech that can be heard. The resulting voice has a robotlike quality, but the words are distinct.

What are the symptoms of the presence of a foreign body in the throat?   A child will be fussy, have coughing and a crowing type of breathing, will appear apprehensive and may have blueness about the mouth and fingernails. Sweating is common. An adult with something caught in the throat will be excited and fearful, unable to speak, and very short of breath. Complete obstruction of the airway leads rapidly to asphyxia with loss of consciousness and blue discoloration of the mucous membranes and nail beds.

What is the treatment? The foreign body should be removed by employing the Heimlich maneuver as described on pp. 194–95. When the object cannot be removed in this manner, the person should be rushed to a hospital, where emergency tracheostomy may be necessary.

What is tracheostomy? Also known as tracheotomy, this operation consists of cutting through the front of the neck below the Adam's apple to make an opening into the trachea (windpipe). A tracheotomy tube is inserted to keep the hole open. In most instances the operation is temporary, and the hole can be sutured up when the immediate problem is over.

When is tracheostomy indicated? It may be done as an emergency when the throat or airway is obstructed or when heavy secretions prevent breathing. It may also be done to aid the breathing of someone in a coma from stroke, drug overdosage or head injury. The victim of a paralytic disease, such as polio or Guillain-Barré syndrome (see p. 303), or one who is having trouble breathing because of cystic fibrosis (see p. 397) or muscular dystrophy (see p. 336), may benefit from tracheostomy. The operation may also be performed during treatment for laryngeal cancer.

11

BRAIN and NERVES

How big is the brain? It weighs about three pounds in an adult and accounts for 2 percent of body weight. Its melon shape is not too different from that of the skull, and it is only slightly smaller than the person's head.

How is the brain structured? The cerebrum consists of two hemispheres, each covered with folds and furrows and resembling cauliflower. Though only a fraction of an inch thick, the gray matter on the outside of the cerebrum governs movement, thought, speech, sensation, vision and most other human activities. It does so by virtue of containing the brain's ten billion neurons, specialized cells that are constantly in touch with what is happening and that are capable of making things happen.

The cerebellum, or "small brain," coordinates body movements. Located in the back of the skull and below the cerebral hemispheres, it is a pear-shaped structure whose functions are still incompletely understood. The brainstem is a knobby extension below the cerebrum and cerebellum. Carrying nerve connections to the spinal cord, with which it is continuous, it controls unconscious activities such as breathing and the height of the blood pressure.

How does the brain work? Somewhat like a computer in that it collects, stores and acts on the information that it continually receives by way of sight, sound, touch, taste and smell. One part of the brain is responsible for

285

initiating movement, another for speech, another for memory and still another for sexual arousal. Coordination of these activities is accomplished by an interplay between the neurons located in the gray matter and the cells that make up the connecting white matter forming the bulk of the brain.

Where is the mind?   Thinking must occur by an interaction among the neurons, but the site of the mind is still unknown. It is thought that the frontal lobes, large structures in the cerebrum, govern thought.

What are nerves?   They are the brain's message carriers to the rest of the body. The twenty-four cranial nerves, twelve on each side, carry messages and receive information from the head and neck. Peripheral nerves come from the spinal cord and carry messages to the neck and lower parts of the body. Sensory nerves from the body and extremities feed their information into the spinal cord.

How do nerves work?   If you decide to get up from a chair, the impulse to do so speeds down the spinal cord and is relayed to the nerves going to the muscles of your arms and legs. As your muscles lift you out of the chair, sensory nerves are telling the brain the location of your body parts.

What tests can be done to study the brain?   The skull X-ray gives information about the bony cage of the brain and about certain structures inside the skull. An electroencephalogram records the brain's electrical activity and is helpful in diagnosing epilepsy. By beaming sound waves into the brain and recording their patterns of reflection, the echoencephalogram helps to tell if one part of the brain is denser than another (tumor), displaced (tumor or hemorrhage), or lacking in structure (cyst or abscess). An arteriogram is done by injecting dye through an artery in the neck and taking X-rays as the dye courses through the vessels in the brain. A tumor or hemorrhage may stand out, and the arteriogram is the best way to detect an enlargement of a vessel. A pneumoencephalogram is done after air is injected into the spinal canal and allowed to pass upward to the brain. It is especially useful in showing the region where the brain attaches to the spinal cord. All of these tests have now assumed a secondary importance to the CAT scan.

What is the CAT scan?   "CAT" stands for computerized axial tomography, and the study combines modern X-ray techniques with computer technology to give, in effect, a view of the brain (or chest or abdomen) that is as good as if you had opened the skull and looked directly at it—without causing any damage.

How is a CAT scan done?   An X-ray beam is sent through one section of the brain a hundred and eighty times with a one-degree change in angle each time. At the end of the reading, the computer creates a three-dimensional image of that area of the brain. An enhanced CAT scan can be done by injecting dye.

What are the uses of a CAT scan?　To detect such things as brain tumor, stroke, brain hemorrhage, hydrocephalus or an area of localized infection (abscess) in the brain.

How dangerous is the study?　A plain CAT scan gives you about as much irradiation exposure as a skull X-ray series. Allergic reaction to the dye occurs in one out of 2,000 persons. A physician should be available to treat an allergic reaction in the event that one occurs.

What's the difference between a neurologist and a psychiatrist?　A neurologist specializes in treating diseases of the brain and nerves, while a psychiatrist specializes in treating mental disorders. Both specialists have completed four years of postgraduate study and have been certified by the American Board of Psychiatry and Neurology. Typically, neurologists have some training in psychiatry, and psychiatrists in neurology. The dual training is necessary because of the overlap between diseases of the mind and those that affect the brain and nerves.

How do you find a good neurologist?　An internal medicine specialist, who usually has had some training in neurology, can treat many brain and nerve disorders. He or she is, in this case, the best person to refer you to a neurologist. If this doesn't work out, ask for a referral from the best teaching hospital in your area.

HEADACHE

What are the causes of headache?　The most common causes are shown in the accompanying chart.

COMMON CAUSES OF HEADACHE

Psychogenic headache
　Depression
　Nervousness
　Tension
Vascular headache
　Migraine
　Cluster headache
Infection

Common cold or flu
Strep throat or fever from any cause
Meningitis or encephalitis (uncommon)
Fatigue
   Eyestrain
   Hunger
   Sleepiness
Hangover
High blood pressure
Stroke or impending stroke
Brain tumor (rare)

What are some frequent locations of headache?   Though overlap may exist, the following are some frequent locations for headache:

· *Tension headache or headache due to fatigue or depression* is most often in the back of the head and the upper neck. It may wrap around the head like a vise or heavy weight and may also be felt in the front or top of the head.

· *Migraine* typically occurs on one side of the head but may involve both sides, and is often accompanied by other symptoms, such as nausea and vomiting.

· *Cluster headache* appears on one side of the head in or behind the eye.

· *Sinus headache* is in the face on either side of the nose and above the eyes; it is worsened by leaning forward.

· *Eyestrain headache* is most severe in the front of the head, is accompanied by tiredness in the eyes and may be associated with tension headache.

· *High blood pressure* headache may occur in any part of the head or feel as if the top of the head were about to blow off. Often it's felt in the back of the head early in the morning just after awakening.

· *Brain tumor* may cause headache in any part of the head. The headache may be mild in its early stages but gets worse as the tumor grows.

What is the most common form of headache?   The most common headache is that due to fatigue, eyestrain or hunger, or the end-of-day headache that reaches its peak in a traffic jam and may be gone five minutes after arrival home. More serious psychogenic headaches from nervousness, tension or depression are of longer duration. They account for eight out of ten headaches severe enough to prompt a medical visit.

How often is sinusitis a cause of headache?   An attack of sinusitis does cause headache, as does obstruction of the nose, but sinusitis is rarely the cause of chronic headache. Often a person with tension or psychogenic headache will attribute the pain to "sinus."

Are certain headache remedies better than others?   Yes, buffered aspirin or acetaminophen is best. These drugs are the standards against which other compounds are measured, and the combination drugs are no better than plain aspirin or plain acetaminophen. Sinus headaches may be relieved by decongestants.

Do you need more than two aspirin tablets?   No, two aspirin or acetaminophen tablets provide the same amount of pain relief as do three or more. The relief should last for three or four hours.

What about using both aspirin and acetaminophen?   For a severe headache this may work, but doing it more than once is not advisable. Persistent headache not relieved by aspirin or acetaminophen calls for a medical visit.

What are the signs of serious headache?   The main ones are:
 · Sudden onset of headache when you've never had it before, or onset of headache that is different from what you've had before
 · Headache following an injury to the head
 · Headache that wakes you up in the morning or during the night
 · Headache accompanied by vomiting, fever or confusion, or one that is increased by coughing or straining or is accompanied by weakness, paralysis or dizziness
 · Headache that does not respond to aspirin or acetaminophen

Does the severity of headache correlate with its seriousness?   Not always. Some of the most severe headaches are those due to migraine. Headache due to a brain tumor or hemorrhage may be mild to severe in intensity. Perhaps the best indicator of a serious headache is one that persists or keeps returning.

What causes migraine?   It is due to a painful dilation of one or more arteries on the surface of the brain or skull. Migraine tends to run in families and to strike a perfectionist, anxious individual.

How common is migraine?   An estimated ten million Americans have migraine.

What are the symptoms of migraine?   The headache is often preceded by a warning—dizziness, flashing dots in front of the eyes or loss of vision in certain of the viewing fields. The headache follows as a sudden, intense pain, usually in one temple, and throbs with the pulsebeat. It may spread to the front or back of the head or include the entire head. It may be mild and last less than an hour, or it may be incapacitating and last several days.

Nausea, vomiting and diarrhea may accompany the attack. The person may be oversensitive to light and noise at this time, and the tendency for the sufferer to seek a quiet room has led to the designation of migraine as "sick headache."

What's the age of onset for migraine?   It usually begins in the teens or twenties, rarely after the age of forty-five. Migraines tend to disappear after age forty.

What may bring on an attack?   Hunger, fatigue, emotional tension, frustration or depression may bring on an attack. Among women, migraine is worse around the time of the menstrual period. The headaches generally leave during pregnancy and are less frequent after menopause. Birth-control pills may worsen migraine or bring on the attacks in one who has never had migraine.

What's the treatment for migraine?   Mild migraine may be relieved by aspirin or acetaminophen or a number of mild to moderate prescription painkillers. Quiet rest in a dark room—especially if the person can fall asleep—may stop an attack. Abortive therapy with the drug ergotamine is attempted when other measures fail. The drug should not be used during pregnancy or by anyone suffering from heart disease or high blood pressure. It works by constricting blood vessels to counteract the dilating effect of the migraine attack. To be effective, it must be taken as soon as possible after the onset of an attack or the premonition of one. Ergotamine is usually given in a combination form with caffeine, and side effects of the preparation include rapid heartbeat, slight nervousness, itching, nausea, muscle pains and tingling in the fingers and toes. Allergic reactions to either drug may also occur.

Can a migraine attack be prevented?   Two out of three migraine sufferers will have fewer attacks after learning to cope with stress in a more effective manner. Psychotherapy may be indicated. Talking through one's inner conflicts at regular intervals may be therapeutic, and setting goals a little lower may help to relieve frustration and promote a sense of well-being.

What about preventive drug therapy?   Preventive drug therapy may be indicated when migraine attacks occur weekly or more often, or when the attacks cannot be aborted by ergotamine. Antidepressants, as well as drugs that are ordinarily used to treat heart disease and to lower blood pressure, have been tried, but these are still considered investigational in the prevention of migraine.

The only drug approved by the FDA for prevention of migraine attacks is also the most dangerous: Sansert. Structurally similar to LSD, it may cause a severe overgrowth of fibrous tissue around the kidneys, heart or liver. Deaths from kidney complications have occurred. In the view of many physicians, the risks of Sansert outweigh its benefits—it should not be used, or if it is, not for more than several months without stopping to see if any of its side effects have occurred.

Is biofeedback useful in treating migraine? It may be if one is capable of the intense concentration required for success at biofeedback. The person learns to concentrate on raising the temperature in a body part such as the hands; as the temperature in the hands goes up, blood is diverted there from the head, thus helping to relieve the pain of migraine.

What is cluster headache? Closely related to migraine, cluster headache is so named because of the tendency for the attacks to come in groups or clusters. It is five times as frequent in men as in women and is often the most severe of the various kinds of headache. An attack begins high in the nose or beneath one eye, remains localized as a severe, throbbing pain, and is accompanied by watering of the nose and eye. An attack may last up to two hours and several may occur in a day. After several weeks of headache, the person may be free from the problem for months. During a cluster, alcohol consumption seems to precipitate an attack.

What's the treatment for cluster headache? The drugs used to treat migraine may be effective. Since histamine plays a role in cluster headache, research has been aimed at desensitizing the sufferer to histamine. The results to date have been equivocal.

What about hangover headache? The best treatment for this headache is prevention, for hangover signals that a person has abused alcohol—or sleeping pills or tranquilizers. Coffee, aspirin and "tincture of time" are the best remedies.

How can I find a headache specialist? By writing the American Association for the Study of Headache, 5252 North Western Avenue, Chicago, Ill. 60625, or the National Migraine Foundation, 2422 West Foster Avenue, Chicago, Ill. 60625. The association or foundation can supply you with the names of headache specialists in your area. You can also consult your internist, friends whose opinion you value or your local hospital.

BRAIN DISEASES

What are the symptoms of brain tumor? Headache is often the earliest symptom. It is worst in the morning or may awaken the person. It tends to get worse during coughing, straining or bending forward. In the early stages it may be relieved by aspirin, but it becomes persistent and isn't relieved by nonprescription drugs. Depending on the location of the tumor, associated symptoms include nausea and vomiting, double vision, loss of vision, weakness in a part of the body, confusion or bizarre behavior. A seizure is sometimes the first symptom of brain tumor.

How common is brain tumor?   About 11,000 persons develop it each year. It accounts for 20 percent of malignancies in children, but only 1 to 2 percent of cancers in adults. Many times a brain tumor is discovered as an incidental finding at autopsy. Presumably the tumor caused either no symptoms or minimal symptoms.

Are symptoms of brain tumor different in children?   The tumor may cause a child's head to enlarge too rapidly or give rise to irritability, lethargy and vomiting in an infant or small child. Headache and visual problems are more apt to occur in an older child.

Can a tumor spread to the brain?   Yes, a fourth of brain tumors begin in another part of the body and are carried to the brain by the blood.

What's the treatment for brain tumor?   Surgery is preferable if the tumor can be removed, but X-ray therapy may be given instead of as well as after surgery. When cancer of the lung, breast or other organ has spread to the brain, the first order of treatment is directed at the primary tumor. Anticonvulsant drugs, steroids and pain relievers are given when indicated. Chemotherapy is sometimes chosen.

What's the chance of a cure?   Caught early, a tumor such as meningioma may be completely curable. The highly malignant glioblastoma multiforme, which occurs in persons over the age of forty, is usually fatal within a year or a year and a half despite treatment. Taking into account the many types of brain cancer, the overall survival is about 40 percent at five years for adults, and 40 percent at ten years for children.

What is stroke?   An injury to the brain occurring when a cerebral artery bursts, clots or becomes obstructed by a piece of material that has lodged in it. Though the symptoms differ, the end result of each of these processes is the same. The area of brain beyond the vessel is deprived of blood flow and dies, and the functions performed by that part of the brain are lost. Dead neurons cannot be replaced, but surviving cells in adjacent areas of the brain may be able to take over their function and allow rehabilitation from stroke.

What are the symptoms of stroke?   A stroke may be quick or slow. The quick form, due to cerebral hemorrhage or blockage of an artery, justifies the name "stroke" or "apoplexy" by the way it shuts off consciousness, produces paralysis or snuffs out life. Headache, difficulty in speaking and dizziness may precede the attack, which often cuts one down during work or exercise. Slow stroke is more likely to begin during the night from a clot that forms in a brain artery. Over hours or days the person experiences weakness progressing to paralysis on one side of the body. Confusion and garbled speech may appear, but the victim often remains fully conscious.

What causes stroke?   Stroke in an older person is usually due to hardening of the arteries. High blood pressure contributes to the process. Fatty plaques build up in the brain arteries and create the environment for clot formation or rupture of the vessel.

Stroke in someone under fifty is more likely due to rupture of a defective artery at the base of the brain. The weak spot in the vessel, a berry aneurysm, is like the blister seen in an inflated inner tube that has a soft spot. Some persons have many such balloonings in the vessels lining the brain, and high blood pressure contributes to the sudden bursting of one of them.

What are the symptoms of berry aneurysm?   The first sign of it may be an excruciating headache accompanied by a stiff neck. The headache is usually the worst the person has ever had—a throbbing, intense pain radiating into the neck. Dizziness and vomiting may occur. The person may lose consciousness abruptly, as in a quick stroke, or experience a mild blackout and quickly regain consciousness.

How is stroke diagnosed?   A doctor can recognize stroke from the history and physical examination of the patient, though it may not be clear whether the cause is a hemorrhage, blood clot or embolus. Berry aneurysm is always suspected when a previously healthy person in his or her twenties or thirties has a stroke. Hardening of the arteries is the usual cause in an elderly person. Stroke in an older individual with no history of high blood pressure may occur when a blood clot or clump of material—known as an embolus —passes to the brain from another part of the body. Meningitis and encephalitis must be ruled out in anyone thought to have a stroke.

A lumbar puncture to obtain a sample of spinal fluid is useful: blood staining of the fluid indicates a bleeding episode in the brain, whereas an elevated white count points to infection. Other helpful tests include the CAT scan and arteriograms.

What's the treatment for stroke?   Bed rest in a quiet room is prescribed, but other measures depend on the cause of the stroke and the inclinations of the attending physician. For the victim of slow stroke, some favor the use of anticoagulants, drugs that slow the blood's tendency to clot, while others doubt their benefit. Blood-thinners are not indicated when the person has high blood pressure or brain hemorrhage, since to thin the blood might favor progression of the stroke. Amicar is a drug that may be helpful in controlling the hemorrhage from a berry aneurysm.

How effective is surgery for stroke?   It's only indicated for proven berry aneurysm, and then only under certain circumstances. After the weakened vessel ruptures, bleeding usually stops within a day or so. Half the victims die within a month of the event; the cause of death is usually recurrent hemorrhage. Surgery is aimed at preventing additional bleeding, but large studies in the United States and England have shown that not all berry aneurysms should be attacked surgically. The surgery itself is inexact. Among the procedures that have been tried are tying off the weakened vessel, repairing it with a graft or metal clip, or leaving the aneurysm in place and filling it with hog's hair bristles shot into it as a method of strengthening it.

The best way to avoid inopportune surgery is to make sure that the stroke victim is under the care of a good neurologist or internist, who can help to judge the need for surgery in consultation with the neurosurgeon.

What's the prognosis after stroke?   Quick stroke due to brain hemorrhage is fatal about half of the time. Slow stroke carries a better prognosis: three-fourths of the victims survive the attack. The great danger in berry aneurysm is recurrent bleeding, since the mortality rate is 40 percent for each bleeding episode. Hemorrhage has recurred as long as twenty years after the first episode, but the longer one goes without additional bleeding, the less likely it is to recur. Prognosis is definitely better when the victim of berry aneurysm never loses consciousness from the hemorrhage.

What's the treatment for paralysis from stroke?   Paralysis is most likely to affect one side of the body and may be accompanied by loss of speech and lack of bladder and bowel control. Early, vigorous retraining will help the person keep what function is left and recover some or all of the use of the paralyzed extremities. When possible, the rehabilitation program should be planned and supervised by a physiatrist, a medical specialist whose field encompasses the disciplines of neurology, orthopedics and physical therapy.

What is a CVA?   The letters stand for *c*erebrov*a*scular *a*ccident, and the term is popular among doctors in speaking of a stroke without having to specify whether it was due to a clot, hemorrhage or embolus.

Will aspirin help to prevent a stroke?   A large study in Canada showed that one aspirin taken four times a day helped to reduce the risk of cerebrovascular accidents in stroke-prone men. The aspirin was not effective in reducing the risk of stroke in women. Obviously, such treatment should be undertaken only with a physician's supervision.

How do you recognize the stroke-prone individual?   Before having a stroke, a person may have attacks of diminished blood flow to the brain. Symptoms during an attack include dizziness, slurred speech or numbness and weakness in the face, hand or leg. The attacks may last minutes or hours and occur several times a day or no more often than once a month. Five percent of persons experiencing these attacks will have a stroke within a year, and these are the individuals who may benefit from aspirin therapy. They should see a physician, however, as soon as such symptoms are noted.

What is multiple sclerosis?   The white matter of the brain consists primarily of a fatty substance, myelin, that covers nerve fibers as well as cranial and peripheral nerves. Certain diseases, among them multiple sclerosis, are characterized by a degeneration and loss of myelin. The brain of a person dying of multiple sclerosis will be speckled with grayish plaques of hard material that have replaced the normal white matter. Though the cause of multiple sclerosis is unknown, an allergic reaction or a viral illness has been suspected.

What are the symptoms?   Weakness of the legs is usually the first symptom, sometimes with associated frequency and urgency of urination. Numbness is a common early symptom. Double vision or impaired vision, lack of coordination, tremor of the hands and mental changes are other frequent symptoms. But the most typical thing about multiple sclerosis is that the symptoms tend to come and go. The person may enjoy months or years of freedom from the disease in between attacks.

Who is most susceptible to multiple sclerosis?   It occurs with equal frequency in men and women, blacks and whites, but is six times more common in those living in the North than in those residing in the South. The disease shows no familial tendency and is most likely to strike someone between the ages of twenty and forty.

What is the treatment for multiple sclerosis?   Steroid hormones and injections of the hormone ACTH have been used with varying success, but there's no known cure for the disease. Care of the person consists of managing problems such as infection, mental difficulties, urinary problems and pain.

What is the prognosis for multiple sclerosis?   An initial attack involving visual loss, pain or urinary difficulties is less ominous than when it causes muscular weakness, tremor and lack of coordination. Some persons die within weeks of the onset of MS, while others have lived for fifty years with the disease. Ten years after the diagnosis is made, half of multiple sclerosis victims are still able to work.

What is Lou Gehrig's disease?   Known medically as amyotrophic lateral sclerosis, this is the disease that struck the great Yankees' first baseman in 1938 and led to his death in 1941. Central to the disease is a loss of the neurons controlling voluntary muscular activity; the neurons are lost in the cerebral hemispheres and brainstem and create a spastic or jerky type of progressive muscular paralysis. Tiny muscle spasms, which look as if there is crawling under the skin, are among the symptoms. The cause of the disease is unknown.

How common is Lou Gehrig's disease?   Each year 3,000 new cases are diagnosed, and at any one time about 10,000 Americans have this condition.

Who is most likely to get it?   It occurs more often in men than in women, and is more apt to strike someone who had polio years earlier. The onset is usually in the forties or fifties, but it may begin as early as the twenties.

What are the symptoms of amyotrophic lateral sclerosis?   Muscle quiverings and weakness are the earliest symptoms. These changes begin in the legs or arms, and sometimes the disease affects primarily the muscles of the face and throat, causing difficulty in swallowing and speaking. Complete paralysis may occur in advanced disease.

What can be done for someone with amyotrophic lateral sclerosis? There's no treatment, and the relentless course of the disease usually leads to death within three or four years of its onset.

What is Tourette's syndrome?   This condition, named for the physician who described it, usually afflicts children between the ages of two and puberty. It causes involuntary muscular movements (tic) of the face, head or limbs and uncontrolled verbal outbursts. The spasms are frequent and rapid. Because the individual may shout or curse, he or she is often thought to have a behavioral or emotional problem rather than a neurologic disorder. Tranquilizers may reduce the tic and control the verbal outbursts.

How common is Tourette's syndrome?   Several hundred cases are known to exist, but it's thought that thousands of children with the condition have not been diagnosed. Information about the condition can be obtained from the Tourette Syndrome Association, Bell Plaza Building, 42-40 Bell Boulevard, Bayside, N.Y. 11361.

296

What is chorea? It is a neurologic condition characterized by involuntary movements of the hands, arms, face and other body parts. Unlike the sudden spasms of Tourette's syndrome, choreiform movements have a continuous, dancing quality. The movements occur at rest, are accentuated during purposeful movement and are absent during sleep.

What causes chorea? It may complicate rheumatic fever or encephalitis, be a manifestation of Huntington's chorea or appear for an unkown reason in an elderly person.

What is Huntington's chorea? It is an inherited disease that causes choreiform movements, mental deterioration and, eventually, death. Half the children of an affected person will show signs of the disease, and the onset is usually between the ages of thirty-five and fifty. No specific treatment is known.

What is tremor? It's an involuntary shaking of the hands, head or other body part. Most noticeable at rest, it often diminishes during purposeful movement.

What causes tremor? Some common causes include fatigue, excitement, nervousness, alcoholism and a benign tremor occurring in older persons. The most frequent cause of persistent tremor is Parkinson's disease, shaking palsy.

What are the symptoms of Parkinson's disease? A person in his or her fifties or sixties notes a gradually increasing tremor in one or both hands. The tremor is a repetitive motion as if the person is trying to snap the fingers. It lessens during purposeful movement and is absent during sleep. Over a period of months to years, muscle movement becomes difficult. The legs feel heavy and stiff. The person loses control of the facial and jaw muscles, speech becomes difficult and drooling may occur. A fixed, emotionless expression is typical of full-blown Parkinsonism. The person lets the head slump forward, shuffles instead of walks, turns with difficulty and needs help to eat or dress.

What causes Parkinson's disease? In most instances the cause is unknown, though it may follow encephalitis.

How common is Parkinson's disease? An estimated one million Americans have it, and 50,000 new cases are discovered each year. The incidence is the same in men and women and in all races.

What is the treatment for Parkinson's disease?   Most of the drugs that are used to treat Parkinson's disease are not very useful and cause a wide range of troublesome side effects, such as dry mouth, blurred vision and rapid heart rate, or restlessness, dizziness, confusion and hallucinations.

Levodopa and, more recently, carbidopa have been hailed as the best drugs yet for Parkinson's disease, though neither leads to a cure. Half of those who take these drugs show a good result, and a third show remarkable improvement. Side effects, however, limit the drugs' usefulness. They may cause depression, confusion, hallucinations, loss of appetite, nausea and difficulty in sleeping. These changes occur in over half of those taking the drugs, and 40 to 80 percent of users develop involuntary movements of the face, trunk or extremities. The movements may take the form of grimacing, yawning or rolling and twitching of the tongue. Many physicians are now limiting the drugs to those persons who don't respond to less toxic agents.

Is surgery useful for Parkinson's disease?   The availability of levodopa has all but eliminated surgical treatment. The once popular operation for Parkinson's disease might be indicated to treat tremor in one arm that persists despite levodopa therapy, or when the drug cannot be used because of the side effects of levodopa. The main drawback to surgery is that it is most beneficial for those who need it least—persons with minimal symptoms of Parkinson's disease.

What's the long-term outlook for one with Parkinson's disease?   In most instances the person can look forward to ten or twenty years of relatively little difficulty before the disease becomes incapacitating.

Can drugs cause a Parkinson-like reaction?   Yes, phenothiazine tranquilizers may cause a temporary condition resembling Parkinson's disease. The person develops choreiform movements, wryneck, restlessness and an involuntary arching of the back. Compazine, a drug used to treat nausea, is frequently responsible for this reaction, and Thorazine, Stelazine and Mellaril may cause it.

What's the treatment for the Parkinson-like reaction?   Stopping the causative drug will bring relief within several days. Symptoms can be controlled more quickly by the use of Benadryl or phenobarbital. Avoid future use of the drug that caused the problem.

What is hydrocephalus?   The word means "water brain," which is accurate to the extent that enlargement of the head occurs from the pressure of too much fluid inside the brain. The condition, which is fortunately rare, is usually diagnosed in the first few weeks of life.

What are the symptoms of hydrocephalus? The baby's head is too large at birth or begins to increase in size rapidly after birth. The soft spot bulges. The forehead stands out. The eyelids are pulled upward so that the whites of the eyes are visible above the iris. The scalp, shiny and with dilated veins, becomes taut from the pressure of fluid inside the brain. The baby is usually irritable, has a thin, high-pitched cry, and may not be able to move the eyes in all directions.

What causes these problems? Each day a pint of cerebrospinal fluid is produced by blood vessels lining the brain. The fluid circulates through a series of brain passageways called ventricles and eventually reaches the spinal canal, where it is resorbed. In hydrocephalus, the flow of fluid through the brain is partially obstructed, and it accumulates and presses outward on the brain.

How is hydrocephalus diagnosed? It can be suspected by alert parents and physicians and confirmed by a CAT scan. A study is then made to localize the site of the defect.

What is the treatment for hydrocephalus? A neurosurgeon places a small tubing through the skull and into the ventricle in the same path that the probing needle took to locate the defect. The tubing is tunneled beneath the scalp to the neck, then guided beneath the skin of the chest until it reaches the abdominal cavity, where it empties its contents. In this way, fluid is shunted around the obstruction so that the pressure doesn't build up inside the brain.

How effective is treatment? Sixty percent of children having the shunt survive for ten years, and a fourth of the survivors have normal intelligence. Those with subnormal intelligence frequently are only mildly retarded and can live at home while attending a self-contained or integrated class at a public school. Seizures may occur but can usually be controlled by medication.

What is epilepsy? A disease causing the patient to have "seizures" or attacks characterized by loss of muscle control, loss of consciousness or altered consciousness, and rhythmic, convulsive movements of the arms, legs or trunk. An abnormal discharge of electrical activity in the brain is responsible for the attack.

How common is epilepsy? There are 4 million known epileptics in the United States, and probably many more persons who have had only one or two convulsions. It is estimated that 5 to 10 percent of children have one or more convulsions, but only 2 percent of them go on to develop epilepsy. According to the Epilepsy Foundation of America, half of epileptics remain seizure-free on medication, while one-fourth have a minimal number of seizures while taking anticonvulsant drugs.

What causes epilepsy?   In nine out of ten persons with recurring seizures, the cause is brain damage. For whatever reason, a scar forms in the gray matter of the brain and becomes the focus for abnormal discharges of electrical activity which trigger the seizures. The spectrum of causes is shown in the following chart:

CAUSES OF CONVULSIONS *(Epilepsy)*

Brain damage suffered at or before birth
Meningitis or encephalitis
Head injury from a blow or auto accident
Hydrocephalus
Brain tumor
Low blood sugar
Deficiency of blood calcium or magnesium
Stroke
Withdrawal from drug addiction
Tay-Sachs disease
Phenylketonuria
Inherited epilepsy
Fever over 103° to 104° F. (39.5° to 40° C.) in a susceptible child

Who is most susceptible to epilepsy?   A child known to have suffered brain damage before, during or after birth is most susceptible. Seizures occurring in a child with mental retardation and spastic paralysis almost always point to brain damage. Children of parents who had febrile seizures (see p. 154) have a greater than average risk of having a seizure during a high fever. Epilepsy may be inherited, but if so, it usually begins before the age of thirty. Sudden onset of seizures in an adult calls for a workup to rule out brain tumor, low blood sugar, drug addiction and other problems.

What are the types of epilepsy?   The four main ones are:
· *Grand mal seizures,* which may accompany brain injury, stroke, hydrocephalus, low blood sugar, high fever, meningitis or brain tumor. The attack may be preceded by an aura—a visual sensation or odor telling that the seizure is about to occur. Momentary excitement is followed by loss of consciousness and generalized muscular spasms. Jerking of the arms and legs lasts for a few seconds to several minutes and is followed by half an hour or more of grogginess before a return to normal.

· *Petit mal seizures,* which momentarily interrupt normal activity, do not cause muscle spasms. Instead, the child's head may droop, turn slowly to one side or be lifted upward as if he or she had decided to peer glassily at the ceiling. Ten or fifteen seconds later the child awakens and may take up the previous activity right where it was left off. It's not unusual for a child having fifty or a hundred such seizures a day to be referred to a psychologist for counseling because of "laziness," "learning disability" or "short attention span." Most children outgrow petit mal seizures by the late teens.

· *Minor motor seizures,* which are also known as myoclonic or infantile drop seizures, interfere with muscular control. During an attack the child may fall down as if paralyzed. Though conscious, the child is unable to control his or her muscles for minutes at a time, and when the seizures occur frequently the condition is incapacitating.

· *Psychomotor seizures* begin in the area of the brain beneath the temple and are characterized by a loss of consciousness in spite of the performance of apparently voluntary acts. The distinguishing thing about the attacks is their bizarre or repetitive nature. The individual may jump up from a chair, take several brisk strides, then return to the chair and repeat this sequence again and again for several minutes. Chewing motions, smacking the lips or picking at the clothing are common. In the course of psychomotor seizures persons have allegedly committed crimes, though it is difficult for the judge and jury to accept this plea on behalf of the defense.

Is it possible to have more than one type of epilepsy?   Yes, the victim of grand mal seizures may also have petit mal and minor motor epilepsy. Sometimes grand mal and psychomotor epilepsy coexist.

How is epilepsy diagnosed?   A neurologist, pediatrician, internist or other physician may make the diagnosis by observing the person during the seizure or listening to a description of the activity. Confirmation of the diagnosis requires an electroencephalogram (EEG). The brain-wave tracing is accurate about 85 percent of the time, meaning that a physician may go ahead with anticonvulsant medication when well-documented seizures have occurred in spite of a normal EEG. Presence of a normal brain tracing after a convulsion is a favorable sign suggesting but not guaranteeing that further seizures won't occur.

What is the treatment for epilepsy?   Anticonvulsant drugs are prescribed to prevent attacks, and during seizure a tranquilizer such as diazepam may be administered by injection. The choice of drug is dictated by the type of seizures and by the side effects of the drug. Most anticonvulsants cause drowsiness and other effects. Treatment should be under the close supervi-

301

sion of a good neurologist, who may have to use a combination of drugs to provide optimum control of the epilepsy.

When is surgery indicated to treat epilepsy? Epilepsy that is due to a brain tumor, cyst or vascular defect may be cured by surgery. In selected persons, removing scar tissue from the brain will cure epilepsy. Information about this and other methods of treatment, educational services, job assistance and professional help can be obtained by writing the Epilepsy Foundation of America, 1828 L Street, N.W., Washington, D.C. 20036.

Is it possible to recover from epilepsy? Yes, children usually outgrow petit mal and febrile seizures, and may stop having grand mal, psychomotor or minor motor seizures. A trial off medicine may be given after the person has passed the age of twenty or twenty-one and been free of seizures for a year or more. Correcting a medical or surgical condition that was responsible for the seizures is also a way of freeing the person from epilepsy.

What is hyperactivity? It is a pattern of disruptive behavior, short attention span, low frustration level and destructiveness that may be noticed in up to 5 percent of elementary school children. It is sometimes known as minimal brain dysfunction (MBD), minimal brain injury (MBI), hyperkinesis syndrome, hyperkinetic syndrome or learning disability.

What causes hyperactivity? Some children with this problem are found to have minimal brain damage with a borderline level of intelligence. Inability to perform fine motor skills may be noted. Most hyperactive children are not retarded or brain-damaged. Their intelligence is normal, their motor skills are not impaired, and they grow out of the hyperactivity at or before puberty. The cause of hyperactivity is still under investigation but suggested causes include vitamin and nutritional deficiency, psychological or cultural deprivation and intolerance of certain foods and food additives.

What's the treatment for hyperactivity? Behavior-modification techniques may help, and the child may do better in a smaller class with less rigid rules of discipline. An elimination diet may be useful when the hyperactivity can be related to certain foods (see p. 407). Ritalin and amphetamine are among the stimulant drugs that have been employed to control hyperactivity, but this treatment is in disrepute for several reasons. The drugs don't work for every child, and it isn't possible to predict which hyperactive children will respond. The Drug Enforcement Administration has classified stimulants as Schedule II dangerous drugs, meaning that the potential for abuse is high. In addition to being habituating, stimulants may depress the child's appetite or interfere with sleep. Certain antidepressant drugs have also been tried and sometimes found useful for hyperactive children, but they, too, involve psychological and physiological side effects that are hazardous.

What's the long-term outlook for the hyperactive child?　Many children seem to outgrow the hyperactivity at puberty, but long-range studies indicate that the individual may have learning and perceptual problems persisting into adulthood. Some psychiatrists believe that the hyperactive child is more susceptible to emotional or psychiatric illness during adulthood. Those who believe that food additives cause much of the problem stress the need for a controlled diet as early as possible in the child's development (see p. 407).

What is narcolepsy?　It's a condition of excessive sleepiness that affects men and women with equal frequency and usually has its onset in the teens or early twenties. It may prove incapacitating. The person may fall asleep after meals or during lectures, or spend the entire day drifting in and out of slumber. The naps bring a short period of refreshment, but drowsiness soon returns. Narcolepsy is not a form of epilepsy, and its cause is unknown.

What is the treatment for narcolepsy?　The person should consult his or her regular physician for an examination and laboratory workup. Stimulants may prevent drowsiness, and an antidepressant with stimulant properties has proved helpful in the treatment of some persons. Referral to a neurologist or psychiatrist may be necessary if symptoms persist.

DISEASES OF THE SPINAL CORD AND NERVES

What is Guillain-Barré syndrome?　This condition, also known as postinfectious polyneuritis and Landry's ascending paralysis, is characterized by fever and a progressive weakness that usually begins in the legs and ascends to the rest of the body. Complete paralysis of all muscles may occur; the paralysis progresses slowly, lasts for several days after it reaches a peak, and usually disappears over weeks or months, though, rarely, a patient may die of respiratory complications.

What causes Guillain-Barré syndrome?　Many persons developed the disease after the swine flu immunizations of 1976, but it may follow an upper respiratory infection and is thought to represent an allergic reaction to the infection.

What's the treatment?　The person should be admitted to the hospital for intensive nursing care and treatment that may include steroid hormones, ventilation therapy and symptomatic measures.

What are the symptoms of spinal-cord tumor?   The tumor may arise from within the cord or from the structures surrounding the cord in the spinal canal. Muscle weakness and a disturbance of bladder or bowel function are early symptoms of a tumor within the spinal cord. Urinary frequency, urgency incontinence—literally having to go so badly that one can't hold it—urine retention and fecal incontinence may occur. A man may become impotent or develop muscle weakness in the legs or arms that progresses to paralysis.

Pain is the most prominent symptom when a tumor presses in on the spinal cord from the surrounding structures. It is a dull ache that gradually worsens until the person will do practically anything to gain relief; many such persons have become addicted to drugs by the time the tumor is diagnosed.

How is spinal-cord tumor diagnosed?   Information from a thorough examination, X-rays, bone scans and the CAT scan may give a strong suspicion of spinal-cord tumor, but a myelogram is necessary to confirm the diagnosis. For this procedure, a small quantity of dye is injected into the spinal canal, and the flow of the dye is monitored by X-rays to identify a tumor.

What's the treatment for spinal-cord tumor?   If possible, the tumor should be removed immediately. X-ray treatment is more likely to be used when the tumor is malignant.

What's the prognosis after treatment for spinal-cord tumor?   Since 65 percent of spinal-cord tumors are benign, the long-term outlook is usually good. A completely paralyzed person may literally regain all functions, and surgery may relieve pain and allow better mobility for years even when all the tumor can't be removed.

What is sciatica?   It's a painful condition due to irritation of a sciatic nerve, the large nerves that run from either buttock down the back of the thigh to the legs. The pain is felt along the distribution of the nerve and is accompanied by a feeling of heaviness in the leg.

What causes sciatica?   The pain may appear after a protracted period of sitting on the nerve, such as during an auto trip. Loss of weight—and hence the protective layer of fat—increases vulnerability to sciatica. Men are more often afflicted than women. A ruptured lumbar disc, to be discussed in the next chapter, is an important cause of sciatica. An infrequent cause is the maladministration of an injection into the buttocks. If the shot is given too low, the drug may be instilled directly into the sciatic nerve, causing sciatica or even paralysis in that leg.

What's the treatment for sciatica?   When no underlying cause can be found, hot tub baths, avoidance of long periods of sitting, and sleeping on a firm mattress will give relief. Aspirin or acetaminophen will relieve pain.

What is Bell's palsy?   A usually reversible paralysis of the muscles in one side of the face. Symptoms may begin overnight. The eye on that side may not close completely, the corner of the mouth sags, and taste perception is altered.

What causes Bell's palsy?   The problem is in the facial nerve that supplies these muscles. It's thought that a viral infection attacks the nerve, causing it to swell at the point where it passes out of the brain through a narrow bony canal. Sometimes Bell's palsy reflects a brain tumor or marks the onset of Guillain-Barré syndrome or infectious mononucleosis.

What is the treatment for Bell's palsy?   An examination is indicated to rule out an underlying disease. Eye drops ("artificial tears") may be needed if the person cannot completely close an eye. By reducing swelling in the nerve, steroid hormones hasten recovery. Even without treatment most people recover completely within a matter of a few weeks, and permanent paralysis is very unusual.

What is tic douloureux?   Lightninglike episodes of stabbing facial pain are the symptoms of tic douloureux, which means "painful tic." Since the pain occurs along the distribution of the trigeminal nerve, doctors speak of this condition as trigeminal neuralgia. Most victims describe the pain as the worst imaginable. It may be set off by talking, chewing, brushing the teeth, stepping into the wind or even touching a certain spot ("trigger area") on the face. Though the pain lasts only a few seconds, attacks that come in clusters may make it seem to last for hours. Each jab of pain causes a facial grimace, hence the name for the condition, which is most common in middle-aged and older persons.

What causes tic douloureux?   The cause is unknown, though brain tumor may mimic the symptoms of trigeminal neuralgia.

What's the treatment for tic douloureux?   An anticonvulsant drug, carbamazepine, may give relief from the pain. Surgery can be done when the intense pain persists despite drug therapy. The nerves carrying the painful spasms must be cut, so it's best to have them injected with anesthetic first to see what the postsurgical numbness in the face will be like. Some persons prefer the pain to the numbness.

PARALYSIS

What is paralysis?   A loss of voluntary use of the muscles. It may occur with or without a loss of the sense of touch in the skin over the muscles.

What causes paralysis most often?   Cerebral palsy, brain damage incurred at birth or shortly afterward, is the most frequent cause in young people, and stroke is the most frequent cause in adults. Infantile paralysis, polio, is now a rare disease, though many adults remain crippled by it.

What are the symptoms of paralysis?   The person may not be able to move a body part or may walk with a limp. The extent of the paralysis determines the degree of disability.

What type of paralysis accompanies nerve disease?   Cutting a nerve will cause the muscles it supplies to go into flaccid paralysis. The muscles wither and become so loose that the affected limb hangs loosely at the will of gravity. Flaccid paralysis may occur following an attack of polio or when a spinal-cord tumor is responsible for the loss of muscle control.

What other type of paralysis may occur?   Stroke or brain damage may give spastic paralysis—the affected muscles are tight, rigid and drawn into a continuous state of contraction. Though the paralyzed muscles shrink in size, some ability to move them may remain. A child with spastic paralysis may learn to walk, though with a scissorlike, awkward gait.

Can muscle disease cause paralysis?   Yes, muscle paralysis may occur as the result of a disease of the muscle itself, as in muscular dystrophy, or of the junction where the nerve attaches to the muscle, as in myasthenia gravis. Muscle disease will be discussed in the next chapter.

What can be done for the paralyzed person?   When possible, the cause of the paralysis is removed. The victim of polio may benefit from leg braces and physical therapy to strengthen those muscles over which control remains. Several weeks of spastic paralysis may create contractures—tendon scars that hold the limb in a spastic posture even if the person later recovers from the paralysis. Prevention of contractures is the goal of early physical therapy for the victim of stroke or cerebral palsy. Surgery is sometimes indicated to free contracted tendons and enable a spastic child to walk with a more normal gait.

Who should treat the victim of paralysis?   A pediatrician, internist or neurologist should diagnose the cause of the condition. Surgery, should it be indicated, is done by a neurosurgeon or orthopedic surgeon, depending on the problem that is to be corrected. The best one to manage the overall rehabilitation of a paralyzed person is the physiatrist, a physician specializing in physical medicine and rehabilitation.

EMOTIONAL PROBLEMS

What is neurosis?   An emotional disability in which a person's behavior gets in the way of a satisfactory adjustment to life. The neurotic is usually able to function in the everyday world. He or she doesn't lose touch with reality. But neurotic people don't function as well as they might because they waste a good deal of their energy in unproductive, self-destructive behavior.

What is neurotic behavior?   An inappropriate pattern of behavior that a person has developed to relieve anxiety. While such behavior may relieve anxiety, at least temporarily, it doesn't solve the underlying problems that cause the anxiety. Compulsions of all sorts, hysterics, phobias and imaginary physical ailments are examples of neurotic behavior. We all have our own forms of such behavior, but when they influence a person's life unduly, that individual is said to have a neurosis.

What causes neurosis?   Neuroses can usually be traced to deep-seated, hidden feelings, such as anger, fear or insecurity, that go back to early childhood. These feelings may have been a natural response to the people and situations the individual faced as a child. To cope with them, he or she has developed certain patterns of behavior—withdrawing from social contact, aggressiveness, overeating, self-effacement. This behavior has then become a habit that has been carried over into adulthood, and the neurotic person uses it to deal with those old feelings as well as other threatening feelings. The behavior, instead of relieving anxiety, serves to keep the person uncomfortable, unhappy or unproductive.

Can neurosis be cured?   Yes. The patient has to learn new, more constructive ways of responding to life's realities and dealing with feelings. The length of time it takes depends on how deeply those behavior patterns are ingrained.

How is neurosis treated?   The course of treatment is often to go back and discover the feelings that prompted the neurosis in the first place—revisiting childhood and exploring the circumstances that taught the person to act the way he or she does. With that knowledge, the neurotic person may begin to separate present reality from the way he or she felt as a small, helpless youngster and realize that such behavior is no longer necessary. The feelings behind the behavior may never be completely lost, but many people can learn not to act on them anymore.

This is the basic approach that much contemporary treatment takes, but there are many variations. Some experts advocate long and intensive psychoanalysis. Others shortcut the analysis and the delving into historical causes. Instead, they focus on problem-solving and behavioral changes. Some believe the patient should be guided into making his own realizations. Others actively direct the patient toward certain insights. Some therapists treat patients individually; others treat people in groups. Some use drugs such as mild tranquilizers to relieve symptoms; others rely on more powerful drugs; still others feel the use of drugs to be unwise. There are all sorts of methods, theories and schools of thought.

How do you find a good psychiatrist?   A qualified psychiatrist is a physician who has finished four years of postdoctoral training in an approved residency program. He or she will be certified by the American Board of Psychiatry and Neurology. The type of treatment offered will depend on the doctor's own approach to mental disease. You can read books on the various methods and then interview the psychiatrists of your choice on the techniques they use. Whomever you choose, you should carefully and regularly evaluate how you are progressing and whether you are satisfied with the improvement you have made.

Who else can treat emotional problems?   A clinical psychologist who has passed a certifying examination is also a qualified psychotherapist, although he or she cannot prescribe drugs or admit a patient to a hospital.

In many states, psychiatric social workers are also licensed to counsel people on emotional problems. Ministers, physicians who are not psychiatrists and laymen may offer counseling on a formal or informal basis, though they have only minimal training in this area.

What is psychosis?   It is another word for insanity—a mental state characterized by a loss of contact with reality. The ability to function in the real world fails, and delusions and hallucinations may take over. The person's personality changes drastically. Whatever the symptoms, he or she will usually show lack of insight into the problem. Some psychoses are temporary, others seem to be permanent, though they remit from time to time.

What are the types of psychosis?   The main long-term ones are schizophrenia and manic-depressive psychosis, but there is also an organic psychosis

308

that results from damage to the brain. Ingestion of alcohol or a drug such as LSD may produce a temporary psychosis known as acute brain syndrome. Psychosis may follow syphilitic infection of the central nervous system or degeneration of the brain, as in senile dementia.

What is schizophrenia?   There is considerable difference of opinion about the categories of diagnosis and what symptoms are characteristic. The most commonly accepted description of schizophrenia is that it is psychotic behavior characterized by change in personality or a sudden worsening of previous symptoms. The individual may withdraw into himself or herself and stop trying to communicate with others. Fright, suspiciousness and moodiness may occur. In a rare instance the person may go into a violent rage and do harm to others. A disorganization of thought patterns is evident when the person speaks. He or she may reply inappropriately to a question, be unable to complete a sentence, or talk in meaningless generalities. The person's behavior may be bizarre as a result of delusions and hallucinations.

What are delusions?   They are blatantly false beliefs that a person sees as truth. The delusion is as vividly real to the psychotic as it is patently inaccurate to others, and may influence that person's behavior and reactions.

What are hallucinations?   They are false perceptions of sight, sound, smell or touch. A schizophrenic may hear voices warning him or her about plots, threats or suspicious individuals. Visual hallucinations are more apt to occur in an acute brain syndrome, such as one that's induced by LSD or other hallucinogenic drugs.

Is there more than one type of schizophrenia?   Yes, though these may be hard to differentiate. Psychiatrists have developed these categories:
· *Simple schizophrenia* is characterized by indifference and withdrawal, but delusions are not prominent.
· *Paranoid schizophrenia* is characterized by delusions of persecution. The person may seem certain that others are plotting against him or her. This is the most common form of schizophrenia.
· *Hebephrenic schizophrenia* may begin during adolescence with bizarre behavior, inappropriate laughter and impulsive, spontaneous outbursts of anger.
· *Catatonic schizophrenia* is characterized by such extreme withdrawal that the person literally stays in one position all the time. Seemingly indifferent, the catatonic schizophrenic is alert to his or her surroundings and may suddenly become violently mobile.
· *Undifferentiated schizophrenia* is what the disease is called when it takes no clearly defined pattern.

What is the treatment for schizophrenia?   Certain tranquilizers are successful in controlling the more dramatic symptoms in most schizophrenics, but they often leave the patient apathetic and functioning both physically and psychologically at a less than desirable level. Drug therapy should be combined with psychotherapy. Convulsive therapy with electroshock treatment is rarely indicated, for many schizophrenics become well enough on drug therapy to live and function in society. Recurrences are common, however, and some individuals require daily supervision in a controlled environment, though not necessarily in a hospital.

What is autism?   Autism is a mental illness of unknown cause that may be noticed during the first year or two of a child's life. It is characterized by withdrawal from the parents and the environment. Because such children shut off external stimuli, they don't develop speech and other abilities. Their behavior may be eccentric and violent. Evaluation and treatment by a pediatric psychiatrist is indicated.

What's the difference between autism and childhood schizophrenia?
Schizophrenia may develop in a child, but usually not till after age five or six. Delusions, hallucinations and a disordered thought process occur. The onset of autism is earlier, and such children don't usually have delusions or hallucinations.

What is actually meant by the term depression?   Depression is a normal emotion following the loss of a close relative or a job; it may occur after failure to meet a life goal or during a disabling (and possibly fatal) illness, such as cancer or stroke. This form of depression is known as exogenous, or reactive, depression. Usually it just has to be lived through, and it is only when symptoms and feelings persist and continue to interfere with function that it can be characterized as an illness.

When depression comes on without apparent cause, it is called endogenous depression and requires medical evaluation. Sometimes periods of profound gloom alternate with periods of extreme elation and frenetic activity. This pattern is seen in manic-depressive psychosis.

Can a drug cause depression?   Yes, the prescription drug, reserpine, is one of a number of drugs that may do this. It is used to treat high blood pressure. Other antihypertensives may also bring on depression. Less commonly, certain tranquilizers used to control agitation may cause depression, and so may progesterone-containing drugs, such as birth-control pills, as well as steroids, such as cortisone. Stopping the drug will usually relieve the symptoms.

How common is depression?　　Serious depressive illness occurs during the lifetime of 1 or 2 percent of persons, but the incidence is as high as 5 or 10 percent in older persons.

What drugs are used to treat depression?　　Three classes of drugs have been employed with success: tricyclic antidepressants, monoamine-oxidase inhibitors and lithium carbonate. The tricyclic drugs relieve the depression of about three-fourths of persons who receive these medications. The recovery occurs slowly during the first four to eight weeks of therapy. In persons who respond, the drug is continued for six to eight months and then slowly withdrawn. Persons who don't respond to a tricyclic antidepressant may get relief from a monoamine-oxidase inhibitor. These drugs may cause side effects, such as liver damage and a sudden rise of blood pressure. The blood pressure response occurs after eating cheese and certain other foods that must be avoided during therapy. Lithium carbonate is excellent for controlling the manic phase of the illness; it may also help during the depressive phase. Lithium therapy must be instituted during a hospital stay so that the dosage can be individualized. Blood levels of the drug must be monitored monthly during therapy. Early signs of a high blood level are nausea, vomiting, diarrhea and a fine tremor of the hands. Extreme care must be exercised in the use of diuretics, which may cause lithium toxicity.

How effective is electroshock therapy (EST)?　　Administered properly, EST is the treatment of choice for extremely severe or suicidal depression when the person doesn't respond to drug therapy or when faster recovery is desirable. The recovery rate following EST ranges from 80 to 95 percent. Improvement begins after two or three treatments (a total of four to seven constitutes a course of EST), and a shorter period of hospitalization is required than for drug treatment of depression.

What are the risks of EST?　　It may cause heart stoppage, an irregularity of the heartbeat or a fracture of the spine or other bones, though fractures are now uncommon because of the use of muscle relaxants. The presence of an anesthesiologist during the shock treatment permits rapid attention to any complications. Temporary confusion and loss of memory of recent events occur following the treatments. One death occurs for each 25,000 courses of EST, so the chances of survival are better than 99.7 percent. The treatment is, however, so dramatic, and is perceived by most patients as so traumatic, that it is being increasingly replaced by drug therapy.

How is EST given?　　It is given in the hospital in much the same way as surgery. The person receives a sedative and a muscle relaxant beforehand and is anesthetized during the actual shock. The electric charge, administered through electrodes attached to the scalp, produces a brief convulsion. Heart activity and other vital signs are monitored so that supportive measures can be taken if necessary. Within a few minutes of the treatment the person awakens and is able to return to his or her room. Treatments are generally given every other day.

What happens after the course of EST? The person is observed in the hospital until the doctor is sure that recovery has occurred. Regular follow-up visits are necessary, and a tricyclic drug is given to lessen the chance of a relapse of depression, which may occur months to years after EST. Occasionally, repeat courses of EST are necessary.

What is the most dangerous complication of depression? Suicide.

SUICIDE

How common is suicide? It is the ninth leading cause of mortality in this country, accounting for 26,000 deaths a year. This is 1.5 percent of all deaths. It is one of the most common causes of death among teenagers, and its frequency is also increasing among younger children.

Who is most likely to commit suicide? More than half of persons who will commit suicide are suffering from a psychotic depression, and alcoholics account for a fourth of suicides. Others who may kill themselves are victims of schizophrenia, another mental illness or drug abuse. Men are three times as likely to commit suicide as women, and it is more common for older persons than for young persons to kill themselves. However, the suicide rate among adolescents is increasing.

Is it true that one who talks of suicide won't usually do it? Not at all. Two-thirds of persons who commit suicide have communicated the intent to others in the hours, days or weeks before the event. Sometimes the threat is indirect and takes the form of a statement such as "If anything ever happens to me, I'm sure you'll carry on."

Will asking about suicidal intent push someone over the brink? No, because the possibility of self-destruction will have occurred to the person long before he or she is asked about it. The depressed person may be relieved to know that others care enough to ask.

What should you do when you think someone is contemplating suicide? The person needs psychiatric help, and should be protected by the doctor and those involved in his or her care. The situation precipitating the suicidal feelings is usually addressed first, to relieve anxiety, before the underlying condition is diagnosed and treated.

DRUG ABUSE

What is drug abuse?   The use of a drug for a nonmedical purpose or the overuse of a prescribed drug. The abuser may be habituated to the particular drug so that he or she doesn't feel normal without it. In a severe instance, addiction may occur.

What is addiction?   It's habituation plus a physical dependence on the drug. The effects of the dependence may not become apparent until the agent is stopped and a withdrawal reaction occurs. Examples of withdrawal include the nervousness and discomfort occurring when one stops smoking, the delirium tremens that may follow an alcoholic's withdrawal from alcohol, and the convulsions that may complicate the withdrawal from barbiturate addiction.

Which drugs are most apt to be abused?   The Federal Drug Enforcement Agency has classified drugs into schedules according to their potential for abuse:
   · *Schedule I drugs* have no universally recognized medical usage and cannot be prescribed without a special permit. Agents in this category include marijuana, heroin and LSD. These drugs have great potential for abuse, though they may be useful in special medical situations. Marijuana, for example, can be used to control the nausea of chemotherapy for cancer.
   · *Schedule II drugs* have medical uses as well as a strong potential for abuse. They can be prescribed, but a written prescription is usually required and no refills are given. Drugs in Schedule II include Demerol, morphine, codeine, most barbiturates, amphetamines and Ritalin.
   · *Schedule III drugs* include sleeping pills, such as Doriden and Noludar, and appetite-suppressant drugs. The potential for abuse exists, and a pharmacist, in most states, will give out no more than a month's supply at a time and up to five refills in a six-month period.
   · *Schedule IV drugs* include agents such as phenobarbital, Dalmane and Valium. The potential for abuse exists, and the doctor must use his or her narcotics number in writing the prescription.
   · *Schedule V drugs* have an abuse potential that is less than those in Schedule IV and consist of certain cough and antidiarrheal preparations.

Is it possible to abuse a drug that is obtained only through a prescription?
   It certainly is. Valium is the most commonly prescribed and probably the most commonly abused drug in America. Many of the millions who take

it are habituated to it. Sleeping pills, such as the barbiturates, soon lose their potency if taken in the prescribed dosage, and the tendency is to take more and more to get the same effect. Soon the person is dependent on the pills for sleep and has withdrawal effects if they are suddenly stopped.

Are nonprescription drugs ever abused?　Yes, the most harmful drug in America is alcohol because it is so widely abused. Cigarettes, whose consumption is also high, contain the drug, nicotine, a central nervous system stimulant that also happens to be addicting.

How common is alcoholism?　It occurs during the lifetime of 5 percent of persons. Five times more common in men than in women, alcoholism affects 10 million Americans. One out of ten persons who takes that first drink will become an alcoholic.

What are the symptoms?　The earliest is the discovery that one associates drinking with having a good time. The use of alcohol to the point of intoxication is a sign of abuse. Though the desired feature of getting drunk may be the drug-induced psychosis, it is an acute brain syndrome that may harm the body and further increase the chances of addiction. The need for a drink during the day or first thing in the morning is a sure sign of drug dependency.

What's the treatment for alcohol abuse?　Hospitalization and detoxification are indicated, but the best chance for long-term help is an organization like Alcoholics Anonymous. The organization stresses that help isn't possible unless the person wants to stop drinking.

12

BONES, JOINTS and MUSCLES

What is a joint?   It is the place where two bones meet, such as at the knee, hip or elbow. Movement of the bones on either side of a joint makes motion possible, and each joint contains a padding of cartilage and a lubricating mechanism of slippery fluid inside a thin sheath known as the synovial sac. Ligaments and tendons help to hold the joint together.

What is a ligament?   A fibrous connection between the bones on any side of a joint. A tear of a ligament is known as a sprain.

What is a tendon?   The cordlike end of a muscle attaching it to bone. Tearing of a tendon creates a muscle strain.

What is arthritis?   An inflammation or irritation of the joints.

What causes arthritis?   Among the causes are cartilage degeneration, as in osteoarthritis; infection, as in gonococcal arthritis; buildup of body chemicals, as in gout; and an inflammation of unknown cause, as in rheumatoid arthritis.

Is arthritis different from rheumatism?   A less specific term than arthritis, rheumatism is the term some people use to describe pain and stiffness in the back, hips or knees. The usual cause of rheumatism is osteoarthritis.

315

Which physician should treat arthritis?   Any medical doctor is qualified to treat mild arthritis, but the person whose symptoms are moderate to severe or who needs long-term care should see an internist or a rheumatologist. An internist is a specialist in treating diseases by means other than surgery. The internal medicine specialist has completed three or four years of postgraduatuate study in this field, and has been certified by the American Board of Internal Medicine. A rheumatologist is an internist or pediatrician who has taken an additional year of training in the diagnosis and treatment of joint diseases. Do not consult an orthopedist for arthritis. The orthopedic surgeon's training and scope of practice do not include medical treatment of arthritis, which should always be attempted before resorting to surgery.

What other physicians or practitioners may treat diseases of the bones, joints or muscles?   A physiatrist is a physician trained in physical medicine and rehabilitation who should be consulted to help someone recovering from stroke, cerebral palsy, muscular dystrophy or disabling arthritis when a strong program of exercise and physical therapy is indicated. A podiatrist is a doctor specializing in the medical and surgical treatment of diseases of the foot. He or she has been trained in a college of podiatric medicine and may have served additional years of postgraduate training. Podiatry is an ethical profession and podiatric physicians are qualified to treat diseases of the feet. An osteopath or chiropractor is sometimes consulted for bone or joint disease.

Is an osteopath a qualified doctor?   An osteopathic physician receives the same training as a medical doctor, though not always quite as rigorous, and is licensed to practice medicine in the same way as a medical doctor. Osteopaths no longer emphasize the treatment of disease by manipulation of bones, and there are osteopathic surgeons and other specialists just as in regular medicine.

What about chiropractors?   Chiropractic has flourished despite lawsuits and other efforts of the medical profession to stop it. This method of treatment owes its success to the laying on of hands or manipulation of parts of the body by the chiropractor, the genuine interest the practitioner takes in his or her patients, and the straightforward explanation that the problem lies in malalignment or disease of the spine. Physicians must admit that they often neglect the person complaining of backache; what sufferer hasn't thought of turning to someone who offers a different approach and even the possibility of relief? The danger of seeing a chiropractor is that serious disease might be overlooked either at the beginning of the treatment or during its course. Once a physician has evaluated and treated the problem, there's no harm in trying a chiropractor provided that medical follow-up with the physician is maintained. Most physicians believe that a chiropractor should not perform X-rays, draw blood samples or perform acupuncture.

ARTHRITIS

How common is arthritis?   It affects 60 million Americans, and 3.5 million of them are disabled by the disease.

Who is most likely to get arthritis?   Women are affected more often than men, and the chances of developing the disease are greater when one has a family history of it.

What are the main symptoms of arthritis?   Pain, stiffness and swelling in the joints are the main symptoms. The onset is usually gradual, and the symptoms are worse first thing in the morning and get better with exercise of the joint. Gout, a form of arthritis, is an exception in that the symptoms begin suddenly and are worsened by exercise.

What produces the symptoms?   The arthritic process irritates the synovial lining of the joint, the cartilage or both. Stiffness is due to the limitation of motion produced by swelling or to mineral deposits within the joint. Pain is caused by the inflammation or by the uneven movement of the joint because of the arthritis.

Which joints are mainly affected in osteoarthritis?   The symptoms are generally worse in the hands, knees, hips and spine. As cartilage in these joints degenerates, the edges of the adjacent bones touch and wear against one another; the friction creates a bony overgrowth known as "spur" formation. It's because of these changes that osteoarthritis is called bony arthritis.

What causes the cartilage degeneration in osteoarthritis?   It is a normal part of aging that occurs in everyone, but when it proceeds much too quickly, it causes arthritis in certain persons. Repeated injury to a joint is sometimes the cause of bony arthritis.

Does osteoarthritis shorten one's life-span?   No.

What's the profile of someone with this disease?   Usually an overweight woman past fifty notices pain in her knees and hips at the end of the day and upon getting out of bed in the morning. The stiffness persists for ten or fifteen minutes until the joints are warmed up, and then recurs later on in the day after activity. Symptoms are worse in cold weather and are relieved by aspirin or a warm bath. The fingers are also stiff and slightly painful each morning, and until they are warmed up, it hurts to make a fist or hold a pen.

What's the long-term outlook for one with osteoarthritis?   In most persons symptoms are minimal until after the age of sixty-five or seventy. Severe involvement of the hips is the most common cause of disability, and this is most apt to occur in the very elderly.

How does rheumatoid arthritis differ from bony arthritis?   The symptoms of osteoarthritis stay the same or progressively worsen, but the symptoms of rheumatoid arthritis may suddenly improve for a lengthy period of time and then just as suddenly reappear and seem worse. Rheumatoid arthritis may affect the person's heart and lungs as well as the joints. Some rheumatoid arthritics also have features of lupus. Because rheumatoid arthritis tends to start at an earlier age and is more likely to cause disability and deformity, it is sometimes known as "crippling" arthritis.

How common is rheumatoid arthritis?   About one in 50 persons will develop it at some time in his or her life. An estimated 5 million Americans suffer from the disease, which occurs three times as often in women as in men.

What's the long-term outlook for someone with rheumatoid arthritis?
Half of the people suffering from rheumatoid arthritis are still able to work and function almost normally after ten or fifteen years of the disease. Ten percent of sufferers will be completely disabled after this length of time of having the disease. Overall, more people are disabled by osteoarthritis than by rheumatoid arthritis; the reason is that the former is ten times as common as the latter.

Does rheumatoid arthritis shorten one's life-span?   Not usually.

What tests are used to diagnose arthritis?   Specific changes may appear on an X-ray of the joints, and blood tests help to support a diagnosis of rheumatoid arthritis. The typical findings are mild anemia, an elevated red blood cell sedimentation rate, and a positive rheumatoid arthritis latex test. The anemia is slight and not usually a problem. The sedimentation rate goes up during a worsening of symptoms and returns to normal during quiescent periods. A positive rheumatoid arthritis latex test may not accompany the disease, though it is usually present, or the test may be found to be positive in someone who has no arthritis. The latex test is based on an immune reaction between antibodies in the person's blood and bits of protein that are present on the latex particles.

318

What are the general measures for treating arthritis? Life stresses should be minimized to allow more rest, exercise and recreation. Good diet and a reduction to normal body weight are helpful. Warming the joints with water, a heat lamp or warm paraffin may prove useful. To preserve joint mobility, a range of motion exercises should be performed daily. The limbering-up exercises consist of moving the arthritic joints repetitively through their full range of motion for five or ten minutes.

What drugs are used to treat osteoarthritis? Aspirin in a buffered or slightly altered form such as sodium salicylate is the preferred treatment. Alternate drugs include acetaminophen, Motrin, Indocin and a newer drug, Clinoril. The purpose of these drugs is to relieve symptoms at the lowest possible dosage, and drug therapy should be combined with the measures mentioned above.

What drugs should not be used to treat osteoarthritis? Strong drugs shouldn't be used to treat a relatively mild, lifelong disease such as osteoarthritis. Codeine and other narcotics should not be taken for relief of pain, for the tendency would be to increase the dosage and run the risk of addiction. Phenylbutazone and oxyphenbutazone may suppress blood cell formation and aren't indicated in the management of osteoarthritis, nor is cortisone.

What drugs are used to treat rheumatoid arthritis? Therapy begins with aspirin or another salicylate, and this is usually sufficient to control symptoms. Your physician may prescribe other nonsteroid, anti-arthritic alternatives to aspirin but many studies show that these newer, more expensive agents are no more effective than aspirin. However, their side effects may be fewer. Steroids, gold or antimalarials may be used when the symptoms of rheumatoid arthritis aren't relieved by other therapy. Cortisone produces the most dramatic relief from pain and stiffness, but it does have serious side effects.

What are the side effects of cortisone? After several months to a year on the drug, one may develop elevated blood pressure, stomach ulcers, sugar diabetes, easy bruisability, trunkal obesity, a moon shape to the face, thinning of the bones and increased susceptibility to infections (see pp. 350–51).

Is there any way that these side effects can be prevented? The current recommendation is that cortisone or prednisone should not be used unless the person with rheumatoid arthritis has severe or disabling symptoms. Even then, safer therapy should be attempted first. If steroids are used, they should be taken in small doses and for periods of only a few weeks or months. Sometimes they are prescribed for use on alternate days. The person must often take antacids to guard against ulcer formation and may need medication to control blood pressure elevation induced by the cortisone.

How useful is treatment with gold and antimalarials?   Gold therapy works in an unknown way to suppress the inflammation of rheumatoid arthritis. It may cause allergic reactions, kidney damage, a severe skin condition known as exfoliative dermatitis, or a reduction in the white blood cell and platelet counts. Many rheumatologists feel it is unsafe; others prefer it to steroids. Antimalarials may relieve the symptoms of rheumatoid arthritis, but since they may cause eye or ear damage, they are not safe for use on a long-term basis.

Is surgery performed for rheumatoid arthritis?   Because the inflammation in rheumatoid arthritis occurs in the synovial lining, the removal of the lining has been advocated as a treatment for the disease. This often works, and many physicians favor surgery for well-established rheumatoid arthritis when the patient's symptoms aren't responding to medical therapy. The person contemplating surgery should discuss it with a rheumatologist and with the orthopedist who will perform the surgery. The patient should ask about the probability of improvement of function and appearance.

Is surgery ever indicated for osteoarthritis?   Yes, when a person can't get around because of a diseased hip, knee or foot, the surgeon can remove damaged bone or totally replace the joint. Hip replacement produces improvement in 90 percent of persons having the operation. The mortality rate of the procedure is 1 percent, and some surgeons prefer that the patient be under age sixty. Replacement of the knee, ankle and shoulder joints is also possible. Information about surgery and other forms of treatment may be obtained by writing the Arthritis Foundation, 1212 Avenue of the Americas, New York, N.Y. 10036.

Is acupuncture effective in treating arthritis?   As far as we can tell, no, though a few patients do claim some benefit, despite the lack of scientific evidence.

What is juvenile rheumatoid arthritis?   Also known as Still's disease, this is the childhood form of rheumatoid arthritis that affects 25,000 children in this country. Symptoms may begin with fever, rash and enlargement of the spleen and liver in a child under four. In an older child the symptoms are similar to those of an adult with rheumatoid arthritis.

What is the treatment for Still's disease?   Aspirin and similar agents are used to relieve symptoms. Prednisone and gold therapy may be used at minimum dosage, but great care must be taken to monitor for the side effects of these drugs.

What's the outlook for a child with rheumatoid arthritis?   In up to 95 percent of youngsters, the arthritis will disappear before puberty. Disease that begins in the teenage years usually continues as the adult form of rheumatoid arthritis.

Who is most likely to develop infectious arthritis?   Bacterial arthritis is most likely to occur in someone suffering from gonorrhea, sickle cell anemia, rheumatoid arthritis, antibody deficiency disease, or a condition requiring therapy with immunosuppressive drugs or cortisone. Infective arthritis also may begin in an artificial joint months after the surgery.

What are the symptoms of infectious arthritis?   They include fever along with pain, swelling and heat in the infected joint. Symptoms progress rapidly, and the joint may be destroyed unless treatment is begun promptly.

What's the treatment for infectious arthritis?   The person should be hospitalized and treated intensively with antibiotics. The diagnosis is made by aspirating fluid from the infected joint. Smears and cultures will identify the causative bacteria so that the right antibiotic can be selected. When treatment is begun within a week of onset, the outlook for complete recovery is good.

GOUT

What is gout?   It is a form of arthritis that occurs in severe attacks and is due to abnormal metabolism of uric acid. A body product formed during the breakdown of cells, uric acid may also be ingested in foods such as liver, kidney and sardines. Normally excreted in the urine, it may build up in the bloodstream and accumulate in or around one or more joints to cause arthritis.

How common is gout?   A million people in this country have it, 95 percent of them men.

What causes gout?   The cause is unknown, though a fourth of persons who develop it have a family history of gout. In these individuals it is thought to be an inborn error of metabolism, and this is also the explanation when gout occurs in the absence of any contributing cause. Secondary gout occurs when the uric acid elevation is due to a blood disease, kidney disease

321

or diabetes, or when the condition occurs, in susceptible individuals, during therapy with a diuretic.

What are the symptoms of an attack?   Gout strikes suddenly in the middle of the night or first thing in the morning, causing excruciating pain, swelling and tenderness in one joint. Most often the attack is in the big toe at its junction with the foot. Other joints in the foot may be affected, or the disease may strike the ankle, knee, wrist or hand. The gouty joint swells, turns red and becomes untouchably tender. The person may also have fever and generalized distress.

What sets off the attack?   It may follow indulgence in drink or rich food, or occur after a trivial injury, such as stubbing the toe, or it may appear with no apparent cause.

Does the person's blood level of uric acid go up during an attack of gout? Yes.

Does everyone with a high uric-acid level develop gout?   No, only one out of six persons with an elevated blood level of uric acid actually develops gout. In fact, medicine given to lower the uric acid may mobilize so much of this mineral that an attack of gout is precipitated.

What's the treatment for gout?   Colchicine is the most effective drug. It is given hourly for six to eight hours, and is so specific in its pain-relieving effect that it may be used to confirm the diagnosis—no other form of arthritis will respond to colchicine. Diarrhea is an unfortunate side effect of colchicine, and it tends to occur before or at about the time the drug relieves the joint pain. Other anti-inflammatory drugs may also be used to control an attack of gout. Without treatment, an attack will last three to five days and subside.

What are the complications of gout?   In long-standing gout, uric-acid crystals may accumulate in the outer ear, the joints of the hands and other body parts. Kidney stones or kidney failure may occur. Complications are more likely to occur in one whose gout began before the age of forty.

How may these complications be prevented?   For the person with true gout, lifelong therapy with drugs that decrease the uric acid is indicated. Treatment for the individual whose gout is secondary to another disease or to drug therapy is aimed at removing the underlying cause.

What is pseudogout?   Occurring usually in a person over sixty, this condition produces a gouty attack of arthritis in one joint. The knee is most often affected, and the condition can be distinguished from true gout by aspirating fluid from the joint and examining the fluid under a polarizing microscope. Crystals of calcium pyrophosphate are diagnostic of pseudogout, and these show up as distinctly different from the crystals of uric acid seen in true gout.

Who is most apt to develop pseudogout?   Persons with diabetes and certain endocrine conditions are susceptible to it, and it also tends to run in families.

What's the treatment for pseudogout?   Aspirin, or one of the nonsteroid anti-arthritic drugs may be used in the treatment of an acute attack, usually with prompt relief. Long-term therapy is not indicated.

NECK, SHOULDER AND ARM PROBLEMS

What causes pain in the neck?   Pain occurring in the absence of injury may be due to arthritis of the spine, a pinched nerve, a slipping of a spinal vertebra, fibromyositis, meningitis or wryneck. Pain following an injury is more likely caused by a whiplash injury or dislocation of the neck.

Is neck pain usually serious?   No. Nine out of ten persons with it don't have a serious problem. Wear and tear on the neck may produce some changes in the vertebrae by middle age, which is also the time when the symptoms of osteoarthritis may begin. Inability to turn the head easily is an early symptom. A dull ache accompanied by a tired feeling may seem to localize in the neck at the end of the day. Stiffness is most prominent early in the morning and when the weather changes. Identical symptoms in a younger person are usually attributed to fibromyositis, an inflammation of the muscles and their linings. "Trigger point" areas of tenderness may be noted in the muscles between the shoulder blades. Fibromyositis is most likely to occur in a tense individual, and is akin to tension headache.

What's the treatment for these conditions?   Heat in the form of a hot bath or shower, hot water bottle or heating pad may bring relief, and aspirin or acetaminophen can be used as necessary. A massage of the shoulder and neck muscles and a program of neck exercises may help.

How can you tell if neck pain is serious?   Pain that shoots down the arm and is accompanied by numbness or a pins-and-needles sensation in the arm or hand is a serious sign: a nerve in the neck may be pinched. Neck pain or stiffness following an injury should be taken seriously, especially if the person cannot move the head or must hold it tilted to one side. Neck pain in association with fever suggests meningitis. Prompt, thorough evaluation is indicated in each instance.

What is a whiplash injury?   A sprain of the neck caused when the head is suddenly snapped backward like the lash of a whip. The injury may occur during an auto accident. A football player may suffer whiplash when hit hard from behind. The damage is to the ligaments and other soft tissues around the cervical spine. Stiffness and dull pain in the back of the neck are the main symptoms.

What's the treatment for whiplash?   The neck is immobilized by having the person wear a cervical collar. Traction of the neck is sometimes used. Young persons respond more quickly than older ones. Muscle relaxants and medication for pain may be used as well as hot pads and massage.

What is wryneck, or stiff neck?   This painful condition is due to spasm in one sternomastoid muscle, the muscle that stands out between the ear and the neck when you turn your head all the way to the right or left. The head is bent to one side and the neck muscle is exquisitely tender to the touch. A child or adolescent may develop wryneck following a respiratory illness or blow to the head or neck. Sleeping in a draft or in an unusual position may cause it. A newborn may have the condition from an injury during a difficult delivery.

How is wryneck diagnosed?   It is diagnosed clinically, but if it persists for more than a day or so or follows an injury, the neck should be X-rayed to rule out a fracture or dislocation of the spine.

What is the treatment for wryneck?   Most patients will respond to muscle relaxants and rest, and should be markedly improved within one or two days. Mild stretching exercises may relieve wryneck in a newborn, and surgery to lengthen the muscle may be necessary to prevent deformity in rare cases.

What is bursitis?   A bursa is a lubricating sac of fluid found between two muscles or between a tendon and bone. Inflammation—bursitis—may follow injury or overuse of the part.

What is tendinitis?   An inflammation of the tendons, most typically in the outer part of the upper arm. The symptoms closely resemble those of bursitis.

What are the symptoms of bursitis and tendinitis?   An attack begins with soreness that is followed by pain which limits use of the muscle. The deltoid muscle that lifts the arm is a common site—the right arm if the person is

324

right-handed. Symptoms may last a week or longer, and recurring attacks are the rule.

How is bursitis diagnosed?   It can be recognized clinically, but a small fleck of calcium may be seen in the deltoid muscle an inch or two below the point of the shoulder or on an X-ray of the arm. The calcium deposit marks the site of the inflammation.

What's the treatment for bursitis?   An injection of an anesthetic, together with a long-acting steroid, can be made into the affected area to produce a dramatic relief of pain. Primary-care physicians, orthopedists and surgeons are able to give the injection, which occasionally causes a shrinkage of tissue or loss of pigment in the overlying skin. Aspirin, heat and rest— the conservative methods of treatment—should be used for a mild attack.

What causes pain in the hand?   Arthritis and injury are obvious causes, and a pinched nerve in the neck may send pain shooting down the arm to the hand. A diabetic may develop hand pain from a form of nerve degeneration, and a frequently overlooked cause is carpal tunnel syndrome.

What is carpal tunnel syndrome?   At the wrist, a nerve to the hand must dip under the tendons through a tunnel of fibrous tissue—the carpal tunnel. In certain persons, usually middle-aged women, the covering tightens and presses on the nerve. Burning pain or a dull ache occurs in the hand at night. The pain is most severe in the thumb, index or middle finger and is unlikely to affect the small finger. Numbness or a feeling of pins and needles may accompany the pain. Driving a car or holding a newspaper may bring on the symptoms, as may bending the hand in against the wrist and holding it there for a minute. Long-standing carpal tunnel syndrome may cause weakness and a withering of the muscles at the base of the thumb.

How is it diagnosed?   Carpal tunnel syndrome can be suspected on the basis of the person's history and confirmed by electrodiagnostic studies of nerve conduction to the hand, which are performed usually by a neurologist.

What is the treatment for carpal tunnel syndrome?   A splint is used to hold the wrist in a neutral position. An injection of cortisone into the wrist at the site of the problem may relieve symptoms for weeks or months, but surgery to relieve pressure on the nerve is indicated if the symptoms persist or return following the injection.

What causes pain in the fingers?   Aside from arthritis, finger pain may be caused by an inflammation of the tendon linings along the underside of the hand. The condition is known as "trigger finger." It occurs most often in a man and usually in the index (trigger) finger. The finger tends to lock in the flexed position and the person experiences pain when it is straightened.

What is the treatment for trigger finger?   An injection of steroid may give relief, though it's best to get by without steroids if possible. Resting the fingers by wearing a hand splint for a week or two may allow the tendons to heal. Surgery to remove the inflamed tendons has been used, but the operation is necessary only in severe cases that do not respond to more conservative therapy.

What else may cause difficulty in straightening the fingers?   Tightening of the fibrous sheath covering the palm of the hand—Dupuytren's contracture—may limit the ability to straighten the fingers. This condition occurs most often in men over fifty. A callus-like nodule forms in the palm, and the tendon sheaths stand out like cords. Eventually the little and ring fingers may close tightly against the palm and resist straightening.

What is the treatment for Dupuytren's contracture?   Steroid injection may relieve the symptoms if done early, but surgery is necessary for severe contracture.

Can a hand that has been severed be sewed back on?   Yes, if it is kept on ice and the person is rushed to a facility capable of doing the surgery. The operation, done by a team of surgeons, is most likely to be successful in a young person.

BACK PROBLEMS

How common is backache?   Half of all adults have it at one time or other, but backache is not a serious problem in most of them.

What are the symptoms of the more common forms of backache?   Osteoarthritis causes a dull backache that is worst in the lower back. Fibromyositis may cause pain in the middle or upper part of the back. It occurs in a younger individual, and the pain is more pronounced during times of tension, fatigue or excessive activity. Back strain may occur after lifting a heavy object or stretching the back, as in reaching down to pick up something. The pain may be sharp and so severe as to interfere with ordinary activities; sometimes it doesn't begin until a day or two after the activity that produced it. Sacroiliac inflammation, occurring usually in women, is responsible for low-back discomfort. The pain is worst first thing in the morning and gradually leaves during the day, though it may return if the person has to sit still for any length of time.

How are these problems recognized?   They can usually be diagnosed clinically, but a back X-ray is needed to rule out a spinal problem. Sacroiliac inflammation can be diagnosed by a bone scan.

What measures are used to treat backache?   Nonspecific remedies include:
· Sleeping on a firm bed or placing a sheet of 3/8-inch plyboard between the mattress and the box springs.
· Reducing to normal weight if one is obese.
· Applying heat to the back in the form of baths, a heating pad or heat lamp.
· Taking aspirin, acetaminophen and/or a muscle relaxant.
· Exercising the back regularly, using a set of exercises demonstrated by a physical therapist or recommended by the physician. By strengthening the back muscles, the exercises reduce pain and improve mobility.

What are the more serious causes of backache?   These include ankylosing spondylitis, abnormal spinal curvature, tumor of the spine or cord (discussed on p. 304) and slipped disc.

What is ankylosing spondylitis?   A form of arthritis limited primarily to the back and occurring nine times as often in men as in women. A man in his teens or twenties notes pain and stiffness in the low back. The onset is gradual, and a peculiar characteristic is that rest tends to bring on the pain while motion relieves it. The pain may awaken the individual early in the morning and leave after he gets out of bed and moves around, and progressive disease produces stiffness of the spine and varying degrees of disability.

What causes ankylosing spondylitis?   Ninety percent of those who have it show a specific white cell antigen pattern, suggesting that a predisposition to develop the disease is inherited. The disease is thirty times as frequent among persons who have a relative with it.

What's the treatment for ankylosing spondylitis?   The person should follow the general measures for treating backache, and anti-inflammatory and analgesic drugs may be used in the treatment, under careful supervision with monitoring for side effects.

What is a disc?   A disc is a specialized shock absorber lying between each of the vertebrae that, collectively, make up the backbone. The disc itself is not as simple as its name implies. It is a complex structure composed of a semisolid inner layer encased in a thick, fibrous ring.

What is a slipped disc? It is a rupture of the inner, semisolid part of the disc occurring in a manner similar to the way that seeds may be squeezed from a grape. The most common site for the rupture, or herniation, is at the lower lumbar spine near where it joins the sacrum.

Who is most likely to have a slipped disc? Over 80 percent of slipped discs occur in men between the ages of twenty and forty. Greater occurrence in men is attributed to their more frequent performance of heavy physical labor requiring bending and lifting.

What are the symptoms of a slipped disc? Low back pain occurs suddenly or gradually following a period of heavy labor or exercise. The pain is worsened by movement and relieved by rest. Typically, it radiates down the back of the thigh in the form of sciatica. The pain may be incapacitating: any movement of the back or legs is unbearable, and the person may not be able to rest except with the legs elevated. An X-ray of the back often shows a narrowing of the space between the vertebrae where the disc has ruptured.

What is the treatment for a slipped disc? Resting flat in bed, except for bathroom visits, for two or more weeks will usually relieve the symptoms. Afterwards the person must guard the back to prevent a recurrence of the painful condition and strengthen it with exercise. The definitive treatment, an operation known as laminectomy, may be performed by a neurosurgeon or orthopedic surgeon, but before undergoing the operation a second opinion should be sought on its advisability.

What is scoliosis? An abnormal spinal curvature that begins during childhood and in a severe case may progress into adulthood to cause backache, breathing difficulties and heart problems. In most instances the curvature is mild and nonprogressive.

Who is most likely to have scoliosis? A family history of the condition is present in a third of those who develop it, but many times the condition occurs for no apparent reason. It is seven times as frequent in girls as in boys and usually is first noticed between the ages of eight and ten.

How is scoliosis recognized? Unevenness in the height of the shoulders is the earliest clue. The abnormal curvature is most pronounced in the upper part of the back, with the convexity usually pointing to the left. One way to identify the defect is to ask the child to bend forward from the waist until the back is parallel to the floor; the child's hands should rest directly beneath the head on a stool or chair. When scoliosis is present, the back will slump more on one side than on the other. School screening programs uncover many instances of scoliosis, and the diagnosis is confirmed by an X-ray of the backbone.

What is the treatment for scoliosis?   No treatment is indicated for a curvature of less than 20 degrees. A Milwaukee brace may be worn to correct thoracic scoliosis of 20 to 40 degrees. More severe angulation calls for surgery, though a 50 percent reduction in the abnormal curvature is all that can be expected. Surgery should be done at a center specializing in this disease, for long-term bracing and follow-up are needed afterward. In every instance, the earlier the scoliosis is detected, the more likely it is that it can be managed successfully.

What precautions should an adult with scoliosis take?   Seek regular medical examinations if there are problems or pain. If one has a severe curvature, genetic counseling may be desirable before considering pregnancy because of the possibility of transmitting the defect to a child. The child of a parent with scoliosis should be examined for evidence of the disease.

What causes swayback?   The lower spine has a normal bend inward toward the abdomen, and an accentuated curvature is responsible for swayback. This, in itself, is not a cause of backache, and no treatment is indicated.

What is the cause of hunchback or humpback?   Tuberculosis used to be a common cause of hunchback, but TB of the spine is now a rare condition. Scoliosis is a more common cause of hunchback. Even more common is the gradual degeneration of the spine which creates "widow's hump." This may occur in an elderly man or woman and doesn't usually require treatment.

LEG AND FOOT PROBLEMS

What causes a limp?   A limp in an adult is often due to arthritis, but the sudden onset of a limp in a child or adult reflects injury or infection in the lower extremity. A persistent limp in a child points to inflammation of a bony center in the leg, muscle weakness from polio or muscular dystrophy, or spasticity from brain damage. Evaluation by a pediatrician and/or orthopedic surgeon is indicated. It is especially important to have the examination done early when a child limps while learning to walk, for the problem could be a dislocated hip.

What are the signs of a dislocated hip?   A painless limp and a lurching gait are the classic signs. The child walks well on the good leg, but has to throw the affected leg out and forward with each step.

Can a dislocated hip be recognized before the child begins to walk?　Yes, a normal infant's legs can be frog-legged out till they almost touch the examining table, and resistance to this movement or a slipping sensation points to dislocation. The frog-leg test should be performed by a pediatrician, family physician or orthopedic surgeon on every infant during routine examination the first few months of life. The earlier treatment is begun for the condition, the less the chances are of a permanent deformity.

What is the treatment for a dislocated hip?　A child under four months of age may be placed in a splint to hold the leg in the frog-leg position. The use of double and triple diapers, though this is sometimes advised, is *not* adequate to achieve the desired results. Treatment started after four months may require the use of a cast. When dislocated hip is not recognized until walking begins, surgery may be necessary to correct it; the operation is usually done between the ages of two and four.

What causes knock-knee?　Knock-knee and bowleg are normal conditions during childhood. A child just beginning to walk is normally bowlegged, but knock-knee becomes more prominent by the age of two or three. The legs tend to straighten out by the time the child reaches school age, but the use of leg braces at night is indicated to treat a severe deformity. An overweight, knock-kneed child needs to lose weight, and may benefit from wearing orthopedic shoes designed to correct the uneven weight distribution.

What makes a child's toes turn in?　This condition, often due to the position of the child's foot in the uterus, usually corrects itself before age one. Rarely, nighttime splinting is needed. Toeing in of a child who has just begun to walk is also usually self-limited, and studies comparing the use of braces to doing nothing have shown no difference in the outcome.

What makes the toes turn out?　This occurs normally in some children and is noticed when the child begins walking. One foot may turn out more than the other. Nighttime splinting may be used if the problem is severe, but the condition usually corrects itself by age six. Children with outpointed toes should be cautioned to avoid sitting spraddled on the floor with the legs splayed out at the knees.

Is flatfoot a permanent condition?　Many more children have flatfoot during infancy than actually turn out to be flatfooted later on. If flatfoot persists past the onset of walking, have the child checked by a pediatrician or orthopedic surgeon. An orthopedic shoe may be needed to relieve leg or foot pain sometimes associated with flatfoot.

What is clubfoot?   Occurring once in a thousand births, clubfoot follows an inherited pattern and varies greatly in severity. The foot is not at all like a club. Most commonly the heel is raised and the toes are pointed down and in as if the baby were about to take a step on tiptoe. Tight ligaments, not a bone deformity, are responsible for the condition.

How is clubfoot treated?   With slight force the foot can be brought into alignment, and straightening followed by splinting should be started in the newborn nursery and continued as long as necessary to correct the deformity. Casting may be necessary when the child is a little older. Half of children with clubfoot eventually need surgery to loosen the tight ligaments that hold the foot out of alignment.

What is the treatment for bunion?   This bony swelling at the base of the big toe represents a partial dislocation of the joint where the toe joins the foot. It is often due to wearing tight shoes, and the best treatment is prevention. Wear shoes that are long enough and wide enough, and avoid high heels, which may contribute to bunion formation. Surgery may be done for a bunion that is unsightly or very uncomfortable.

What's the treatment for ingrown toenails?   Nails that grow into the soft flesh on either side of the big toe can cause pain and frequent infections. The risk of infection can be lessened by applying antibiotic ointment to either side of the toenail after cutting and cleaning. It is not necessary to cut the nails straight across, but persistent difficulty with ingrown toenails may require a surgical procedure to remove the burrowing part of the nail. The operation can be done in a surgeon's or podiatrist's office and gives long-term relief.

SPORTS INJURIES

What is tennis elbow?   An inflammation of the outside of the elbow caused by overstressing the joint, as in playing tennis, throwing a ball ("Little League elbow"), or using the arm for an unaccustomed activity, such as sawing, chopping or hammering. The basic problem is that the forearm cannot stand the abnormal strain. Each impact is absorbed by the elbow and may create inflammation.

What are the symptoms of tennis elbow?   Pain begins following exercise, and it may be so severe as to make lifting a fork or turning a doorknob difficult. Heat and swelling may be noted in the elbow.

What's the treatment for tennis elbow?   The arm must be rested for a week or two, though it should not be placed in a cast. Injection of a steroid

331

hormone may relieve pain but the possible side effects should be carefully considered. Wearing a brace on the forearm may prevent a recurrence. The best preventive measure is to learn how to hit the ball without straining the elbow—easier said than done, if you have this problem.

What is baseball finger, or jammed finger? When a ball—a basketball, football, soccer ball or baseball—strikes a fingertip, severe pain occurs immediately and the finger swells and is difficult to move. The injury can vary from a mild strain to ligament tear or a fracture, and X-rays must be done to determine the extent of injury. In most instances a fracture isn't present and the ligaments aren't torn.

What's the treatment for baseball finger? Treatment consists of applying ice to reduce swelling and taking some aspirin or acetaminophen to relieve pain. The finger should be splinted lightly either by taping it to the adjacent finger or by using a metal splint. When the injury is severe or if the problem persists, an orthopedist should be consulted.

What is trick knee? It is a knee made unstable by an injury such as torn cartilage suffered while playing football. Cartilage doesn't heal as readily as bone, and torn cartilage may give trouble for life. The ligaments in the knee may be lax from the same injury, and weakness of the knee muscles may contribute to instability. Suddenly, while running, climbing stairs or changing position, the person has severe pain along with locking or collapse of the knee.

What's the treatment for trick knee? A painful locking episode may require emergency medical attention. In a less severe instance, aspirin or acetaminophen will give relief. A period on crutches may be necessary. The need for surgery depends on the degree of disability; the person who prefers to get by with conservative management can usually do so. The modern tendency is to operate immediately after a severe knee injury to preserve the stability of the joint.

What about dancer's knee? This condition is most apt to occur in a young woman engaged in ballroom dancing, ballet or gymnastics. Suddenly, while the leg is bent, severe pain, swelling and limited motion occur in the knee, and the kneecap is found to have slipped to the outside.

What causes dancer's knee? A woman's thighs slant down and in from her relatively wide pelvis, and the muscles join the kneecap at an angle. Resting in the ligament from the thigh muscles, the kneecap is in a position to be jerked out of alignment during dancing or other activities.

What's the treatment for dancer's knee?   The kneecap can be pushed back into position, though this is apt to be painful. Ice will help to relieve swelling, and the causative activity must be avoided while the knee is strengthened through exercise. Recurrent dislocation of the kneecap requires surgical correction. The ligament holding the kneecap has to be tightened, and the person must stay in a cast for eight weeks after the surgery.

Can you do without the kneecap?   Yes, and it is sometimes removed as treatment for a severe fracture of the kneecap.

What causes runner's knee?   Pain, stiffness and swelling characterize this condition, which comes from a wearing effect of the thighbone against the kneecap. Malalignment of the structures in the knee is often responsible, and faulty weight-bearing by the foot may contribute to the problem.

What's the treatment for runner's knee?   Symptoms, usually occurring in a hard-core jogger doing over fifteen miles a week, are relieved by temporarily cutting down on mileage. Exercises to strengthen the thigh muscles may help, and an orthopedist or podiatrist can prescribe wedges (shoe inserts) to shift the weight-bearing in a way that may prevent runner's knee.

What causes pain in the ankle after running?   Inflammation of the Achilles tendon can cause soreness and pain at the back of the ankle and in the heel. Among the causes are overtraining, neglecting to wear good shoes and failing to do stretching exercises before running.

What's the treatment for ankle pain?   Butazolidin will relieve the symptoms, but it's better to stop running for a week or two and let the tendon heal on its own. When you start back, do hamstring and calf-muscle stretching exercises before each run. Wear good jogging shoes with an added heel lift to prevent stretching of the Achilles tendon. Run on a flat surface or downgrade, go less than your previous distances and build back up slowly. If you develop ankle pain again, seek help from a physician with a background in treating running injuries.

The too-quick medical advice for many running injuries is to give up the sport. You may be able to locate a sympathetic physician in your area by writing the American Medical Joggers Association, Box 4704, North Hollywood, Cal. 91607. Another source of information is *Runner's World Magazine,* Box 366, Mountain View, Cal. 94040.

What are shin splints?   This is a sharp discomfort in the shins developing in one just starting a running program or in ice skaters. The pain is usually felt when the exercise has just begun, and it may leave after a sufficient period of warming up.

What causes shin splints?   Microscopic areas of hemorrhage are thought to occur between the shin bone and its fibrous covering. These reflect the stress of an uneven pull between the relatively strong muscles in the back of the leg and the relatively weak muscles in the front.

What can you do for shin splints?   Wear good jogging shoes or skates, and if you are jogging, make sure that you land flat-footed with each step and not on your toes. Begin a program of exercises to strengthen the muscles in the front of your leg. One method is to sit on a table with your legs hanging down. Add sand to an empty one-gallon paint bucket, hook the handle over your forefoot, and do five to ten curls with each foot. Gradually increase the weight and the number of repetitions, and continue the exercises for several weeks.

What's the treatment for ankle sprain?   This injury occurs when the foot strikes the ground unevenly and is forced inward. Pain and swelling are immediate, and it may not be possible to walk on the foot. For a mild sprain, resting for a day or two with the leg elevated will bring relief. Ice should be applied in the early stages, but hot baths will bring relief after the first day. Wrapping the foot with an elastic (Ace) bandage may relieve symptoms when walking is attempted.

Severe sprain causes a lot of swelling and the person can't put any weight on the foot. X-rays are indicated to rule out fracture or ankle dislocation. Treatment consists of resting with the foot elevated for ten days to two weeks, or the use of a plaster-of-Paris walking cast and crutches for a quicker return to a normal routine. Complete recovery from a severe sprain may take several months.

How is a fracture treated?   A break in the ankle or any bone elsewhere will heal on its own when the bones are held in alignment by a cast. Reduction, or aligning of the bones, can almost always be done without surgery. A bump from bony overgrowth appears at the site of the fracture during healing, but it will eventually leave and the healed bones will look completely normal to the eye and by X-ray.

BONE DISEASES

How does a bone infection occur?   This infection, osteomyelitis, may follow a direct penetrating wound but is more often the result of germs reaching the bone through the bloodstream. The thighbone and knee are frequent sites, and *Staphylococcus aureus* is responsible for 85 percent of such infections. Occurring more often in boys than in girls, the infection is most common in children between the ages of five and ten. The onset is sudden, with chills and fever. After several days tenderness and swelling appear over the involved bone, which may by then show through X-ray the changes of infection.

What's the treatment for osteomyelitis?   Caught early, the infection can be controlled by penicillin or another antibiotic. Infections more than several days old may require drainage of pus and removal of dead bone by surgery, so early hospitalization and intensive therapy are indicated.

What are the symptoms of bone cancer?   Pain is felt deep in the bone and swelling may occur around it. Symptoms often develop quite rapidly, and the usual site is the thighbone, leg bone or upper arm bone.

Who is most susceptible to bone cancer?   It is most apt to occur in an adolescent or older teenager.

What is the treatment for bone cancer?   Osteogenic sarcoma is the most common tumor, and the treatment is amputation of the affected limb followed by chemotherapy and X-ray therapy. The other form of cancer, Ewing's sarcoma, is usually treated by X-ray therapy and chemotherapy.

What is the outlook for someone with bone cancer?   The prognosis is best for Ewing's sarcoma, and three-fourths of persons treated for the disease are still alive with no evidence of cancer three years later. Of those treated for osteogenic sarcoma, 6o percent are alive and apparently free of cancer two years later.

What causes osteoporosis, thinning of bone?   It is a natural part of aging that occurs in most persons beyond the age of sixty, though it seems to be more of a problem in women. Evidence points to a loss of calcium and protein content in the thin bone, but the cause for the loss remains unknown. Persons with thin bones have been found to consume less calcium than is normal or to absorb a smaller amount of what is ingested.

What are the symptoms of bone thinning?   Backache may result from pressure on nerves as the vertebrae lose their strength and are squeezed together. In severe cases, as the person becomes shorter the ribs may touch the pelvic bones. Fracture of the hip or other bones is likely to occur if the person falls down.

What can be done for thinning of the bones?   An increase in calcium intake and exercise form the basis of therapy. Since it would take a quart

335

of milk a day to provide the needed calcium, many persons prefer calcium supplements. Vitamin D may be given along with the calcium to improve its absorption. Sodium fluoride is sometimes prescribed, but its use is controversial because it is suspected of causing the bone to be brittle. The person must be followed closely for symptoms of excessive calcium intake, such as nausea, vomiting, weakness and unusual thirst. The side effects of estrogen replacement therapy are probably greater than the benefits it offers in the treatment of bone thinning.

MUSCLE DISEASES

What is muscular dystrophy?   It is an inherited degeneration of muscles occurring mainly in boys. Symptoms usually begin between the ages of two and six.

What are the symptoms of muscular dystrophy?   The child may begin to walk normally, then gradually weaken and have a tendency to waddle. Running is not possible and climbing stairs is out of the question. Some children walk on tiptoe or hop around, and all have trouble getting up after falling. A typical sequence is for the child to put his hands on his knees and get into a stooped position, then gradually raise himself by literally climbing his hands up his legs until he's standing.

Do the muscles appear small?   The muscles may be large early in the disease. Later, they diminish in size.

What happens as the disease progresses?   By the time of adolescence the child may be unable to walk. Respiratory infections become a problem, and survival beyond the age of thirty is unusual. In certain forms of muscular dystrophy, delayed onset and slower progression are seen.

What's the treatment for muscular dystrophy?   A cure has not been found, but physical therapy and the use of braces and other devices have helped to maintain the mobility of children with this disease. Financial aid is available through the local Muscular Dystrophy Association, and you can obtain the address and phone number of the office nearest you by writing the Muscular Dystrophy Associations of America, 810 Seventh Avenue, New York, N.Y. 10019.

How good is genetic counseling for muscular dystrophy?   It offers the best chance for controlling the disease. With an enzyme study it is often possible to tell if a woman carries muscular dystrophy; it is also possible through amniocentesis to tell if a fetus has the disease, so that an abortion can be performed if the parents wish it.

What causes muscle weakness in an adult?   Fatigue, the flu or any febrile illness may cause muscle weakness, as may certain neurologic conditions or stroke (see Chapter II). Two less common causes are myasthenia gravis and polymyositis.

What is myasthenia gravis?   A rare disease occurring most often in women of about forty and characterized by weakness of the eyelids, face and other muscles. The weakness comes in spells separated by weeks or months. During an attack the person's eyelids droop and he or she may see double. Difficulty in chewing, swallowing, speaking clearly or breathing may occur. Progressive disease may lead to death, but more often the person has a long and chronic course with relatively stable symptoms.

What's the treatment for myasthenia gravis?   Drug treatment may relieve the symptoms. The use of plasmapheresis is the newest treatment and seems to be very successful. Removal of the thymus gland, a small gland below the thyroid, may be indicated for one who doesn't respond to drug treatment. Two-thirds of those who have the operation note an improvement in symptoms. Cortisone has been used successfully in the treatment, but both surgery and hormonal treatment require careful consideration and expert medical care.

What is polymyositis?   A progressive muscular weakness of the hips, shoulders, back and neck suggests this condition, which affects women twice as often as men and usually begins between the ages of forty and sixty. Pain and tenderness may be noted in the weak muscles. Sometimes a rash appears on the face or trunk.

A fourth of women and over half of men with this condition have an underlying cancer of the prostate, intestine, lung, uterus, breast or ovary. The muscle condition is thought to represent a reaction to the tumor, and removal of the cancer may cure the polymyositis.

What's the treatment for polymyositis?   A workup to rule out cancer is indicated. Steroid hormones, administered under close supervision, may relieve polymyositis that is not associated with an underlying cancer.

13

DIABETES
and GLANDULAR
PROBLEMS

What are glandular problems?   The endocrine glands, which produce hormones, include the thyroid, the parathyroid, adrenal and pituitary. When these or other hormone-producing organs fail to function properly, a disease may occur.

What do the endocrine glands normally do?   They help to regulate many body functions by controlling such things as temperature, blood pressure, growth rate and sexual development. The glands work by releasing hormones into the circulation.

What is a hormone?   A hormone is a chemical substance that serves as a stimulus to many body systems. Insulin made in the pancreas is necessary for sugar to get from the blood into the cells. Without it, diabetes develops. Growth hormone made in the pituitary is necessary for body growth. Without it, dwarfism occurs. Thyroid hormone regulates the speed of energy production by the body's cells. Without it, all body processes slow down. The adrenal hormones, such as cortisone, help to control blood pressure. Hormones released by the brain help to initiate and maintain testicular development in a boy and menstrual cycles in a girl.

Can other organs make hormones?   Yes, the ovary and the testicle, in addition to making eggs or sperm, produce the sex hormones. The kidneys,

338

pancreas, liver and intestinal tract also secrete hormones in addition to their other functions.

What are the symptoms of endocrine disease?　　In a child, excessive growth or inadequate growth may reflect an endocrine disease. Failure to develop sexually may represent an endocrine problem as may precocious puberty. Kidney stones may occur in someone with overactivity of the parathyroid glands. Loss of energy and intolerance of cold are symptoms of thyroid deficiency, while weight loss, nervousness and a tremor of the hands occur with thyroid excess. Too much insulin can cause low blood sugar and blackout spells, while too little insulin may lead to increased appetite, unquenchable thirst and excessive urine output—which are symptoms of diabetes.

Who should treat endocrine disease?　　A general physician may spot the problem, but a specialist should give treatment. A pediatrician or a pediatric endocrinologist should manage a child with an endocrine problem, and an internist or endocrinologist should take care of an adult. An endocrinologist is a physician who has had subspecialty training in treating glandular problems.

DIABETES

What is diabetes?　　The condition occurring when sugar can't get from the bloodstream into the body cells at a normal rate. As it builds up in the blood, the sugar spills into the urine to create high urine output and a greater body need for water. The problem typically begins as a pancreatic failure to produce enough insulin, but diabetes is a diverse process that may eventually affect the kidneys, nerves, eyes and other body structures.

What causes diabetes?　　It may be inherited or related to obesity. Ethnicity plays a role: diabetes occurs in up to half of members of certain American Indian tribes and is rare in Eskimos and Orientals. In susceptible persons, therapy with thiazide diuretics or steroid hormones may elevate the blood sugar and create a condition indistinguishable from diabetes.

How common is diabetes?　　It occurs during the lifetime of 4 percent of women and 2 percent of men. Nine out of ten cases occur in adults, though the disease affects one out of every 500 to 1,000 schoolchildren. Diabetes is the sixth leading cause of death in this country.

Who is most susceptible to diabetes?　　An overweight person beyond the age of forty who has a family history of it. A child born to one diabetic parent has a one-in-four chance of becoming diabetic. When both parents are diabetic, the risk is even higher, and some authorities believe that all such children will be diabetic.

Is the onset of diabetes related to age?   To some extent, yes. It may occur in a child under the age of ten, but most children with diabetes develop it at about the age of puberty and carry the condition into adulthood. It may also first appear during pregnancy. Most instances of adult-onset diabetes occur after the age of forty, and the risk of getting it increases with each year of age. Half of persons in their eighties have high blood sugar, though this may not have the same significance as diabetes in younger people.

What are the symptoms of diabetes?   Increased appetite, insatiable thirst and high urine output are the classic symptoms which are more likely to occur in a child diabetic than in an adult with the disease. Sometimes coma is the first obvious sign of diabetes. A tendency to have urinary infections or the rash of yeast (candidiasis) may indicate diabetes. Bearing a child weighing over ten pounds is suggestive of the disease, and some diabetics first learn of the diagnosis after a routine blood test.

What test indicates diabetes?   A urine test for sugar may be used to screen for the disease, but the definitive test is one that shows that the blood sugar is higher than normal. The sugar may be greatly elevated or the abnormality may be so slight that a glucose tolerance test is needed to make the diagnosis.

What is a glucose tolerance test?   A way of stressing the body to expose a latent or mild case of diabetes. The test is based on the inability of the diabetic to pass a load of sugar (glucose) into his or her cells. The test is done first thing in the morning on an empty stomach. After a blood sample is taken, the person drinks a glass of flavored water containing 100 grams of glucose. Blood sugars are measured every hour, and the normal response is a mild increase with a return to normal in two to three hours. A diabetic will show a steep rise in blood sugar persisting for two or more hours.

Does a known diabetic need to have a glucose tolerance test?   No, it's a waste of time and money for someone with a moderately elevated blood sugar to have this test. When a doubt about diagnosis exists, many doctors prefer to measure the blood sugar two hours after the person has eaten a meal. The food takes the place of the glucose load, and a sizable elevation in blood sugar is diagnostic of diabetes.

Can diabetes be diagnosed in any other way?   Diabetes is more than an elevation of glucose. Specific changes may be noted in tissue obtained by skin, muscle and kidney biopsy or in the vessels that can be seen coursing

340

across the retina. It is possible when these findings are present to say that the person has diabetes even when his or her blood sugar happens to be normal. A more accurate term would be "prediabetes," as most such persons will eventually develop an elevated blood sugar.

What is the treatment for diabetes?   To a great extent, treatment depends on the diabetic's weight, age, dietary habits and general health. There are two main types of diabetes: unstable and stable. The unstable diabetic tends to be a younger person who is not overweight and who is prone to having attacks of ketosis, a body condition where fats are broken down excessively and appear in the urine in the form of acetone and other ketone bodies. Severe ketosis may lead to diabetic acidosis, a potentially fatal condition that will be discussed later. The stable diabetic tends to be someone beyond the age of forty who is overweight and not prone to attacks of ketosis.

In either instance, dietary control of the disease should be attempted before resorting to pills or insulin. Recent evidence indicates that dietary control is possible in 90 percent of stable diabetics and in many persons with unstable diabetes. Sometimes a decision is made to admit the person to the hospital for the institution of strict dietary control.

What type of diet is indicated?   The total caloric requirements can be estimated by multiplying one's desirable weight by ten, and correcting for activities such as exercise, which will, of course, require an increase in calorie intake. The meals should be divided into breakfast, lunch and dinner, with an afternoon and bedtime snack. Carbohydrates may comprise up to 40 or 50 percent of the total calories, but one should avoid sugar and sweets, which are very concentrated forms of carbohydrates. The intake of proteins and fats is about 60 to 100 grams of each per day, depending on the person's needs. In each instance, dietary counseling is necessary, and it is essential that the person learn to measure and weigh food portions accurately.

When is insulin therapy needed?   It is more apt to be needed by an unstable diabetic, and in any instance, insulin therapy versus dietary control should be discussed thoroughly at the outset. Sometimes it is necessary to seek a second medical opinion. It is generally recognized that doctors have been too quick to resort to insulin or pills to treat stable, maturity-onset diabetes.

Why the difference in the likelihood of insulin therapy for stable versus unstable diabetes?   One whose diabetes begins before adulthood may have an actual deficiency of insulin due to failure of the pancreas to produce enough of this hormone. Thus, insulin shots in conjunction with dietary therapy may be necessary. It is more likely that the obese, adult-onset

341

diabetic has a normal or elevated insulin level. The problem here is not an inadequate production of insulin by the pancreas but a resistance to its effects. In this situation the insulin resistance is related to obesity, and weight loss will lessen it or reverse it completely. Since not every obese person becomes diabetic, the problem of insulin resistance is more likely to occur in one who has inherited a tendency to have diabetes.

What benefits can the obese adult-onset diabetic expect from weight loss?
The disease can be controlled by gradual weight loss and it is possible that all signs of diabetes may leave if the person reduces to his or her desirable weight. Studies have shown that a beneficial effect occurs from the very beginning of weight loss. Ideally, the person should lose a pound or two a week under close medical supervision until the desirable weight is attained.

Is exercise good for the diabetic?   Yes, exercise has been called "invisible insulin" because it has an insulinlike effect. In addition to helping the person lose weight, the activity helps to lower the blood sugar. A juvenile or adult diabetic taking insulin must learn to lower the dosage before the exercise or to eat a little extra to avoid low blood sugar. Walking, jogging, swimming or any other enjoyable exercise is helpful, but an obese person who is not used to exercise should begin the program gradually and under the direction of a physician.

How does one learn to use insulin?   The doctor who prescribes it or a nurse under his or her direction should show the person how to give himself or herself an injection. It is desirable but not necessary to start insulin therapy during a hospitalization, and the actual dosage has to be worked out carefully between patient and physician. A diabetic should take classes and read about the disease to be aware of the many things that may alter insulin requirements. Contact the American Diabetes Association, 600 Fifth Ave., New York, N.Y. 10017, for very useful information.

How effective are the pills used in the treatment of diabetes?   The sulfonylurea drugs, such as Orinase, Diabinese and Dymelor, have been in use since the late fifties and have a proven ability to lower the blood sugar when the person is unable to control the diabetes by losing weight. They work by increasing insulin output from the pancreas. The pills are not indicated unless diet control and exercise have failed to lower the blood sugar.

Do the pills have side effects?   Yes, they may cause rash, nausea, indigestion, liver problems and a depression of the blood-forming tissues. The most dangerous effect is a severe, sudden lowering of the blood sugar to produce unconsciousness that may last up to several days. The reaction is most apt to occur when the person takes aspirin, alcohol, blood-thinning drugs, Butazolidin or a sulfa drug, such as Gantrisin, along with the diabetes pill. Fatalities have resulted from this drug-induced lowering of the blood sugar.

Do the diabetes pills cause heart disease? In a large study it was determined that the person who takes sulfonylurea drugs runs a greater risk of heart disease than do age-matched diabetics not taking these drugs. Many physicians dispute these findings, as do some pharmaceutical companies.

Does the urine have to be checked regularly? It should be checked daily or several times a week to see if it contains sugar, unless the diabetes is so mild that sugar never appears in the urine. Tes-Tape, Diastix or Clinistix can be used for this purpose. These products are available in drugstores. In uncontrolled diabetes, the patient may spill acetone, and a similar dipstick can be used to test for it. Acetone is a product of fat breakdown and its presence in the urine should be reported to the physician immediately. Results of the urine checks should be recorded and shown at each medical visit.

What other measure is indicated for the diabetic? The person should wear a bracelet or necklace from the Medic Alert Foundation, P.O. Box 1009, Turlock, Cal. 95380. The bracelet will identify the diabetic and give a number that can be called in case the person is unconscious from an injury or from a complication of diabetes. The person who receives the call will look up the diabetic's record and inform the caller of specifics in his or her medical history.

What are the other problems encountered by diabetics? Diabetics are more susceptible to infection, heart disease, vascular disease and a condition affecting the retina that may cause blindness. As discussed in Chapter 16, kidney disease and kidney failure are more frequent among diabetics. Certain of the body's nerves may stop functioning normally to cause impotence, diarrhea, numbness in the arms or legs, or a loss of sensation in the knee or ankle joints. Fortunately, these complications are not universal, and when they do occur, it's usually after years and years of the disease.

Hypoglycemia, a sudden lowering of the blood sugar, is a complication that may occur in someone taking insulin therapy. A more serious complication is diabetic acidosis representing a relative deficiency of insulin. Before the discovery of insulin therapy in the 1920s the person with severe diabetes often developed progressive acidosis leading to coma and death.

How is hypoglycemia recognized? This condition is also called insulin shock. When the blood sugar drops to less than half of its normal level, the person develops a typical pattern of sweating, rapid heartbeat, hunger, headache and the sensation of graying out or faintness. Loss of consciousness may occur suddenly like a blackout spell or be preceded by irritability, personality changes, slurred speech and staggering gait. Persons with hypoglycemia have been arrested on suspicion of drunkenness.

In what situations is hypoglycemia most likely to occur?   This situation occurs from taking too much insulin or from failure to eat regularly after the insulin has been taken. For the individual who is on NPH or Lente insulin therapy, hypoglycemia is most likely to occur around four in the afternoon following insulin injection that morning and with insufficient food during the day. The effects of NPH or Lente insulin reach a peak about eight hours after the injection and this, coupled with the insulinlike effect of exercise, produces the afternoon blackout, or "insulin reaction." Hypoglycemia at night may cause nightmares.

What is the treatment for hypoglycemia?   Frequent insulin reactions mean the dose of insulin is too high. The person should take less insulin or adjust caloric intake. A snack before an exercise session may head off a reaction, and candy or fruit juice should be kept on hand to ward off a reaction when symptoms first appear.

What is functional hypoglycemia?   For poorly understood reasons, hypoglycemia may also occur in persons who do not have diabetes. Known as functional hypoglycemia or rebound hypoglycemia, the condition may be triggered by the ingestion of coffee, tea, alcohol or aspirin. The person notes rapid heartbeat, nervousness, sweating and weakness. Because of its catchall symptoms, functional hypoglycemia is often overdiagnosed. In rare instances, liver disease or an insulin-secreting tumor of the pancreas is responsible for hypoglycemia.

What is the treatment for functional hypoglycemia?   Adjustment of the diet will usually control functional hypoglycemia. The diet should be high in protein, low in carbohydrate and sufficient in fat to meet the person's caloric needs. All sugar, as well as coffee, tea and alcohol, should be avoided.

How is diabetic acidosis recognized?   This condition occurs most often in an unstable diabetic when the disease gets out of control. The symptoms include thirst, nausea, weakness, increasing urine output and gradual loss of consciousness. For days or weeks beforehand, the person will have had large amounts of sugar and acetone (ketones) in the urine, which is why measuring these substances and reporting increases to the doctor is one way to avoid diabetic coma.

In what situation does diabetic coma most often occur?   It usually develops following emotional stress, lack of attention to diet or after an infection. Diabetics who are sick may stop eating and mistakenly believe that they don't need insulin. Actually, in the presence of an acute infection they may need as much or more than they normally would. Stopping the insulin injections leads to increased breakdown of body fats, creating acidosis and, with it, nausea and vomiting. The excessive amount of sugar being spilled into the urine greatly increases urine output, leading to more dehydration and a worsening of acidosis. This progressive series of events may follow the abrupt, deliberate cessation of insulin injections. Juvenile diabetics, in particular, very often impulsively stop their insulin therapy and they need especially careful supervision.

What's the treatment for diabetic acidosis?   The diabetic should seek medical help during any illness resulting in a drop in fluid or food intake. Adequate fluid intake is a must. The person's friends and relatives should be aware of the need for medical help to prevent acidosis when the person cannot help himself or herself. When acidosis or coma does occur, it's a medical emergency requiring immediate hospitalization and intensive therapy with insulin and fluids. Untreated, it is invariably fatal. Even with treatment the mortality rate is as high as 5 or 10 percent.

Should diabetics seek genetic counseling?   Yes. There is a strong possibility that the children of two individuals with this disease will be diabetic. A more usual situation is when other relatives of the prospective parents have diabetes, and genetic counseling may help in assessing the risks.

What is diabetes insipidus?   Insatiable thirst and a voluminous urine output characterize this condition, which may begin so suddenly that the person is aware to the hour of its onset. Most of the time the cause is unknown, but it may follow a head injury or arise from a tumor in or around the pituitary gland, or it may occur in certain families. Both sexes are affected, and the onset is usually during the teens or early twenties.

How does it differ from sugar diabetes?   High urine output is a feature of both conditions, but whereas the urine of a regular diabetic may contain sugar, the urine of one with diabetes insipidus does not contain sugar.

What is the deficiency in diabetes insipidus?   The deficiency is one of antidiuretic hormone, an important substance produced in the pituitary gland that acts on the kidney to cause it to conserve water. In its absence, as much as five or ten quarts of urine may be passed each day. Obviously, this large amount of fluid must be continually replenished by drinking vast quantities of water. Depriving the person of fluid for even half a day may throw him or her into shock and lead to death.

What is the treatment for diabetes insipidus?   The high urine output can be controlled by injecting the deficient hormone every one to three days or by taking antidiuretic hormone daily in the form of a nasal spray. Hormone therapy must be continued indefinitely, though sometimes the condition subsides spontaneously and further therapy isn't needed.

THYROID PROBLEMS

What is the thyroid?   It is a gland at the base of the neck, below the Adam's apple, situated on either side of the windpipe and connected across it by an isthmus.

What does the thyroid do?   It makes thyroid hormone, a substance that regulates body metabolism. Each cell in the body is like a tiny factory that converts nutrients into energy. Thyroid hormone regulates the speed at which the job, such as burning sugar or amino acids to produce energy, is performed. Too little hormone—hypothyroidism—causes a slowdown in body processes, and too much hormone drives the cellular machinery so fast that hyperthyroidism develops. An imbalance in the production of thyroid hormone can also create a goiter.

What is goiter?   Enlargement of the thyroid due to overgrowth of the hormone-producing parts of the gland. The goiter may begin during childhood and grow throughout life, but the condition is most common in women beyond the age of fifty. An estimated 2 to 4 percent of people in this country have goiter. The incidence is much higher in places where a severe dietary deficiency of iodine exists.

What is the connection between iodine and goiter?   Iodine is needed to produce thyroid hormone, and a deficiency of iodine requires the thyroid to enlarge in an attempt to use more efficiently what iodine is available. The addition of iodide to table salt supplies enough of this element to prevent most persons from developing goiter.

What other factors may cause goiter?   Goiter may result from an inherited defect in thyroid function, thyroid inflammation, an inability to utilize iodine from the diet or the lifelong consumption of rutabagas, turnips, cabbage and other foods that are said to favor goiter formation. Since pregnancy causes the thyroid to grow, multiple pregnancies may contribute to goiter.

How big does a goiter become?   It's usually big enough to be seen with the naked eye as a bulge in the neck that rises during swallowing. Some goiters have reached the size of a grapefruit, but this is unusual.

What are the complications of goiter?   A huge one may press inward on the neck to cause difficulty in breathing or swallowing. Hoarseness may occur. Sometimes one area of a goiter will turn into thyroid cancer, but this is rare. Sometimes a goiter is accompanied by the production of too much thyroid, producing the condition known as hyperthyroidism (Graves' disease).

What are the symptoms of hyperthyroidism?   The feeling of being warm, palpitation, nervousness, weight loss, prominence of the eyes and excessive sweating are the main symptoms. Others include diarrhea, blurred vision, weakness, fatigue, tremor of the hands and scanty or missed menstrual periods.

Who is most likely to develop this condition?   At greatest risk is a woman between the ages of twenty and forty who has a goiter, a family history of thyroid problems and who recently went through a period of emotional stress, usually involving the death of a loved one, a divorce or other major separation. The stress doesn't cause the hyperthyroidism, but it may bring out the symptoms of the disease in a susceptible person.

How is hyperthyroidism diagnosed?   The pulse rate is above ninety at rest. The person may have a fine tremor of the hands or a "thyroid stare" created by bulging of the eyes or spasm of the eyelids. Often the whites of the eyes can be seen above the iris and the person has difficulty looking upward or sideways. A goiter is usually present. The palms are moist and the skin has a wet, velvety texture. All in all the person seems to be burning up from within, and the increase in glandular activity can be confirmed by laboratory studies.

What is the treatment for a hyperactive thyroid?   The three choices are drugs, radioactive iodine and surgery. No unanimity of opinion exists as to which is preferable. The antithyroid drugs are propylthiouracil and methimazole. Both drugs may cause rash, hair loss and a depression of the blood-forming tissues. The drugs must often be taken every eight hours and don't always work. Propranolol, a drug used to treat heart disease and high blood pressure, has been found useful in controlling the symptoms of hyperthyroidism, though it does not affect the underlying condition.

The administration of radioactive iodine requires only that the person

347

swallow a measured amount of it. The thyroid gland takes up the radioactive mineral, which destroys many of the overactive cells. The problem is that too large a dose may destroy too much thyroid tissue. At least half of persons treated with radioactive iodine develop thyroid insufficiency and have to take thyroid hormone from then on.

Radioactive iodine is most frequently used for older patients, while surgery to remove part of the gland is the most common therapy for younger persons. Medication must be given to prepare the patient for surgery, and the aim is to remove enough tissue to cure the overactivity but to leave enough to support normal thyroid function. Usually, the person treated with surgery doesn't have to take thyroid hormone therapy.

What are the complications of hyperthyroidism? The most dramatic is an overwhelming crisis known as thyroid storm. Often triggered by an infection, it consists of severe weakness, fever, vomiting, disorientation, rapid heartbeat and even heart failure. Emergency hospitalization and intensive treatment are necessary to save the person's life.

Commonly there is a slight protrusion of the eyes, but at times this can be quite severe, with drying of the eyes, inflammation, inability to shut the eyes at night, and a condition where each eye looks in a different direction.

A serious complication, "malignant" exophthalmos, can be recognized by the rapidly progressive protrusion of one or both of the person's eyes. The eyes appear inflamed and double vision usually occurs. This condition endangers the eyesight, and management may include steroid hormones or X-ray therapy to lessen the swelling in the eye muscles. Surgery is sometimes performed to decompress the orbits, or eye sockets. Treatment should be coordinated between an endocrinologist and an ophthalmologist.

Is hyperthyroidism during pregnancy dangerous? The risk is that the fetus may develop hypothyroidism and be born a cretin. Harm to the fetus is unlikely when thyroid-suppressing drugs are given in small dosage. The thyroid may be removed during the fourth, fifth or sixth month of pregnancy when the woman doesn't respond well to drug therapy. In most instances the surgery is well tolerated, though abortion may occur as a result of exposure to the anesthesia and the stress of the operation.

What are the symptoms of hypothyroidism? They are opposite to the symptoms of hyperthyroidism and include sluggishness, cold intolerance, hoarseness, dry skin and irregular bowel function. Others are puffiness of the face, thickening of the tongue, slow speech and coarsening of the hair. This condition develops ten times as often in women as in men, and the onset is usually after age forty.

348

What's the treatment for thyroid failure?   Taking thyroid hormone by mouth will control the symptoms of the disease. To avoid stressing the heart, it is necessary to start with a low dosage and gradually build up to the full amount needed for maintenance therapy. With most forms of medication, the entire dose can be taken once daily.

What causes cretinism?   Thyroid failure occurring during fetal development causes cretinism.

What are the symptoms of cretinism?   The cretin has an above-average birth weight, a large tongue and a hoarse cry. The baby is very sensitive to cold and may appear sluggish or have swelling in the face or extremities. The child suffers from a delay in physical and mental development, but thyroid therapy will allow normal development.

Are cretinism and Down's syndrome related?   Because the signs of cretinism resemble those of Down's syndrome, the two conditions were often confused before the sixties, when it became possible through chromosome studies to diagnose mongolism with certainty. One still finds references to the "cure" of Down's syndrome by the administration of thyroid hormone. The hormone will cure cretinism but not mongolism.

How dangerous is a lump in the thyroid?   The great majority of lumps are not cancerous, but the person who discovers one in the thyroid or neck area should have it investigated. About half of the time the lump is part of a goiter. Perhaps one in ten lumps will be malignant, and this is more likely when the lump occurs in a child, a man or someone who received X-ray therapy to the neck during childhood.

What's the treatment for a lump in the thyroid?   Surgery is indicated if cancer cannot be ruled out, and the entire gland may be removed if the lump is found to be cancerous. Radioactive iodine is used to treat severe forms of thyroid cancer, and most persons must also take thyroid hormone. Even after treatment the person's condition must be checked regularly.

What's the long-term outlook for someone with thyroid cancer?   Treatment of the most common form of malignancy, papillary cancer, gives a ten-year survival rate of 80 to 90 percent. Some persons are alive thirty years and more after the diagnosis and are considered cured. A rare, rapid-growing form of thyroid cancer carries a mortality rate of 80 to 90 percent during the first year after it is diagnosed.

What are the parathyroid glands?   These pea-sized glands in the back of each of the four corners of the thyroid control the body's calcium balance.

This mineral, which is important to bone strength and normal nerve function, is regulated precisely by the parathyroid glands.

What are the symptoms of parathyroid disease?   Overactivity of one or more of the glands—hyperparathyroidism—causes an elevation of the calcium level in the blood, resulting in kidney stones, weight loss, vomiting, bone pain and abdominal pain. A tumor in the gland—adenoma—is responsible for these symptoms. Underactivity of the parathyroids leads to an abnormally low calcium level, producing muscle cramps, spasm of the hand muscles and numbness and tingling around the mouth. The usual cause is accidental removal or injury of the parathyroids during thyroid surgery. Symptoms begin a day or two after the operation.

What's the treatment for parathyroid disease?   Surgical exploration of the neck with removal of the parathyroid adenoma is indicated for hyperparathyroidism. In many instances hypoparathyroidism occurring after thyroid surgery corrects itself spontaneously in a few weeks or months. In the meantime it can be controlled by treatment with calcium tablets and vitamin D.

ADRENAL PROBLEMS

What are the adrenal glands?   The two adrenals sit atop the kidneys and make cortisone and other steroid hormones that are important in regulating blood pressure, blood volume, body minerals and certain aspects of sexual development. Normal adrenal function is necessary for the body to respond to stress.

What causes excess adrenal activity?   For reasons that are not entirely clear, the glands may enlarge and begin overproducing steroid hormones. Less commonly a benign or malignant tumor of one of the glands is responsible for the overactivity. Spontaneous adrenal overactivity, known as Cushing's disease or Cushing's syndrome, is four times as frequent in women as in men and may begin following a pregnancy.

What are the symptoms of Cushing's syndrome?   The symptoms of cortisone excess are given below:
 · Round face ("moon face")
 · Protuberant abdomen
 · Fat chest and back
 · Buffalo hump of upper back
 · Purple stripes on body
 · Weakness and backache

350

- Thin arms and legs
- Loss of muscle mass
- Thinning of the skin
- Easy bruisability
- Menstrual irregularities
- Impotence
- High blood pressure
- Diabetes mellitus ("sugar diabetes")

Can these symptoms be produced by taking cortisone? Yes, long-term therapy with cortisone, prednisone or a similar drug may produce symptoms that are identical with those of Cushing's syndrome.

What's the treatment for Cushing's syndrome? A thorough investigation is needed to make the diagnosis and hospitalization is indicated to analyze the situation fully. The treatment is controversial. Surgery and irradiation, as well as medical therapy, are all in use. Depending on whether both glands must be removed, the person may have to take replacement steroid hormones afterward.

How does drug-induced Cushing's syndrome affect the adrenal glands?
The adrenal glands of one who takes cortisone or prednisone for more than a few weeks begin to lose their natural ability to make hormones. After several months of such therapy, the person may become truly dependent on steroid therapy for life.

Can drug-induced Cushing's syndrome be prevented? It can be eliminated by withholding steroid hormone therapy, but in certain instances the advantages of the therapy outweigh the disadvantages. The tragedy is when steroids are given and continued even when not indicated, as in treating osteoarthritis, mild rheumatoid arthritis or asthma that could be controlled with safer medications.

What happens when the adrenal glands stop functioning? The symptoms of adrenal failure, known as Addison's disease, include weakness, low blood pressure, nausea, headache and fever. Unable to respond normally to stress, the person may become critically ill following what would be an uncomplicated injury or infection in a normal person.

What causes Addison's disease? Tuberculosis of the adrenal glands was once the main cause. More likely now is a spontaneous withering of the adrenals due to a self-destructive (autoimmune) process. A temporary loss of adrenal function may follow long-term steroid therapy, and it takes about a year for the adrenals to regain their normal function.

351

How is Addison's disease dignosed?   The physical findings and lab studies confirm the diagnosis of classic Addison's disease, which is so rare that most physicians will never see a case of it. The most helpful finding in a white person is the presence of brown areas of pigment inside the mouth, around the nipples and at scars and pressure points on the body. One person described the dark pigmentation as being "like a suntan that didn't wear off."

In one who has received steroid therapy, the diagnosis of adrenal insufficiency is often made at surgery or following an injury or infection when the blood pressure drops unexpectedly and won't come back up despite replacement of fluid and blood volume or treatment of the infection with antibiotics. The past history of steroid therapy confirms the suspicion of adrenal failure. Adrenal supplementation may be necessary during periods of stress, such as surgery, for up to a year after steroid therapy has stopped.

What's the treatment for adrenal insufficiency?   When the deficiency is recognized after an injury or during an infection, injectable steroid hormones must be given to support the person's blood pressure. In less urgent situations, replacement therapy with oral steroid hormones may be indicated. The dosage must be carefully monitored by close medical supervision for the patient's lifetime if the glands are permanently destroyed or until the adrenals begin to function normally on their own.

What precaution should someone with adrenal insufficiency take?   The person should wear a Medic-Alert bracelet telling of the problem so that the treating physician can give steroid hormones to support the blood pressure in the event of a serious illness or emergency.

What other problems may be due to adrenal malfunction?   Certain rare tumors other than those producing Cushing's syndrome may cause high blood pressure. These are discussed in Chapter 15.

PITUITARY PROBLEMS

What is the pituitary?   It is an olive-sized gland at the base of the brain. Better protected than any other structure in the body, it is the master gland controlling all others. Among its secretions are hormones that regulate the activity of the thyroid and adrenal glands and the ovary and testicle. The gland also secretes growth hormone, and an excess of this substance produced by a pituitary tumor may cause giantism which begins during childhood or acromegaly which occurs in adults. These conditions are relatively rare.

What are the signs of giantism?   The person begins growing excessively during childhood and may suffer from headaches and visual problems.

In giantism, how much growth is possible?   The height may approach nine feet. Robert Wadlow of Alton, Illinois (known as the "Alton giant"), weighed nine pounds at birth and sixty-two pounds at one year of age. At the age of eight he was six feet tall and weighted 169 pounds. He eventually reached a height of eight feet and eleven inches, and his maximum weight was 491 pounds. He died in 1940 at the age of twenty-two. This much growth is now unlikely because of better methods of treating pituitary tumors.

What are the signs of acromegaly?   Overgrowth of soft tissues produces broadening and thickening of the hands and feet. The tongue and internal organs enlarge. The jaw grows outward so that the bottom teeth lie outside the top ones. Growth of other facial bones produces a coarsening of the features. These symptoms may occur slowly and subtly, and may only be obvious when the person's appearance is compared with that in an old photograph. Diabetes, visual problems and menstrual irregularities may occur. The symptoms usually develop in the twenties or thirties and become very obvious in the forties.

What is the treatment for acromegaly or giantism?   The tumor is removed surgically or controlled by X-ray therapy; often the two methods are combined.

What causes dwarfism?   Underfunction of the pituitary gland beginning during childhood may cause dwarfism. The child lags far behind normal standards of growth, but pituitary dwarfs are of normal intelligence. The administration of growth hormone will allow normal development if the condition is diagnosed early enough. Pituitary dwarfism is very rare. Shortness of stature is usually inherited and is no cause for alarm.

Does pituitary failure ever occur in adults?   Yes, it may result from hemorrhage into a woman's pituitary gland at the time of delivery. The affected woman has no breast milk, doesn't return to having menstrual periods, and notes weakness, loss of weight and disappearance of body hair in the months after the baby is born. Cold intolerance, coarsening of the skin and absence of sweating may occur. These changes can be reversed by giving replacement therapy with sex hormones, cortisone and, if indicated, thyroid hormone, but such individuals will remain infertile.

Pituitary insufficiency that is not related to pregnancy is most often due to a tumor that destroys the gland. Treatment of the tumor, which may occur in a man or a woman, is to remove it or to control its growth by X-ray therapy.

OBESITY

What is obesity?   It is fat, or an excess of body weight, amounting to 10 percent or more of the predicted normal weight for the person. In an adult this usually amounts to fifteen pounds or more of fat, and the person with problem obesity generally is forty or fifty pounds overweight.

What's the difference between overweight and obesity?   The increased weight in obesity is due to an excess of fatty tissue. An athlete may be overweight as the result of an excess of muscle tissue without having an increase in body fat. The most reliable test for obesity is to measure the thickness of the skin fold along the upper back part of the arm; this fold should be less than three-eighths of an inch thick.

Is obesity a glandular problem?   Not that we know of. Most persons with thyroid insufficiency are not obese. Most obese persons do not have a thyroid problem.

What causes obesity?   It develops when the person's energy intake in the form of food exceeds energy expenditure in the form of exercise. Allowed to persist, the imbalance creates obesity and is often a lifelong problem.

Are there any factors that contribute to obesity?   Yes. Among them are:
  · Obesity tends to run in families. Fat adults have fat children—because of eating patterns that are learned in the family.
  · Obesity during childhood is thought to cause an increased number of fat cells to develop, though there is some evidence that fat cells can multiply in adults too. An overweight infant or child is three times as likely to be an obese adult as is the child whose weight remains normal. The person whose obesity begins during adulthood develops larger-than-normal fat cells.
  · Women are more likely to become obese than men.
  · The incidence of obesity increases with age.

How common is obesity?   In the United States, 30 percent of men and 40 percent of women are twenty pounds or more overweight. This represents a third of our population: 75 million people! It is the greatest health problem in this country.

What are the health problems an obese person may develop?   The obese person is four times as likely to develop diabetes as one whose weight remains normal. Other problems that occur in greater frequency among the obese are heart disease, high blood pressure, stroke, lung problems, varicose veins, hemorrhoids, blood clots in the legs and to the lungs, slow wound healing, and rashes and skin infections. The psychic problems are obvious—they include being shunned by society in general and by sexual partners in particular, difficulty in finding employment, difficulty in finding clothing, and a feeling of being left out of many vigorous activities.

Can weight reduction be successful for the obese?   Reducing is the only way to remove the risks of obesity, but the five-year success rate from problem obesity is less than 10 percent, meaning that nine out of ten persons who are obese will remain so.

Why is it so hard to lose weight?   One explanation is the emphasis on short-term rather than long-term weight loss. It is not enough to remove a certain number of pounds and then resume previous eating habits, for the weight will come right back. One has to change the pattern for life—a very difficult thing to accomplish.

What is the best diet for losing weight?   It consists of eating foods from the four basic groups, but eating less of them. The "diet" is really a life plan of eating less.

What about fasting?   This is not an effective way to keep weight down and it may endanger your health. Too stringent dieting of any sort brings the risk of the loss of protein, including muscle, in addition to the loss of fat.

How good are quick-weight-loss diets?   These diets primarily accomplish weight loss of water, not fat, and may endanger the health of certain persons.

How do you lose fat?   Each pound of fat contains 3,500 calories of stored energy that has to be burned off in excess of caloric intake. The best way to burn fat pounds is to combine exercise with a reduction in food intake.

Which exercise is best for the obese individual?   Walking is an activity that can be done easily and regularly, for fifteen to thirty minutes, two or three times a day. A thirty-minute walk each day, coupled with no increase in food intake, could lead to a pound a month of weight loss. Obese people should not begin to exercise strenuously until they lose some weight, and even then, the exercise program should be launched under a physician's guidance.

What about diet pills?   They have no long-term benefit in helping one lose weight. Many of them have serious side effects and are a danger to your health.

Should you undergo surgery for obesity?   No. Jaw-wiring, intestinal bypass and surgical removal of fat are risky treatments that not only have serious side effects but are not certain to cure the problem. These procedures have largely fallen into disrepute.

What's the best word of caution about obesity?   It is easier to prevent than to correct. A fat baby is not a healthy baby, so don't overfeed during infancy. Don't use food as a reward at any time of life, especially during childhood. Develop a lifetime program of exercise. Develop a lifetime habit of assuaging desires in ways other than through food intake.

14

DISEASES
of the
BLOOD and VESSELS

What are the components of blood?   Cells account for 40 to 45 percent of blood, and the rest is a watery substance known as plasma, which contains glucose, minerals, amino acids, fats and soluble proteins. Among the last are the clotting factors that can precipitate out of the blood to form a clot.

What are the kinds of blood cells?   Red cells give the blood its color. They carry and exchange oxygen and carbon dioxide between the lungs and the body tissues. The blood also contains a variety of white cells which are important in fighting infection, in antibody formation and in certain other types of body defenses. Platelets are cellular fragments that circulate in the blood like white blood cells. Containing several clotting factors, they gather at a site of injury and squeeze out these substances to initiate and maintain a clot.

Where is blood made?   The plasma, or the liquid part of the blood, comes from body fluids, and blood cells are made in the bone marrow, the hollow part of most bones.

What may go wrong with the blood?   The most common problem is anemia, a lower-than-normal red blood cell count. The white blood cells may be harmed by a drug or chemical, creating increased susceptibility to infection. Bleeding problems may occur when the blood doesn't clot properly. Cancer of the blood is known as leukemia, and usually also involves the bone marrow.

Who should treat a blood disease?   A family physician may diagnose anemia or a deficiency or increase of white cells or clotting elements, but determining the cause of the problem usually requires the services of a specialist. Referral to a hematologist is indicated when the problem is serious. The hematologist holds Board certification in internal medicine or pediatrics, as well as in the subspecialty of hematology, the diagnosis and treatment of blood diseases.

ANEMIA

What is anemia?   The word is used to describe the presence of a low red blood cell count.

What is the normal red cell count?   Each cubic millimeter of blood normally contains about 5 million red blood cells.

Are the normal values the same for men and women?   No, the "normal," or average, count for a woman is said to be slightly lower than for a man: 4.5 million as opposed to 5 million cells per cubic millimeter of blood. Women tend to have lower blood counts than men, but the reason is periodic bleeding due to the menstrual flow. In fact, this means that many women are mildly anemic. The still lower "normal," or average, count for a child is 4 million cells per cubic millimeter, reflecting the widespread iron deficiency anemia that is so common during childhood.

Does living at high altitude affect your blood count?   Yes, people living in Denver or Salt Lake City normally have a higher red count than those living at sea level. The greater number of red blood cells is the body's way of compensating for the rarefied air at high altitudes.

What is the percentage of red cells in the blood?   Normally, 40 to 45 percent of the blood's volume. Known as the hematocrit, this is the measurement by which doctors usually describe the blood count.

How low is the hematocrit in anemia?   For an adult, a hematocrit of 35 to 40 represents mild anemia, one of 25 to 35 signifies moderate anemia, and one of less than 25 indicates severe anemia. These limits are somewhat arbitrary, and one person may tolerate anemia better than another.

What is the blood count during pregnancy?   During the first months of pregnancy the hematocrit ought to remain over 36. Some dilution occurs as the blood volume expands late in pregnancy and the normal lower limit is then a hematocrit of 33 or a hemoglobin of 11.

What is hemoglobin? It is the iron-containing protein molecule of which red blood cells are made. The "heme" pigment gives red cells their color. A normal man will have a hemoglobin of about 15, and a normal, nonpregnant woman will have a hemoglobin of about 14. The numerical value refers to the number of grams of hemoglobin per 100 milliliters of blood. As a general rule, the hemoglobin tends to be about one-third of the hematocrit.

What are the symptoms of mild anemia? The person with mild anemia developing over months or years may have no symptoms. The body just compensates, which may be why physicians are reluctant to call slight anemia abnormal, especially if no symptoms are reported. Following treatment with iron therapy, the person may feel better than before and recognize the existence of symptoms that had been accepted as "normal." Among these are loss of energy, fatigue or a dull headache, mild breathlessness and a pounding heart after climbing a flight of stairs.

What symptoms do moderate to severe anemia cause? Moderate to severe anemia causes fatigue to the point where the person feels dead tired. He or she may become short of breath after walking a block or two. The mouth and eyelids turn pale, and pallor and a waxy hue may be striking features in a white person whose complexion was previously ruddy. In severe anemia, congestive heart failure may occur.

Under what circumstances does anemia develop? Anemia may result from bleeding; defects in the production of red cells, as from iron deficiency, infection or cancer; or an increased rate of red cell destruction, as in sickle cell anemia. Certain drugs may produce anemia, and some illnesses, such as kidney failure, infection and cancer, may decrease production and also increase destruction of red cells.

Can mild bleeding lead to anemia? Yes, menstrual bleeding causes a loss of two or three ounces of blood a month, and that's a pint and a half to two pints a year. The main cumulative effect is iron loss. Each pregnancy also extracts iron from a woman's body, and she may not get enough iron in her diet to make up for these losses.

How common is iron deficiency? It is the most common cause of anemia in the world. Even when the low "normal" limits mentioned earlier are used, 10 to 30 percent of women in this country have it. As many as half of pregnant women develop iron deficiency, and in children the deficiency is especially frequent during the first few years of life when the main food is milk.

Are there any special symptoms of iron deficiency?   In most instances there are no discernible symptoms other than, possibly, fatigue. Some people develop unusual dietary cravings, such as a desire for clay, corn-starch or ice. The craving may be noted during the anemia, leave following iron therapy, and reappear if the blood count drops again. A desire for ice and ice water may be tied to the swelling and tenderness of the tongue and the rawness in the throat that may occur with severe iron deficiency.

What is the treatment for iron deficiency anemia?   Iron tablets, in a dose prescribed by a physician, should be taken three or four times a day during or just after meals and with a snack at bedtime.

How long should the therapy continue?   The tablets should be taken long enough to return the blood count to normal and then for an additional several months.

Why continue the iron after the blood count is back to normal?   Iron deficiency anemia doesn't develop until one's iron reserves have been used up. These reserves, found in the blood and bone marrow, are the last to be replenished during iron therapy. The purpose of taking iron for a few extra months is to return storage levels to normal.

Is it necessary to determine the cause of iron deficiency anemia?   Yes, because the anemia is a sign of disease rather than a disease itself. In most instances the cause is fairly obvious: excessive menstrual bleeding, multiple pregnancies or a poor diet. With no history of bleeding, the anemia could represent slow, unrecognized blood loss into the stools from a cancer of the intestine or from other abdominal problems. Iron therapy would correct the anemia while allowing the real problem to continue. This is especially true when iron deficiency occurs in a man. In the absence of an obvious source of bleeding, the possibility that the man has a cancer of the bowel should be investigated.

Should people without anemia take iron tonics?   They shouldn't, unless a blood count indicates that anemia is present and other diseases have been ruled out.

Should a woman with mild anemia take iron tablets?   Yes, provided the cause of the anemia is known and the iron therapy makes her feel better. Ferrous sulfate taken orally may help to prevent a recurrence of anemia from excessive menstrual bleeding. The iron therapy should be coupled with periodic medical checkups and blood counts.

What should be done about iron deficiency in the young?   A breast-fed baby may need iron supplements in the form of liquid drops, prescribed by a physician, starting at about six months if breast-feeding continues to be the main source of nutrition. The bottle-fed baby should receive an iron-enriched formula. Anemia occurring during infancy or childhood should be evaluated by a pediatrician.

What are the side effects of iron tablets or liquid?   They upset the stomach of about 10 percent of persons who take them. Indigestion, nausea and abdominal pain or cramps are the main symptoms. Lowering the dosage will usually give relief. Iron taken by mouth may turn the stool black or gray.

When are iron injections indicated?   Only if the person cannot absorb or tolerate iron in tablet form. Sometimes these injections are used to correct a very severe iron deficiency and to avoid the need for blood transfusions, but this treatment is rarely necessary.

Why should caution be exercised in giving iron injections?   Because the injections may cause a fatal allergic reaction in a small percent of those receiving them. Other side effects include fever, severe lowering of the blood pressure, pain in the muscles and joints, rash and nausea. A distressing and permanent brownish or black discoloration of the skin may appear at the site of the injection.

What foods are rich in iron?   Most foods contain some iron, but liver, lean meat, iron-enriched bread, eggs and raisins are rich sources. Spinach, contrary to Popeye, does not contain much iron and may interfere with the absorption of iron from other foods.

Can too much iron harm the body?   Yes, excessive iron that gets into the body via iron that is injected or taken orally, blood transfusions or the diet can create the condition called hemochromatosis. Some persons have an inherited defect causing them to absorb too much iron from the diet, and alcoholics show an increased susceptibility to hemochromatosis. Besides causing diabetes, liver problems and heart failure, the extra body content of iron may tint the skin of a white person a bronze or slate-gray color.

What's the treatment for hemochromatosis?   When the person can tolerate it, repeated bleedings of a pint of blood every week or two is the best way to remove iron from the body. Treatment with the drug desferrioxamine is sometimes helpful in removing extra iron from the body, but the drug itself may cause serious side effects.

What other nutrient deficiencies may cause anemia?   Deficiency of folic acid, a vitamin that is present in green vegetables, liver and other foods, may cause anemia. Those apt to develop the deficiency are alcoholics with a poor diet, pregnant women whose folic acid requirements are increased, persons suffering from poor intestinal absorption, and those taking anticonvulsant drugs, such as phenytoin or mephenytoin. The anemia can be prevented by taking folic acid tablets during pregnancy or while on anticonvulsant therapy. Folic acid deficiency may occur in women taking the Pill, but not so often that routine folic acid supplements are needed.

What is pernicious anemia?   This condition is rare in young people, and is more common in those beyond the age of sixty. The tendency to develop it is inherited, and the anemia is due to a deficiency of vitamin B_{12} caused by an inability of the stomach to absorb it. The individual with pernicious anemia lacks stomach acid and therefore has a higher-than-average susceptibility to stomach cancer. Therapy with vitamin B_{12} injections will correct the anemia.

How often should B_{12} injections be given?   Once a month is adequate to treat pernicious anemia.

Do B_{12} injections have any other use?   Apparently not, though they are frequently prescribed for nervousness, fatigue, a tingling sensation, numbness or leg cramps. The claimed benefit is the strong placebo effect that these bright red injections have.

What is aplastic anemia?   An anemia that results from bone marrow failure. A reduction in white blood cells usually is part of the disease. It is fatal in half the patients who get it.

What may cause aplastic anemia?   It may follow exposure to ionizing radiation, such as an atomic explosion. Ingestion or inhalation of benzene, benzol, chlordane, DDT, Lindane and chemicals inhaled in glue sniffing may cause aplastic anemia, as can certain prescription drugs.

What prescription drugs may cause this complication?   Chloramphenicol, made as Chloromycetin and as Amphicol, is far and away the worst offender. Other causative drugs are phenylbutazone, oxyphenbutazone, sulfisoxazole, gold therapy and phenytoin. Some drugs, such as those used to treat leukemia or to prevent the rejection of a transplant, have a known cell-killing effect and may produce aplastic anemia.

Why is chloramphenicol so dangerous?   Though the risk of developing aplastic anemia after taking chloramphenicol is only one in 20,000 to 30,-000, every person receiving the drug develops a temporary bone marrow suppression. Moreover, the drug may be prescribed when safer drugs would work as well. The only indications for chloramphenicol are serious infections, such as meningitis and typhoid fever, where the patient is in the hospital and tests have shown that a safer antibiotic won't work. Routine prescription of the drug for mild infections is to be avoided.

What are the symptoms of aplastic anemia?   Low-grade fever, frequent infections, weakness and fatigue develop. These symptoms represent a deficiency of both red and white blood cells. A bone marrow examination is necessary to confirm the diagnosis.

What is the treatment for aplastic anemia?   All previous drug therapy must be stopped. Androgen, which resembles the male sex hormone, may reverse the bone marrow failure. Blood transfusions are used to keep the red cell count at a level that will permit ordinary activities.

The most promising form of therapy for aplastic anemia is a bone marrow transplant. This procedure is still experimental, and is most likely to be successful when a close relative can donate compatible bone marrow.

What is thalassemia?   Thalassemia is an inherited defect in the production of hemoglobin, and thus of red blood cells. Also known as Mediterranean anemia, it occurs most commonly in those of Mediterranean background. The mild form, thalassemia minor, occurs in those who inherit and carry the trait. The worst form, thalassemia major, is a tragic disease appearing in children born to parents both of whom carry the trait.

What are the symptoms of thalassemia major?   Severe anemia develops by the age of one. The infant's spleen and liver enlarge, and jaundice may occur. Despite transfusions and other measures, death usually occurs during childhood.

What are the symptoms of thalassemia minor?   The person may have a normal life-span and no symptoms, or note slight weakness and susceptibility to fatigue. Because, on examination, the red cells may resemble those of someone with iron deficiency, most people with thalassemia minor are given iron therapy before the correct diagnosis is made by hemoglobin electrophoresis, a test that shows the components of the red cells. Failure of an apparent iron deficiency anemia to respond to iron signals the possibility of thalassemia minor.

Why is it important for carriers to be identified?   One reason is that the person who is identified as a carrier can avoid potentially harmful and unnecessary iron therapy; another is that the child whose parents both carry the thalassemia trait has a one-in-four chance of having thalassemia major.

What causes sickle cell anemia?   It is an inherited defect in hemoglobin formation. Because red cells of the affected person tend to collapse into a crescent shape, or sickle, the cells move sluggishly through the small vessels of the body. Kidney problems and increased susceptibility to infections occur. Anemia develops as a result of the red cells dying much more quickly than they should.

How common is sickle cell anemia?   It affects one in 500 black persons in the United States, but the carrier state—the sickle cell trait—affects 8 percent of American blacks.

What are the symptoms of sickle cell trait?   Because sickle cell trait doesn't cause anemia, the person usually has no symptoms. However, attacks of bleeding into the urine may occur, and severe abdominal pain may appear during flights above 10,000 feet in an unpressurized airplane. Life expectancy is normal.

How serious is sickle cell anemia?   Symptoms develop before the first birthday. The child has frequent and severe infections, as well as attacks of pain and fever. The anemia is severe enough to require frequent transfusions. Antibiotics are given to control infections, but death may occur during childhood. Survival beyond early adulthood is rare.

How is the carrier state detected?   The carrier state and the actual disease are diagnosed by blood tests and hemoglobin electrophoresis.

What are the chances of someone with sickle cell trait passing it to a child?
    If the person's spouse was normal, half the children would be carriers of sickle cell trait, but none of them would have the actual sickle cell disease. One out of four children born to two persons carrying the sickle cell trait would, however, have sickle cell anemia. Half of the children born to two carriers would also have sickle cell trait.

What are the chances of someone with sickle cell anemia passing it to his or her child?   If the person's spouse was normal, each child would carry the sickle cell trait. If the spouse had the sickle cell trait, half of their children would have sickle cell anemia and half would have the sickle cell trait. If both parents had sickle cell anemia, all of the children would have the disease.

What is spherocytosis?   A rare, inherited defect of the red cells. Unable to secrete sodium normally, the cells swell to a globular form (spherocyte) and are broken down by the spleen so quickly that anemia develops. Removal of the spleen is an effective means of therapy.

What is autoimmune hemolytic anemia?   A self-destructive process occurring when a person develops antibodies against his or her own red blood cells. It may accompany lupus erythematosus or lymphoma, a condition resembling leukemia. Therapy with Aldomet (methyldopa), a drug given to treat high blood pressure, may also produce this form of anemia. Treatment with prednisone is usually effective, but removal of the spleen is sometimes indicated. When Aldomet is responsible, the person should switch to an alternate form of antihypertensive therapy.

TOO MUCH BLOOD

Is it possible to have too many red blood cells?   Yes, in the condition known as polycythemia the hematocrit may be as high as 75 or 80 percent. A hematocrit above 55 is considered abnormal, and one above 60 or 65 may produce sluggish blood flow due to thickness of the blood.

What causes polycythemia?   Secondary polycythemia may result from an inadequate oxygen supply to the cells, as in a child with a severe heart murmur or an adult with emphysema or chronic bronchitis. The increased production of red cells is the body's way of attempting to supply more oxygen to the tissues, but the sluggish circulation caused by a very high hematocrit actually interferes with oxygen delivery.

Primary polycythemia, known as polycythemia rubra vera, is a form of chronic leukemia characterized by an increased production of red cells, white cells and platelets. Men are affected twice as often as women, and the onset is usually after the age of forty-five.

What are the symptoms of polycythemia?   Headache, dizziness, weakness and blurred vision occur when the hematocrit is very high. A tendency toward excessive bleeding from a cut is noted. A white person with primary polycythemia has a ruddy complexion and may note intense itching after taking a hot bath or shower. Sometimes a dull heaviness is felt in the left upper abdomen from an enlarged spleen.

What's the treatment for polycythemia?   The cause, if any, should be corrected, and radioactive phosphorus injections are the usual treatment for polycythemia rubra vera. This is one of the few instances where bloodletting is still used. In an adult, the bleeding of a pint of blood is indicated when the hematocrit rises above 65 or so.

LEUKEMIA AND RELATED CONDITIONS

What is leukemia?   It is a malignancy of the blood that takes many different forms. It may be acute or chronic. It's different in children than in adults. It differs depending on the type of cell that is predominantly affected. The common denominator of all leukemias is a block in the production or maturation of white blood cells.

Are other blood cells also affected?   Yes, anemia and a low platelet count accompany the leukemic process and account for many of the symptoms.

What causes leukemia?   For the majority of patients the cause isn't known. An increased incidence of the disease is seen following exposure to nuclear irradiation or X-ray therapy, and repeated contact with benzene or therapy with chloramphenicol, phenylbutazone or cell-killing drugs may increase the risk of developing leukemia. A lot of evidence points to an infectious cause.

Does leukemia run in families?   Certain families show a greater incidence of leukemia than would normally be expected, but this may indicate an infectious rather than an inherited cause for the disease. When one of a pair of identical twins develops leukemia, the other twin has one-in-six chances of also developing the disease—a risk that is tremendously higher than for the general population. Persons with a chromosomal defect, such as Down's syndrome, are more susceptible to leukemia than are normal individuals.

How common is leukemia?   An estimated 20,000 people in this country develop leukemia each year.

What are the symptoms of leukemia in a child?   Frequent infections occur because of the lack of an adequate number of normal white blood cells. Because of the associated anemia, the child may feel tired and weak. Nosebleed and easy bruising may result from the lack of blood platelets. Sometimes abdominal pain occurs from an enlarged spleen.

Among children, who is most likely to develop leukemia?   The disease is twice as common in whites as in blacks, is slightly more common in boys than in girls, and is more likely to strike the first child than a subsequent one. The period of greatest risk is between the ages of one and five, and most children are about four years old at the time the diagnosis is made.

What is the treatment for childhood leukemia?   A combination of prednisone and cell-killing drugs is usually chosen. Though these drugs may cause serious side effects, the trade-off is between the risks of drug therapy and the risks of the disease without treatment.

How good is the treatment for childhood leukemia?   It produces a five-year survival rate of 50 percent, and the average survival is three to five years. This is in contrast to the dismal results in 1950, before these drugs were available, when the average survival was two or three months and most patients were dead within a year.

Can childhood leukemia be cured?   Those involved in therapy of leukemia are now using the word "cure" to apply to children who have survived beyond five years after the diagnosis was made, and who continue to have a remission from the disease. A remission is the disappearance from the blood, bone marrow and other organs of all signs of the disease.

How does leukemia in adults differ from that in children?   Leukemia in a child is almost always of the acute variety. Adult leukemia may be acute or chronic, but adults with acute leukemia don't respond as well to therapy as children with this disease do.

What are the symptoms of leukemia in an adult?   Often the symptoms are those of anemia: tiredness, headache and breathlessness after mild exertion. The leukemia is discovered during routine evaluation of the anemia. In other instances the first sign of the disease is prolonged bleeding from a cut or the menses, or a tendency to have frequent infections.

What's the treatment for adult-onset leukemia?   A combination of cell-killing drugs is usually given, and the choice of drugs depends on the type of cell that has gone awry to produce the disease. The victim of acute leukemia may survive for a year or eighteen months after treatment, while survival for five years or more is possible after the treatment of chronic leukemia in an adult.

What diseases may resemble leukemia?   Other cancers involving the blood or lymph nodes are multiple myeloma, Hodgkin's disease and lymphoma.

What is multiple myeloma?   A form of bone-marrow cancer affecting the plasma cells and usually occurring in persons over the age of fifty-five or sixty. The malignant plasma cells make abnormal antibodies and tend to crowd out the cells that make normal antibodies. As a result, the person has a greater susceptibility to infections such as pneumonia. Progressive

367

anemia causes fatigue and shortness of breath. Bone destruction by the malignancy may be devastating. The bones in the back may lose their support and collapse, producing a loss of several inches in height and the excruciating back and leg pain of pinched nerves.

How frequent is multiple myeloma?   It strikes about 9,000 persons in this country each year.

What is the treatment for multiple myeloma?   A cell-killing drug, melphalan, has given the best results. In persons with a variant of myeloma, macroglobulinemia of Waldenström, it may be necessary to remove the excessive quantities of antibodies from the blood. X-ray therapy is sometimes used to halt the destruction of bone.

What's the prognosis for someone with this disease?   The average survival after treatment for multiple myeloma is three or four years.

What is Hodgkin's disease?   It is a cancer of the lymph glands, the network of infection-fighting nodes found throughout the body but concentrated in areas such as the groin, under the arms and on the back of the neck. Cancer in the glands is also known as lymphoma.

What are the symptoms of Hodgkin's disease?   Often the first symptom is a painless swelling due to an enlarged lymph gland along the back of the neck or in the armpit. Fever, sometimes quite high, may occur each afternoon or night. Weakness, fatigue and generalized itching are early symptoms.

How frequent is Hodgkin's disease?   About 7,000 Americans develop it each year. It is more common in men than in women and in whites than in blacks.

What is the treatment for Hodgkin's disease?   A combination of prednisone and cell-killing drugs is usually chosen. X-ray therapy may be given in addition to, or instead of, drug treatment, and the spleen may be removed.

What's the prognosis for Hodgkin's disease?   Considerable progress has been made in treating this disease in recent years. The five-year survival is now 70 percent, and the ten-year survival is 50 percent. Older persons do less well than the young, and those having the disease in the abdominal organs do worse than those in whom only a few neck or armpit glands are involved.

368

What about other forms of lymphoma?   Lymphoma other than Hodgkin's disease strikes about 20,000 persons a year, and the treatment and prognosis are similar to that for Hodgkin's disease.

IMMUNE DEFICIENCY

What is immune deficiency?   An increased susceptibility to infection due to a lack of antibodies, white blood cells or both.

What causes immune deficiency?   It may accompany aplastic anemia, leukemia or lymphoma, or arise from therapy with the cell-killing drugs used to treat cancer or to prevent rejection of a transplant. Several forms of the disease are inherited and begin during childhood.

How can you tell if a child has an immune deficiency?   The child is subject to repeated infections, usually beginning during the first year of life. (Most children with repeated infections do *not* have this condition.) Growth and development may be retarded.

Which infections are most likely to occur?   Frequent colds and runny nose do not point to immune deficiency. The deficient child is more likely to have skin infections, ear infections, pneumonia and bronchitis.

What is the treatment for immune deficiency?   Treatment should be under the direction of an immunologist, and may include antibiotics, gamma globulin injections and measures designed to keep the child in a relatively germ-free environment. The most promising form of therapy is bone-marrow transplantation.

What is bone-marrow transplantation?   After tissue typing to determine the best donor from among the child's siblings and parents, the bone marrow is withdrawn from the donor by repeated aspiration from various sites. The marrow is then infused into the recipient's abdominal cavity, where the cells are absorbed. Drug and X-ray therapy may be needed to ensure the transplant's success. Other than soreness and the effects of general anesthesia, the bone-marrow donor suffers no ill effects and soon the bones are replenished with new marrow.

How successful is bone-marrow transplantation?   The procedure is successful in one out of four children in whom it is performed to treat immune deficiency. Without marrow transplantation, some children with immune deficiency die during the first few years of life, while others may survive to adolescence and beyond, depending on the type of condition and its severity.

BLEEDING DISORDERS

What causes blood to clot?   Clotting occurs when the blood is in contact with injured tissue and a soluble protein, fibrinogen, precipitates out of the blood to form the insoluble product fibrin. Platelets and the clotting factors must be present in normal amounts for clotting to occur.

What is hemophilia?   The victim of this disorder is a bleeder for whom even a small cut can create a serious problem. Lacking an essential clotting factor, a protein called antihemophilic globulin, the person's blood doesn't clot normally.

What causes hemophilia?   In most instances it is inherited, though occasionally the disease appears in one with no family history for it. Classic hemophilia is passed as a sex-linked disease. Each son of a woman carrying the trait has a fifty-fifty chance of having hemophilia, and each daughter has a fifty-fifty chance of being a carrier.

What are the symptoms of hemophilia?   Serious bleeding may be noted early in life, as when circumcision is performed. Large bruises appear following slight injury, as when the infant falls down. Prolonged bleeding is noted after cuts, dental extractions or surgery, and spontaneous, painful bleeding into the abdomen or the joints is common. It's not unusual for bleeding to stop soon after an injury and then recur and persist from the same site a day or so later. A poorly understood facet of the disease is that the bleeding tendency is worse at some times than at others.

What is the treatment for hemophilia?   The missing clotting factor is given periodically in the form of a frozen or powdered concentrate and the patient himself can learn to give the infusions. Therapy should be initiated and managed by a hematologist; help may be obtained from the National Hemophilia Foundation, 25 West 39th Street, New York, N.Y. 10018.

How can hemophilia be prevented?   Prior to having children, persons with known hemophilia in their families should seek genetic counseling. When a woman is already pregnant and the risk is fifty-fifty that a son may be affected, amniocentesis can be done to determine whether the fetus is a male.

What else may cause a bleeding problem?   A deficiency of platelets may cause easy bruising, prolonged bleeding from a cut or spontaneous hemorrhage. The most common problem is ITP—idiopathic thrombocytopenia

370

purpura, which is the medical term for a platelet deficiency of unknown cause.

What are the symptoms of ITP?   Quite suddenly, bruises and pinpoint dots of hemorrhage appear on the body, usually at pressure points and on the arms and legs. Bleeding from a cut may last much longer than normal.

What causes ITP?   In a child it often follows an infection such as measles, sore throat or a cold. Previously healthy, the child develops the symptoms mentioned above, and may also have bleeding from the nose, kidneys or bowels. Children from two to six are the most susceptible.

What is the treatment for ITP?   Prednisone is usually chosen, and removal of the spleen may be curative in those who don't respond to steroid therapy.

Can drugs cause a platelet deficiency?   Yes, and among the drugs that may cause it are diuretics such as Esidrix, Oretic and Diuril, antibiotics such as tetracycline, erythromycin and penicillin, and other drugs such as aspirin, phenobarbital, codeine and quinine. The platelet deficiency may occur immediately or not till after months or years on the drug.

What is the treatment for drug-induced platelet deficiency?   All drugs should be stopped. Further treatment should be given by a hematologist after he or she has performed additional blood studies and a bone-marrow examination.

What are some other causes of susceptibility to bruising?   This problem may occur for unknown reasons in a woman beyond the age of fifty. The bruises appear on the hands and arms and are more of a cosmetic than a medical problem. Bruising increases, in general, with aging because of the thinning of the skin and the loss of support for the blood vessels. Among the drugs that may cause easy bruising are aspirin, phenylbutazone, Indocin and Clinoril. By weakening the blood vessels, cortisone therapy may cause easy bruising. Vitamin C deficiency may cause easy bruising, but this is rare except in an elderly person whose diet is deficient.

What's the treatment for easy bruising?   A blood count and platelet count should be done, and if these are normal, no specific therapy is indicated other than to stop any drugs that may be responsible and make sure the person is getting a nutritious diet.

DISEASES OF THE VESSELS

What is an artery?   It is a vessel leading from the heart and carrying blood to the tissues. Arteries have muscular walls that propel blood along toward the various body organs.

What is a vein?   A vein is a thin-walled structure that returns blood to the heart from the tissues.

What can go wrong with the arteries?   The most common problem is arteriosclerosis, or hardening of the arteries. The hardening reflects the accumulation of calcium in the arteries, but the cause for this condition is unknown. It does occur as a natural part of aging, but factors that favor early onset or acceleration of arteriosclerosis are smoking, diabetes, high blood pressure and an inherited tendency to have this condition. Certain studies show that a long-term exercise program coupled with a low-fat diet may retard the development of arteriosclerosis.

What are the dangers of arteriosclerosis?   One is stroke (discussed on p. 293), which is more common beyond the age of sixty. The middle-aged person with arteriosclerosis is more likely to have an obstruction of blood flow to the lower extremities. Progressively narrowed, the arteries become incapable of carrying enough blood to the legs. The condition is known as arterial insufficiency or peripheral vascular disease.

What are the symptoms of peripheral vascular disease?   Pain is noted in the calves during walking, and the pain is relieved by rest. This symptom progressively worsens. Indolent leg ulcers may appear because of poor blood flow to the skin, and a man may become impotent from a reduction in blood flow to the penis. The toes and feet are liable to become gangrenous after an infection or injury.

What is gangrene?   It refers to death of tissue in one part of the body, usually the limb, as the result of the loss of the part's blood supply, an infection or a combination of these.

What is the treatment for arterial insufficiency?   A progressive exercise program may stimulate the growth of additional arteries to carry blood to the legs. Cessation of smoking and better control of diabetes and high blood pressure may help. Drugs are sometimes used, with limited effectiveness. When surgery is necessary, one of the techniques used is to restore blood supply by using a Teflon or Dacron graft to bypass the worst area of obstruction. Sometimes one of the patient's own veins is used as the bypass. The surgery is somewhat risky, doesn't always work as well as expected, and is usually not resorted to until medical therapy has failed.

Amputation is necessary if gangrene develops, but the opinion of an internist should be sought before submitting to surgery. As little tissue as possible should be removed.

What is Buerger's disease?   It is a form of arteriosclerosis occurring usually in men between the ages of twenty and forty-five and causing coldness in the feet or hands, severe pain in the legs during walking, and the appearance of small ulcers on the toes or hands. Inflammation of the veins may also occur.

What is the treatment for Buerger's disease?   Most persons with the disease smoke, and giving up this habit is the first and most important step in therapy. Nicotine causes arterial spasm that accentuates the underlying problem. Drug therapy consists of products whose purpose is to dilate the arteries, but most of these are of little value. Sympathectomy, an operation to cut certain nerve fibers, may reduce the spasm of blood vessels and improve the symptoms of Buerger's disease. First, a nerve block should be performed to determine whether the operation will produce a definite benefit. A patient with advanced Buerger's disease may need arterial reconstruction or amputation.

What other problems may affect the arteries?   A blood clot may form depriving the area supplied by that artery of its circulation and causing gangrene. Another problem is the development of an aneurysm, a ballooning of the walls of an artery. It is most frequent in people over fifty and occurs in 2 or 3 percent of the population. It most often affects the abdominal aorta, the main artery carrying blood to the lower body.

What is the danger of an aneurysm?   The main danger is that it may burst, leading to sudden death from internal bleeding.

What's the treatment for an aneurysm?   The dilated part of the artery can be cut out and replaced with a graft of knitted Dacron. This is major surgery that should be performed by a cardiovascular surgeon in a large center who has had much experience in such operations.

What are varicose veins?   They are large veins that stand out from the skin, carry blood sluggishly and are prone to develop clots. They are most often found in the legs and may cause aching, tiredness and swelling. They not only are a great inconvenience, but can also give rise to undue hemorrhage after a wound.

What causes varicose veins?   The cause is unknown, but the predisposing factors are pregnancy, obesity, chronic constipation, an inherited tendency to develop varicose veins and a job that requires standing in one position all day. One in three women can expect to have this problem with varicose veins, but it occurs in just one out of ten men.

How do varicose veins develop?   Blood is squeezed through the veins by the contraction of leg muscles, and a series of one-way valves directs flow toward the heart. Varicose veins begin when these valves become incompetent, allowing blood to be forced backward as well as forward during muscle squeezing. Damage to the valves of the deep leg veins allows blood to be pumped to the superficial veins. The latter become swollen, tortuous and visible.

What is the treatment for varicose veins?   When the swollen veins are mainly a cosmetic problem one can get relief by wearing support stockings and avoiding garters or girdles, which tend to impede blood flow from the leg veins. Support hosiery should be drawn on before getting out of bed and left on all day. The legs should be rested in an upright position as often as possible. Weight loss and an increased content of dietary roughage to relieve constipation may help. If swelling of the legs is a problem, restriction of salt or the use of a mild diuretic such as hydrochlorothiazide three times a week is indicated. Varicose veins that develop during pregnancy often improve or disappear after the baby is born. When the problem is severe, surgery or sclerotherapy may be necessary.

What is involved in sclerotherapy and surgery?   In sclerotherapy, a procedure developed to avoid surgery, the place where the superficial and the deep veins meet is injected with an agent that closes off the connection. The injections are performed at all such sites and the leg is covered for several weeks. Good results are reported by surgeons expert in this procedure, though the sclerosing agent may irritate the surrounding skin if the injection is not performed properly.

Vein stripping, an operation done under general anesthesia, is a much more radical measure. A rod is passed through the vein from the foot to the groin. The surgeon applies a buttonlike tip to the end of the rod and pulls the rod—and the vein—out of the leg. After the operation the leg is wrapped with Ace bandages for six weeks. Nine out of ten persons report long-term relief from the surgery.

What causes a clot to form in the veins?   Among the causes are thrombophlebitis (an inflammation of the veins), varicose veins, Buerger's disease, birth-control pills, estrogen therapy, an intravenous injection or an illness that forces prolonged bed rest, particularly after surgery. Clot formation in the veins of the leg is more common than clot formation elsewhere in the body; clots in the pelvic region are likely to be serious.

What are the symptoms of a clot in a leg vein?   Pain, heat and tenderness develop over the vein if it is just beneath the skin, but fever, leg pain, tenderness in the calf and swelling of the leg are the symptoms of deep-vein thrombophlebitis.

What is the main risk of a clot forming in the veins?   The clot may break loose and pass to the lungs to obstruct blood flow through this vital part of the body. It is likely that all persons have small clots that pass to the lungs and never cause symptoms. A very large clot could cause serious problems, but fortunately, this is a rare condition.

What is thrombophlebitis?   It is an inflammation of part of a vein associated with clot formation in this section of the vessel.

What is the treatment for thrombophlebitis?   Warm soaks and elevation of the arm or leg will usually relieve superficial thrombophlebitis. Phenylbutazone therapy may be used for several days if the symptoms are severe. The individual with thrombophlebitis in a deep vein requires hospitalization. Blood-thinning drugs, or anticoagulants such as heparin, are often used to dissolve the clot.

A large clot that has passed to the lungs may have to be removed immediately by chest surgery. More often, anticoagulants and oxygen therapy are sufficient. It may be necessary to close off the main veins from the legs when these are known to be the source of clots that have passed to the lungs. A device can be inserted into the lower veins of the abdomen that permits blood but not clots to flow toward the heart and lungs.

Can thrombophlebitis be prevented?   In many instances, yes. Some physicians advise wrapping the legs with elastic bandages during an illness requiring bed rest or in the days following surgery, but this has become a controversial procedure. Aspirin or a mild anticoagulant drug may be used postoperatively to prevent clotting. Early activity after surgery has helped to reduce the risk of thrombophlebitis. Removal of varicose veins may lessen the risk of clot formation.

15

HEART
and
LUNG DISEASE

What does the heart do?   The heart pumps blood. It has no other function, yet all other organs depend on it to receive oxygen and nutrients through the bloodstream.

What is heart disease?   It refers to anything that interferes with the pumping action of the heart, including a disease of the heart valves or the heart muscle or the stopping of the blood supply to the heart. When the term "heart disease" is used without qualification, it usually means coronary artery disease. Coronary artery disease that is severe enough to shut off blood flow to one part of the heart may cause a heart attack (see p. 382), or "coronary."

What are the coronary arteries?   They are the vessels that carry blood to the heart muscle itself. They arise from the aorta, the main vessel carrying blood from the heart to the body, and branch into two vessels on the front and one on the back of the heart. Through these arteries the heart is able to get back for its own use fully 5 percent of all the blood that it pumps.

What is coronary artery disease?   It is a narrowing of the coronary arteries so that one or both become unable to carry blood to the heart at the normal rate. The usual cause is coronary atherosclerosis—a buildup of fatty plaques in the walls of these two vital arteries. Complete obstruction of a coronary artery is known as coronary occlusion.

How common is coronary artery disease?   It is the most common cause of death in the United States, accounting for 700,000 deaths a year. Diseases of the heart and vessels kill a million Americans a year. Heart disease is so prevalent that almost every other person can expect to die from it.

Who should treat heart disease?   The best-qualified physician is the cardiologist, an internal medicine or pediatric specialist with an extra year or two of training in the diagnosis and treatment of heart disease. A fully qualified specialist will have Board certification in cardiology.

RISK FACTORS FOR HEART DISEASE

Can coronary artery disease be prevented?   The process of coronary narrowing develops slowly over several decades, and can be influenced by one's lifelong habits of eating, exercise and other things known as risk factors for heart disease.

What are the risk factors for heart disease?   These factors, as developed in a long-term study in Framingham, Massachusetts, are shown in the accompany chart.

RISK FACTORS FOR CORONARY ARTERY DISEASE

Major factors
Smoking
Diabetes
High blood pressure
High serum cholesterol
Enlarged heart

Minor factors
Family history of heart disease
Poor handling of stress
Lack of exercise
Obesity
Male sex
Age above forty
Use of birth-control pills

Can an individual's risk be assessed?   Yes, by measuring the presence or absence of each of the risk factors, a physician can predict with some accuracy an individual's chances of having a heart attack during the next six years. A Coronary Risk Handbook is available from the American Heart Association, 7320 Greenville Avenue, Dallas, Tex. 75231.

Which of the risk factors is most important? No one knows, but it is apparent that the more risk factors a person has, the greater the risk of heart attack. The factors occur in groups. Risk increases with age. Obesity is a contributor to diabetes and high blood pressure. High blood pressure may cause the heart to enlarge. Many obese persons also have a high serum cholesterol which contributes to the risk of heart attack.

What is the difference in risk between men and women? Under the age of forty-five, men have thirteen times as many heart attacks as women. Between the ages of forty-five and sixty-two, a man's heart-attack risk is double that of a woman's. After the age of sixty-two, the rate of heart attacks is the same in men and women.

What can be done to lower the risk of heart attack? Some of the factors —age, sex and family history—cannot be changed, of course, but most of the others can. The general measures to lower heart attack risk are:
· Stop smoking (or don't start).
· Reduce to and stay at normal body weight.
· Exercise regularly and vigorously enough to elevate the heartbeat and make the lungs work.
· Reduce dietary intake of saturated fats.
· Seek treatment for high blood pressure, diabetes or high cholesterol.
· Choose a form of birth control other than the Pill.

Why is diet important in lessening heart-attack risk? The fatty plaques that build up in the coronary arteries are composed of cholesterol and other saturated fats, the same fats found in butter, animal fat, eggs, whole milk and shortening. By avoiding these products it is possible to lower one's level of cholesterol and reduce the risk of heart attack.

Which diet is best? Fats account for 45 to 50 percent of the calories in an average person's diet; a healthier diet would contain less than 40 percent of calories as fats. The fats would consist mainly of unsaturated substances, which, when broken down, are not as likely to contribute to cholesterol and similar products. Whole grains should supply more of the calorie intake, as should vegetables and roughage of all kinds.

It is helpful to trim the fat off meat, to use margarine instead of butter, to drink low-fat rather than whole milk and to cook with unsaturated cooking oil.

How effective are pills to lower the cholesterol?   The most popular cholesterol-lowering drug in current use is clofibrate. It doesn't work in the hereditary form of elevated cholesterol and is no better than good diet management in other forms. Many people taking it develop nausea or diarrhea, and more serious side effects include depression of the blood count, baldness, gallstones, liver damage and irregularities of the heartbeat. It should not be used until dietary measures have been tried.

What form of exercise is best in preventing heart attack?   It hasn't been conclusively proven that any particular form of exercise will lessen the risk of heart attack, but it is apparent that the risk is increased by the lack of exercise of the "aerobic" type which elevates the heartbeat and speeds the rate of breathing. Walking briskly, jogging, swimming, cycling or performing physical labor several times a week seem to be helpful.

Are joggers immune from heart attack?   The risk of heart attack is three times less among those who exercise regularly than it is among those who don't, but joggers still have heart attacks, sometimes during or right after a run. Do not start a jogging program if you are severely overweight or if you are over forty and haven't had a cardiovascular examination in recent years.

How does exercise help the heart?   It increases the heart's efficiency: the resting pulse of a person in good condition is ten or twenty beats a minute slower than the pulse rate of a sedentary person. The slower rate allows the exerciser's heart to rest longer between each beat. By contrast, the heart of the nonexerciser has to work harder and is therefore under a greater strain. Probably the best benefit of exercise is its association with other health habits. The person in good condition is less inclined to smoke or be overweight, and is more likely to follow healthy eating patterns. Exercise may lower the blood pressure, thus alleviating another risk factor.

Does personality have anything to do with heart-attack risk?   Probably so. The aggressive, time-oriented achiever who does everything at a hurry-up pace is more coronary-prone than the individual who tends to take it easy and let things slide. However, the first type might also be more likely to take up an exercise program and be less likely to be obese than the second. All else being equal, one who can find happiness and slow down enough to enjoy life is going to be healthier than one whose life is filled with stress and frustration. Coronary risk factors mirror all aspects of one's life.

379

CORONARY HEART DISEASE

What tests are used to diagnose coronary heart disease?   A coronary arteriogram is a test that uses an injection of dye and a camera to record the condition of the coronary arteries. It is fairly dangerous and should be used only when surgery is contemplated. Certain blood tests may also be useful, but the electrocardiogram (EKG, or ECG) is the standard test. By picking up and amplifying the electrical discharges created as the heart contracts, the EKG machine can tell something of the heart's size, the regularity of its rhythm and the adequacy of its blood supply.

Can heart disease be present in spite of a normal EKG tracing?   Yes, the tracing may be normal even in someone with severe heart disease. Many instances are on record of a person having a normal checkup, EKG included, then having a heart attack the next day.

What can be done to make the EKG study more reliable?   Stress testing was created for this purpose. By placing the heart under stress, exercise accentuates any inadequacy in blood flow and may bring out characteristic changes on the EKG.

How reliable is stress testing?   It is reliable in diagnosing coronary disease about 90 percent of the time, but treadmill testing is generally acknowledged to be much more effective as a diagnostic tool in men than in women.

Is the stress test ever dangerous?   Yes, heart attacks and deaths have occurred during stress testing. A stress test is not indicated when the resting EKG is abnormal, when a heart attack is suspected or has occurred in the last three months, or when the person has severe symptoms suggestive of heart disease. Resuscitation equipment and a physician who knows how to use it must be available during the stress testing.

Are there any warning signs of heart disease?   Yes, angina pectoris is a type of chest pain that points to coronary artery disease. It doesn't occur in all persons with heart disease, but those who have it may be lucky in the sense that it warns of a progressive inadequacy of blood supply to the heart. The pain itself only occurs during times when the heart isn't getting enough blood to meet its needs.

What are the symptoms of angina pectoris?   The pain is felt as a dull ache or heaviness beneath the breastbone during activity, especially if the person is exposed to cold. Stopping to rest relieves the pain. It reappears when the activity is resumed and lets up again upon rest. This pattern is so typical that it becomes familiar to the angina sufferer, who quickly learns how much activity he or she can tolerate without pain. Excitement or eating a heavy meal may also bring on the pain.

Does the pain of angina always occur in the chest?   No, the pain may radiate to the left shoulder and down the arm. Sometimes it goes to the jaw or to the right shoulder and arm. Sometimes it is felt only in the arm, shoulder, neck or jaw.

What is the most typical thing about angina?   The victim of angina will describe a tight, constricting discomfort, a "squeezing" pain. The pain doesn't cut off the wind and is not related to breathing.

What's the treatment for angina?   The time-honored treatment is nitro-glycerin. Placed beneath the tongue, the small white tablet is absorbed rapidly and acts to improve blood flow to the heart and relieve the chest pain. Amyl nitrite and related drugs have an effect that is similar to but longer-lasting than that of nitroglycerin. Propranolol, where it is tolerated, is being increasingly and effectively used to treat angina.

Does whiskey help relieve angina?   No, it tends to make it worse.

What general measures may help to relieve angina?   Control of high blood pressure, reduction of weight for the obese and cessation of smoking are musts. A program of gradually increasing exercise may also help. The walking program should be done under the supervision of a cardiologist experienced in exercise therapy. With slow conditioning, the person is able to tolerate greater amounts of activity without having angina.

What is the long-term outlook for someone with angina?   The person is more likely to have a heart attack than someone of the same age and sex who doesn't have angina, but in many instances the condition remains stable year after year. The prognosis is worse in diabetics and those in whom angina develops prior to age forty.

What about surgery for angina?   The coronary bypass operation, which is performed by the heart surgeons, is one option for the person with severe angina who doesn't respond to conservative therapy. Using a vein taken from the person's leg, the surgeon attaches one end to the aorta, then stitches the other end to a patent section of coronary artery close to the heart. The vein thus bypasses the obstruction in the coronary and sends more blood flowing to the heart.

How effective is coronary bypass surgery?   Most persons who have the surgery notice much less angina afterward, but some studies have shown that the bypass operation doesn't prolong life expectancy. The operation is risky and expensive. Its principal use is in the relief of the symptoms of angina.

What are the risks of coronary bypass? The mortality rate from the operation is 4 or 5 percent, meaning that one in twenty persons having the surgery won't survive it. A fourth to a half of those who do survive have a heart attack following the surgery.

What steps should someone contemplating coronary bypass surgery take?
Seek the services of a good cardiologist and try a program of drugs and other measures before submitting to surgery. Seek a second opinion from another cardiologist or surgeon. If you're sure you want the surgery, have it in a center where many such operations have been done and where you have ascertained that the operative mortality rate is less than 4 or 5 percent.

What is a heart attack? In medical usage, the term is synonymous with a myocardial infarction. The myocardium is the heart muscle, and infarction refers to death of tissue from a loss of its blood supply.

How does a heart attack occur? When a coronary artery or one of its branches is blocked completely, a part of the heart muscle is deprived of its blood supply. The resulting death of heart muscle causes a heart attack. The symptoms of the heart attack depend on how much muscle has died and on whether the infarction involves any of the vital nerves that control the heartbeat.

What are the classic symptoms of heart attack? In a "textbook case," severe, crushing chest pain appears beneath the breastbone and persists despite anything the person can do to relieve it. Nitroglycerin doesn't help. Rest doesn't help. Moving around doesn't help. The person breaks out in a cold sweat and may experience a feeling of impending death. The unrelenting pain may persist for hours or gradually diminish on its own if one survives the attack.

What other symptoms may suggest a heart attack? The pain may not be so severe. Frequently the coronary occlusion creates a dull ache or burning pain in the upper abdomen or lower chest that is attributed to indigestion, or the person may write off the discomfort as a bad attack of angina. One in four persons with heart attack does not have pain, and diabetics are more likely to have painless heart attack.

How often does a heart attack cause sudden death? It is estimated that half of persons with a heart attack die before reaching the hospital. The first two or three hours after the attack are the most critical. The danger is that the heart attack may interfere with the normal heart rhythm to cause ventricular fibrillation, a fluttery, ineffective quivering motion of the heart muscle.

When is sudden death most likely to occur?   Immediately after the attack and during the first two or three hours of chest pain.

What should you do when you suspect someone is having a heart attack?
    Notify the Emergency Medical Service and have the person transported by ambulance to the emergency room of a hospital capable of caring for coronary patients. In the event the person collapses, administer CPR as described on p. 191.

What are the three don'ts in dealing with a heart attack?   Don't presume that chest pain is due to indigestion. Don't delay seeking help in the hope that the pain will soon leave. Many deaths occur during the first critical hours before a decision is made to go to the doctor. Don't waste time trying to locate your doctor if you don't reach him or her the first time. If the pain is serious enough to bother you, the physician at the emergency room will want to examine you immediately.

What treatment is given at the hospital?   Diagnosis comes first, and can usually be made with an EKG tracing. The person should be placed in a Coronary Care Unit so that heart and other functions can be continuously monitored. Drug treatment consists of morphine or Demerol to relieve pain, as well as other medicines as needed to improve heart function or treat a complication.

What are the complications of a heart attack?   The most common one is arrhythmia, an irregularity of the heart's rhythm. It may consist of a few extra beats each minute or represent a life-threatening disturbance in the heartbeat. Drugs are administered intravenously to control the arrhythmia. Sometimes the chest must be shocked with an electrical instrument known as a defibrillator; following the shock the heart's normal rhythm may return. At other times a small machine known as a pacemaker has to be used to control an irregular heartbeat. A severe and prolonged drop in blood pressure and congestive heart failure (a reduction in the heart's pumping ability) are serious complications requiring drug therapy. Rupture of the heart may occur a week to ten days after the attack, and it is the only complication that is more common in women than in men. However, heart rupture occurs in only one out of twenty persons dying from heart attack.

What are the chances of recovery from a heart attack?   A person who reaches the hospital quickly has a good chance of surviving the attack, and

383

a majority of physicians believe that care in a Coronary Care Unit will increase the survival rate. Two-thirds of those who leave the hospital after a heart attack are still alive five years later, and a third are still alive ten years later.

Can a heart attack be treated without hospitalization? In selected instances the person may do as well at home as in the hospital. The problem is in predicting which patient will have a complication and, for this reason, hospitalization is very important.

How soon after a heart attack can the patient be up and around? As recently as the early sixties the treatment for heart attack was an ironclad six weeks in bed. Now much earlier activity and discharge are the rule. Bed rest for the first two or three days is customary until pain is gone and complications have cleared or been shown not to exist. Bathroom privileges or use of a bedside commode may begin on the second or third day, progressing to walking in a week or so. Most persons can be discharged two or three weeks after the attack.

Are blood-thinning drugs useful in treating a heart attack? Earlier return to activity has greatly reduced the need for these drugs. Their main use is to prevent blood-clot formation, and clots aren't likely to form in an ambulatory individual. It is doubtful that long-term use of blood thinners offers an advantage greater than the risks of such therapy.

When is recovery from a heart attack complete? The official recovery period is three months. The person with a mild, uncomplicated attack may feel fully recovered in half this time, but shouldn't return to work until at least two months after the attack, taking into consideration the type of work and the severity of the attack.

Will vigorous exercise reduce the risk of another attack? Just as for the individual who has not had a heart attack, regular exercise is beneficial. However, the person who has had a heart attack should never begin an unsupervised exercise program, because the tendency is to progress too fast and to strain the heart. Modest amounts of swimming, cycling, brisk walking or slow jogging may be advisable *under medical supervision.* Of course, the best time to start an exercise program is before you have a heart attack.

What is heart failure? It is a condition resulting from a reduction in the heart's pumping ability. Because the heart enlarges, has to beat faster to keep up with the body's needs and may not work efficiently enough to keep blood from backing up into the lungs, the condition is sometimes referred to as congestive heart failure. Among the causes are heart attack, long-standing high blood pressure, or an infection of the heart muscle known as myocarditis (see p. 386).

What are the symptoms of heart failure?   The person may become breathless after walking a short distance or lying flat in bed. Sometimes shortness of breath occurs in a sudden and frightening attack in the middle of the night. Swelling may be noted in the feet, ankles and legs.

What's the treatment for heart failure?   Prescription diuretics can be used to rid the body of extra fluid. Salt restriction also helps, as does bed rest. The most effective treatment, however, is digitalis. The main action of this drug is to slow the heartbeat and strengthen the heart's force of contraction.

Are heart transplants still done?   The only surgeon continuing to do this very complex operation with any regularity is Dr. Norman Shumway of Stanford University. As of 1978, more than half of the last seventy-two patients who received a new heart at Stanford had survived for five years or more.

Under what situations should one consider a heart transplant?   The ideal candidate is someone under the age of fifty-five with a good body and a bad heart. One shouldn't consider a transplant unless the heart disease is so serious that death is likely in a fairly short time without a transplant. A third of persons seeking transplant die before a suitable donor can be found.

What is the main problem with heart transplants?   The rejection reaction, an inherent body tendency to reject tissue that is foreign to it. Drug control of this reaction has accounted for much of the improvement in recent survival.

Has there been any progress in the use of the artificial heart?   A satisfactory artificial heart for long-term use in a human has not yet been developed, though calves have been kept alive for six months and more with an artificial heart. Left-ventricular assist devices are occasionally used to temporarily aid the heart's pumping action when heart failure has occurred.

HEART INFECTIONS

What types of heart infection may occur?   In order of frequency they include infection of the lining of the heart (pericarditis), the heart muscle itself (myocarditis) and the heart valves (endocarditis).

How does pericarditis develop?   Among the possible causes of acute pericarditis are a cold or the flu, and it is probably caused by a virus. A man between the ages of twenty and fifty is the most susceptible, but the condition also occurs in women in this age range and in persons over fifty.

What are the symptoms of pericarditis?   Chest pain beneath the breastbone develops over a period of several hours and has a "sticking" or sharp quality. The pain, which may radiate to the shoulder, is usually worsened by swallowing or lying down and relieved by sitting up.

What is the treatment for pericarditis?   A thorough medical examination is indicated to rule out heart disease or noninfectious causes of pericarditis, such as rheumatoid arthritis or kidney disease. When the pericarditis is thought to be caused by a virus, the treatment is symptomatic. Aspirin or acetaminophen is given for pain, and the person should remain at home resting until the main symptoms are over. Spontaneous recovery usually occurs in a couple of weeks.

What is the cause of myocarditis?   Usually a virus, but the diagnosis is difficult to make. Diphtheria may cause myocarditis. The condition also may sometimes occur in joggers who resume running too quickly following a cold or the flu.

What are the symptoms of myocarditis?   The person may develop congestive heart failure with shortness of breath, rapid heartbeat and swelling in the feet and legs. Rarely, myocarditis causes sudden death due to heart stoppage.

What is the treatment for myocarditis?   Hospitalization is indicated when the diagnosis is suspected, and the treatment includes digitalis, diuretics, salt restriction and bed rest. Steroids are sometimes advocated in the treatment, but the problem is in knowing whether the heart failure is due to myocarditis or to another problem. Biopsy of the heart has occasionally been performed, but the risks of this procedure far outweigh any benefits.

Under what conditions does a heart-valve infection occur?   The heart valves are susceptible to infection when they have been injured by past disease. Rheumatic heart disease, syphilis and other illnesses that may cause heart murmur are predisposing conditions.

How do the germs reach the valve?   They may enter the bloodstream from a contaminated needle or an infection in the throat or other part of the body. Often the cause is tooth extraction or a minor procedure, such as the passage of an examining instrument, the cystoscope, through the urethra. Drug addicts who use unsterile needles are particularly prone to the illness.

What are the symptoms of heart-valve infection? Fever and a generalized sickness similar to the flu occur, but the symptoms hang on past the time they would have stopped in the case of the flu. Chills and night sweats are typical, and shortness of breath and swelling of the feet are other symptoms. The most incriminating sign of infected heart valve is the appearance of petechiae, small dots of hemorrhage on the skin. They represent small bits of infected material that have broken off from the main clump of infection in the heart, and they may occur in showers that literally cover the body or they may be limited to the palms, the face or the upper chest and neck.

What is the treatment for heart-valve infection? Hospitalization is indicated, and the first step is to make an accurate diagnosis based on culturing the germ from the bloodstream. Penicillin is the most useful drug, but a very high dose is needed and it usually is given intravenously around the clock. Other drugs may be given along with penicillin or instead of it. Treatment has to be continued for at least three to six weeks.

What is the mortality rate for heart-valve infection? Without treatment the infection is invariably fatal. With early treatment the chances for survival are about three out of four. The long-term outlook is not so good, as only half of persons cured of a valve infection are alive and well five years later. Some develop another such infection and die, and some die from heart damage created by the original infection.

Can heart-valve infections be prevented? The risk of infection is less if a patient with a heart murmur caused by a structurally damaged heart takes penicillin the day of a dental or surgical procedure and for several days thereafter.

HEART MURMURS

What is a heart murmur? It is an abnormal heart sound that can be heard through the stethoscope or, sometimes, with the naked ear. The significance of the murmur is that it may reflect a disease of one of the heart valves.

What are the heart valves? They are thin flaps of tissue that regulate the flow of blood through the heart. The tricuspid and pulmonic valves are in the right side of the heart; the mitral and aortic valves are in the left side of the heart.

What does a murmur sound like? The normal heart sounds are a *lub-dub, lub-dub* created by the opening and closing of the heart valves. A murmur is a hissing or blowing sound that obliterates the *lub-dub* or creates a *lub-hiss-dub.* The vibration from a loud murmur can be felt to the left of the breastbone as a sensation somewhat like that felt by the fingers while stroking a purring cat.

What produces this sound?   A murmur is created by turbulent blood flow across the valve. A damaged valve may be responsible for the turbulence, but most murmurs are "innocent" and don't reflect a disease of the heart valves.

How common is an innocent murmur?   Innocent murmurs account for nine out of ten heart murmurs. The frequency is greater during childhood, but it is not unusual for an adult to have an innocent murmur.

What is the most common cause of a significant murmur?   Congenital heart disease is the most common cause, and conditions such as rheumatic fever, syphilis and an injury or infection of the heart are other, less common causes of murmur.

What is meant by congenital heart disease?   It is a disease of the heart that is present at birth. It may cause severe problems, such as a "blue baby," or be so mild that it goes unrecognized until adulthood or is discovered as an incidental finding at autopsy after a long life. It may affect the heart valves, cause a hole between the heart chambers, or disrupt the normal attachment of vessels to the heart.

What causes congenital heart disease?   Contributing factors during pregnancy include German measles, the flu, drug ingestion or exposure to X-ray. Some types of congenital heart disease run in families, though not usually in a predictable manner. Premature birth favors ventricular septal defect, and the condition known as patent ductus arteriosus is more common among infants born at high altitudes than in those born at sea level.

Does a heart murmur interfere with a child's growth?   An innocent murmur won't, but one due to congenital heart disease may. One type of murmur, aortic stenosis, can be quite dangerous unless it is diagnosed and treated.

What's the danger from aortic stenosis?   Because the stenotic valve is too small to permit the heart to pump a normal amount of blood into the arteries, the person is subject to blackout spells, angina and sudden death. The disease is five times as common in men as in women.

Should the child with a heart murmur be allowed to play ball?   The person with aortic stenosis should definitely not be allowed to participate

388

in athletic competition until the defect has been corrected. A mild problem with the mitral valve might not keep someone from playing football or basketball. An innocent murmur should not prevent athletic competition. In each instance the cardiologist should make the determination.

What follow-up treatment is indicated for a child or adult with a murmur?
The person should be followed by a cardiologist at regular intervals. Symptoms indicating a need for further tests and treatment include shortness of breath, swelling of the legs, chest pain and the blue discoloration resulting from cyanosis, a reduction in the oxygen content of the blood. In these instances it may be necessary to perform cardiac catheterization.

What is cardiac catheterization? It is a diagnostic study in which an incision is made in the groin or arm and a catheter is inserted into the artery or vein. The long, narrow tubing is advanced until it reaches the heart. By injecting dye through the catheter and taking X-rays, the physician can tell if the person has a hole in the heart, an abnormal connection between the great vessels or an obstruction to blood flow. The purpose of diagnosing the exact defect is to determine if surgery may be indicated.

How risky is cardiac catheterization? The risk to an adult is one death per 1,000 studies. In seriously ill children with congenital heart disease the risk is two deaths per 100 studies.

What does heart surgery consist of? The person is anesthetized and may be subjected to cooling measures to lower the body's oxygen needs. A heart-lung bypass machine is employed to keep blood flowing to the tissues during surgery. This allows the heart to be stopped, opened and fixed. The operation may consist of removing a faulty valve and replacing it with an artificial one, or of repairing a hole in the heart with sutures and a graft of material. When the operation is complete, a shock is used to start the heartbeat and the person is taken off the heart-lung pump.

How risky is heart surgery in an adult? The overall mortality rate is 5 percent. Elderly persons withstand surgery less well than young adults, and a person with a disease of only one valve has a better chance than when two or more valves are faulty.

How risky is heart surgery during infancy? The overall mortality rate is 10 percent. The risk is greatest when the child has cyanosis, for defects that create this problem are harder to correct. Surgical risk must be balanced against the natural history of the heart disease, which may carry a mortality rate of 100 percent during the first few years of life.

What accounts for the risk of surgery?   The mortality rate depends on several factors, but an important one is the length of time the patient is left on the heart-lung machine. The greater the skill of the surgeon, the shorter the operation and the better the chance of survival. A patient should know beforehand that he or she is having as little surgery as is feasible and should seek the services of a top surgeon to perform the operation.

What precaution should be taken before signing the operative permit?
Seek the advice and the referral of a good cardiologist who will consult with the surgeon on procedure and results. Ask the surgeon to explain to you *exactly* what he or she will do. Find out what is wrong with the heart and stress specifically that you wish as little surgery as possible consistent with your condition. Do not, if you can avoid it, sign a permit for the surgeon to do "anything deemed necessary" once the operation begins. You may not be able to avoid signing this statement, and if you have confidence in the choice of surgeon, this may not be a problem. Of course, the surgeon may encounter unforeseen conditions while the operation is taking place and you should feel enough confidence in his or her judgment that the procedure will be in your best interests. If you have the choice, you may wish to specify that the surgeon—not an associate—will perform the surgery, but this may not be financially feasible.

IRREGULARITIES OF THE HEARTBEAT

Is it normal for the heart to skip a beat?   Yes, this may happen in a healthy person and is no cause for alarm unless the skipping becomes frequent or causes discomfort. Anger, nervousness and the use of cold remedies may cause skipped beats. Other contributors are smoking and the use of coffee, tea or drugs containing caffeine.

What causes very rapid beating of the heart?   Nervousness and exertion can cause it, but rapid thumping of the heart may accompany an irregularity of the heartbeat such as atrial tachycardia or atrial fibrillation. The arrhythmia may be continuous or occur in episodes lasting minutes or hours.

What is atrial fibrillation?   Normally, a special area of heart muscle in the right atrium fires off impulses at a regular rate of about seventy a minute. In atrial fibrillation, this pacemaker loses control and the entire upper heart beats with an ineffective quivering motion. It sends rapid impulses to the ventricles, which beat irregularly and at a rate that is faster than normal.

What causes atrial fibrillation?   It is usually due to coronary artery disease or rheumatic heart disease, though hyperthyroidism and high blood pressure may cause it.

What is the treatment for atrial fibrillation?   The irregularity can usually be corrected by treatment with digitalis or other drugs. In some instances a surge of electricity is applied to the chest in the same way that defibrillation after cardiac arrest is accomplished. The shock is followed by a normal heartbeat, but the person must still take drugs to prevent a recurrence of the irregularity.

What is atrial tachycardia?   Most common in young people, this is an extremely rapid heartbeat that tends to occur in attacks lasting from several minutes to several hours. The attack, or paroxysm, begins and ends abruptly. Contributing factors include fatigue, smoking, emotional stress or too much coffee or alcohol. Most persons with paroxysmal atrial tachycardia do not have heart disease and eventually recover from this irregularity.

What are the symptoms of atrial tachycardia?   The person may be unaware of the rapid heartbeat, or it may be noticed as a fluttering or pounding in the chest. Dizziness and faintness may occur, but are unusual.

What causes atrial tachycardia?   It is caused by a sudden overactivity of the heart's pacemaker. During an attack the heart rate is usually around 180 to 200 beats a minute, but the beat is completely regular. Why some persons develop this problem is not understood, though it is known that certain measures may help prevent an attack.

What is the treatment for atrial tachycardia?   The attack can often be terminated by taking a deep breath and bearing down—the Valsalva maneuver. Gagging or inducing vomiting may stop an attack. A physician may be able to abort an attack by the use of a technique known as carotid sinus massage or by drug therapy. Prevention of an attack may be possible by avoiding tobacco, alcohol and stimulants such as coffee or tea, and by getting plenty of rest. Tranquilizers are sometimes prescribed for nervous individuals who are prone to attacks of atrial tachycardia. Digitalis, propranolol and quinidine are among the drugs that are occasionally necessary to prevent frequent or troublesome attacks of atrial tachycardia.

HIGH BLOOD PRESSURE

What is blood pressure?   It is the force with which blood is pumped through the arteries.

How is blood pressure measured?   Usually with a sphygmomanometer, a cuff with attached pressure gauge that is placed around the upper arm and inflated until blood flow through the main artery has stopped. By listening below the cuff with a stethoscope as pressure is slowly released, the examiner can tell when blood begins to flow through the artery again. Correlation of this point with the reading on the pressure gauge will give the blood pressure.

What is the normal blood pressure?   The reading of 120/80 appears in many books as a normal blood pressure. Pressures that are higher or lower than this, however, may also be normal. The systolic, or top, pressure (120) corresponds to the maximum pressure in the arteries at the time of the heartbeat; the diastolic, or lower, pressure (80) corresponds to the brief period of rest in between heartbeats. The upper limit of normal is usually set at 140/90.

Is blood pressure apt to vary with activity?   Yes, it is lowest at night during sleep and tends to go up during exercise, excitement or nervousness. For example, the visit to the doctor may create enough stress in a susceptible person to affect the reading. Most blood pressures determined in doctors' offices are, in fact, higher than the person's ordinary levels.

What is the healthiest blood pressure?   The healthiest pressure seems to be the lowest one you can achieve while comfortably going about your normal activities.

Which is worse, systolic or diastolic elevation?   An increase in diastolic pressure (the lower number in the reading) is generally taken as worse than an increase in systolic pressure, but some doctors dispute this. Claiming that elevation of either reading is equally bad, they point out that most persons with high blood pressure have systolic *and* diastolic hypertension.

What is hypertension?   It is the medical term for high blood pressure.

What are the risks from hypertension?   High blood pressure is the culprit in most instances of heart attack, angina pectoris, stroke, congestive heart failure and early onset of arteriosclerosis. Hypertension can damage the kidneys and cause the heart to enlarge. The risks from elevated blood pressure are even greater if the person also smokes, is diabetic or has a high serum cholesterol.

How frequently does high blood pressure occur?   It affects 20 percent of adults—40–50 million Americans. One out of four medical visits by adults is for high blood pressure or a condition resulting from it. About half the people who turn out to have high blood pressure during screening examinations are unaware of having the disease.

Who is most susceptible to developing high blood pressure?   Susceptibility is greater in blacks than in whites, and in obese persons than in those of normal weight. High blood pressure tends to run in families, but not always in a predictable pattern.

What are the symptoms of high blood pressure?   Headache in the back of the head first thing in the morning is the most common symptom. Dizziness, shortness of breath or blurred vision are among the symptoms that may occur. But many persons with high blood pressure have absolutely no symptoms until the condition has caused heart, kidney or brain damage. This is why hypertension is known as "the silent killer."

Are all cases of high blood pressure alike?   No, the general forms of the disease are primary and secondary hypertension. Primary, or essential, hypertension is responsible for four out of five instances of high blood pressure. Its cause is unknown, but heredity and obesity are the main contributors. Secondary, or curable, hypertension may be caused by a tumor of the adrenal gland, disease of the kidney, a kink in the aorta or the use of birth-control pills.

Why make a distinction between primary and secondary forms?   If a definite cause can be found, its removal may cure the high blood pressure. Moreover, some of the causes of secondary hypertension are tumors whose removal may be lifesaving. In these instances the high blood pressure is a symptom of an underlying disease.

What's the treatment for high blood pressure?   The treatment for primary hypertension may include a modification in life style and the use of an antihypertensive drug or a combination of them. These drugs have been classified according to the way they work, and depending on the severity of the condition, are given singly or in combination to regulate the blood pressure. Surgery may be indicated where a correctable disorder is found.

How long does it take to arrive at the correct drug therapy?   Usually two weeks on each drug are needed to assess the response to it, so several weeks are required to start a drug, check its effect on the blood pressure and then possibly add other drugs. The goal is to reduce the blood pressure to normal while causing the fewest possible side effects.

Are other measures ever helpful?   Yes, it will help to stop smoking, reduce to normal weight and restrict the intake of salt in the diet. Reduction of stress is also important. Regular exercise is capable of reducing the blood pressure of many persons, and taken together, these measures may obviate the need for drug therapy in certain individuals. Follow-up medical observation is indicated in any event.

How much salt restriction is necessary?   The person who isn't exercising and perspiring a great deal needs only a gram of salt a day, yet the average American diet contains five grams. Those who add salt to food at the table may get ten or twenty grams a day. The incidence of high blood pressure seems to be directly related to high salt intake. The first step is to keep to a minimum the use of salt in cooking, to avoid the use of salt at the table, and to avoid or limit the consumption of salted crackers, chips and foods preserved in brine.

How does exercise lower the blood pressure?   It causes sweating and the loss of salt from the body. It helps to reduce weight and prevent obesity. Probably the most important effect of exercise is an activation of natural blood-pressure-lowering reflexes. The relaxation that follows a period of exercise seems to be effective in reducing tension and promoting emotional well-being.

What's the long-term outlook for someone with high blood pressure? Caught early and treated appropriately, high blood pressure is compatible with a normal life-span. Among the consequences of untreated high blood pressure are enlargement of the heart, heart attack, stroke and kidney damage.

LUNG DISEASES

What do the lungs do?   In conjunction with the muscles of the chest, the lungs work like a bellows to draw air in, where its oxygen can be removed, and to blow it out along with the waste product, carbon dioxide.

What are the diseases that may affect the lungs?   The most frequent serious lung problem is pneumonia (see p. 170). Chronic forms of lung disease include tuberculosis (p. 171–72), bronchiectasis, chronic bronchitis, asthma (p. 156), emphysema and cystic fibrosis. Lung cancer is the most common form of cancer in men and is a leading cause of death in the United States. The most common respiratory illness is bronchitis associated with a minor respiratory infection (see p. 169).

What are the symptoms of lung disease?   The main one is coughing, and the cough is sometimes productive of blood-tinged or overtly bloody sputum. Other symptoms of lung disease include wheezing, shortness of breath, chest pain, cyanosis and weight loss.

What causes coughing?   It may occur as a symptom of virtually any lung disease, including lung cancer, but it usually reflects an infection of the lungs such as bronchitis. Smoking, a cold and postnasal drip are other causes of coughing.

What causes coughing with bloody sputum?   Tuberculosis and lung cancer are the leading causes, but the phlegm may be tinged with blood in congestive heart failure, bronchiectasis, chronic bronchitis or a bleeding disorder.

What are the general measures for treating a cough?   When the cause of a persistent cough is not known, a medical examination is indicated. The problem can usually be pinpointed by a physical examination, chest X-ray and sputum culture. Treatment is directed toward the underlying cause.

CHRONIC LUNG DISEASES

Who should treat lung diseases?   A general physician, pediatrician or internist is capable of treating most lung problems. The person with a chronic condition, such as bronchiectasis or emphysema, should see a pulmonary disease specialist, an internist who has had one or two years of additional training in treating diseases of the lungs.

What is bronchiectasis?   A chronic infection of the lungs associated with widening of the small air passageways and the accumulation of phlegm and pus in them. The condition may follow an episode of pneumonia or tuberculosis. Measles or whooping cough during childhood may predispose to bronchiectasis years later.

What are the symptoms of bronchiectasis?   The main symptom is sputum production the first thing in the morning and the last thing at night. The sputum tends to have a bad odor because of the bacteria in it. Half of persons with bronchiectasis note blood-tinged sputum on occasion. Lung hemorrhage with coughing of sizable quantities of blood is possible. Recurrent bouts of pneumonia or bronchitis may occur.

What's the treatment for bronchiectasis?   The sputum has to be drained from the lungs by postural methods such as leaning off the bed for ten minutes twice a day. Mist inhalations prior to postural drainage may help to raise the secretions. Antibiotic therapy may be given for long intervals to suppress infection. When only one part of a lung is affected by bronchiectasis, the removal of this segment of lung may cure the person.

What is chronic bronchitis?   Smoking is the usual cause for this condition, which is characterized by a cough and the production of small amounts of phlegm. Other sources of lung irritation include smog, noxious fumes in a factory, and pollen and other material to which the person is allergic. The tendency in recent years is to group severe chronic bronchitis in the same category as emphysema and call the condition "chronic obstructive respiratory disease." Doing so helps to explain why the symptoms of chronic bronchitis are similar to those of emphysema and why the treatment for the two conditions is similar.

What is emphysema?   It is a chronic lung disease created by overdistention of the tiny air sacs (alveoli) that permit oxygen to pass into the blood. Many of these air sacs burst to create large, functionless "holes" in the lungs, and the person has increasing difficulty blowing off carbon dioxide wastes from the body. The lungs of someone with advanced emphysema are inelastic, overexpanded and spotted with areas of infection.

What causes emphysema?   The cause is unknown, but the most important factors are an inherited tendency to develop the disease coupled with a long-term habit of smoking. The deficiency of a substance that inhibits lung enzymes has been blamed for the destructive processes of this disease.

What are the symptoms of emphysema?   Symptoms usually begin after the age of forty-five and consist of progressive shortness of breath and productive cough. Characteristically, the person has trouble blowing air out of the lungs. Wheezing, similar to that seen in asthma, may occur. Distention of the lungs may create the classic "barrel chest" of emphysema.

What is the treatment for emphysema?   The person with chronic obstructive pulmonary disease needs a program of antibiotics, ventilation therapy and the avoidance of lung irritants. Quitting cigarettes is the key to successful therapy for many individuals. Wheezing, if it occurs, can be treated with the same measures used for asthma (see p. 156). Early treatment of respiratory infections is important, because these may quickly become severe in someone with chronic lung disease. It is important to note that the "holes" of emphysema do not heal themselves. Treatment is aimed at preventing further lung damage.

What's the prognosis for someone with chronic obstructive lung disease?
The five-year survival after onset of symptoms is 70 percent, and the ten-year survival 50 percent.

What causes cystic fibrosis?   It is an inherited disease affecting the sweat glands and internal body organs such as the lungs and pancreas. The lungs produce a thick, tenacious phlegm that is hard to cough up, and the pancreas may fail to function properly in the digestion of food. One in twenty persons carries the trait, and one in every 2,000 babies is affected. Someone with a family history of the disease is at greatest risk, and cystic fibrosis is much more common in whites than in blacks or Orientals.

What are the symptoms of cystic fibrosis?   Symptoms often begin during infancy, but the onset may be delayed till adolescence or early adulthood. A cough and respiratory infections occur. Though the infections respond to antibiotic therapy, they do so slowly and, often, after complications such as the collapse of a part of the lung. Attacks of wheezing and shortness of breath may resemble those seen in asthma. Diarrhea and failure to thrive represent the pancreatic manifestations of the disease. Excessive amounts of sodium and chloride are excreted into the sweat.

What is the treatment for cystic fibrosis?   Antibiotics and inhalation therapy are useful in controlling the disease. A bedside vaporizer to moisten the air during sleep is helpful, and so is the use of mist, such as acetylcysteine, to liquefy viscid phlegm in the lungs. Persons with poor digestion can be treated with pancreatic extracts. Financial help and information can be obtained by writing the National Cystic Fibrosis Research Foundation, 3379 Peachtree Road, Atlanta, Ga. 30326.

What's the long-term outlook for someone with cystic fibrosis?   Half of persons with this disease in childhood survive past age eighteen. Some patients live to middle age.

What step should be taken by persons with a family history of this disease?
They should seek genetic counseling to determine their risks of having an affected child or another affected child.

LUNG CANCER

What is the incidence of lung cancer?   It is the leading cause of cancer death in the United States, and if it were ranked separately, it would be the fifth leading cause of death overall. It kills almost 100,000 persons a year in this country, three-fourths of them men. Every five minutes someone dies of lung cancer. Since 1964 the number of cancer deaths has doubled and the rate of lung cancer in women has tripled.

What causes lung cancer?   Though there may be other causes, such as air pollution, the Surgeon General of the United States has accumulated overwhelming evidence that smoking is the primary cause of lung cancer. A light smoker has a sevenfold increase in risk for lung cancer; a moderate smoker's risk is twelve times greater than average; a heavy smoker is twenty-four times as likely as a nonsmoker to develop cancer of the lung. Carcinoma of the lung is rare in a woman who doesn't smoke.

At what age does lung cancer occur?   Usually after the age of forty, and the risk goes up with increasing age in someone who smokes.

What are the symptoms of lung cancer?   In order of frequency: cough, cough productive of blood, shortness of breath and wheezing, weight loss and chest pain. Sometimes the cancer is recognized when it causes bronchial obstruction leading to a bout of pneumonia. Rarely, an enlargement of the tips of the fingers and the fingernails, known as clubbing of the nails, is an early sign of lung cancer. Hoarseness, headache and the appearance of hard nodules at the base of the neck behind the collarbone may reflect spread of the cancer.

What is the treatment for lung cancer?   Surgical removal of the tumor is the only effective treatment. X-ray and chemotherapy are given when the tumor is inoperable.

What's the prognosis for someone with lung cancer?   Only 8 percent of persons with this cancer survive for five years, and the mortality rate is about 50 percent during the first six months after the cancer is diagnosed. The poor prognosis reflects the rapid growth of lung cancer as well as the tendency for early symptoms to be overlooked or denied.

What is the single most important way to prevent lung cancer?   Don't smoke, or if you do smoke, quit. A man or woman who smokes should have an annual chest X-ray and should seek a medical examination at the first onset of the symptoms mentioned above.

What is the current status of lung transplants?   This form of organ transplantation has not proved successful. Thus far the patient who survived the longest following transplantation was a man in Belgium who lived for ten months.

16

DISEASES
of the
ABDOMINAL
ORGANS

What are the abdominal organs?   These organs in the abdomen include the stomach, intestines, pancreas, liver, gall bladder, spleen and kidneys. They are responsible for digestion of foods, processing of nutrients and removal of wastes. Disease may affect any of these structures, but stomach or intestinal disease is the most common and lends itself most readily to medical diagnosis.

What is an upper GI series?   "GI" stands for gastrointestinal, and this series of X-rays shows up the esophagus, stomach and small intestine. Its most frequent use is in testing for the presence of an ulcer in the stomach or in the duodenum, which is the first part of the small intestine.

What about the barium enema?   Barium is passed into the colon through an enema tube and its progress up the colon is monitored by X-rays. The barium enema is useful in evaluating intestinal bleeding, lower abdominal pain, a change in bowel habits or any symptoms suggestive of cancer of the colon.

What other tests are available for diagnosis of stomach or intestinal disease?
It is possible to look directly into the stomach or intestine through a lighted instrument known as an endoscope. The examination can be done through the mouth or through the rectum. A flexible tube, the fiberoptic

endoscope, is now in use. It can bend to conform to body anatomy and, at the same time, allow the examiner to visualize the internal anatomy. Biopsies may also be taken, photographs made and even the removal of polyps performed through the endoscope.

Who should treat a disease of the abdominal organs?   Mild problems can be managed by a family physician, internist or pediatrician. A serious problem with the intestines, liver, gall bladder, stomach or pancreas may warrant consultation with a gastroenterologist, an internist with this subspecialty. The person with kidney disease should be treated by an internist, pediatrician or a nephrologist, who has had a year or two of additional training in treating kidney diseases. The spleen, though it is in the abdomen, is really an appendage of the blood; the individual who has an enlarged spleen or any problem with this organ should seek the services of a hematologist (see p. 358). These specialists may be consulted in severe illnesses, but the primary-care physician is competent in many of these areas.

ESOPHAGUS AND STOMACH

What is the esophagus?   The food pipe, a ten-inch conduit from the mouth to the stomach.

How do you know if something is wrong with the esophagus?   The symptoms of an esophageal problem include the sensation that something is stuck in the throat, a burning sensation beneath the breastbone—"heartburn"— and chronic indigestion or vomiting. Since the back of the throat is continuous with the esophagus, food may get stuck there and create a problem requiring first aid.

Who is most likely to get something stuck in the throat?   Four out of five instances of this problem occur in children under fifteen. An older person who wears dentures is also susceptible. By interfering with normal sensations in the mouth, dentures may lead to attempts at swallowing before the food is ready to go down.

What may get stuck in the throat?   The most common object is a ball of food that's too big to go down. Less often it's a bone or sharp object swallowed by a child. The person becomes aware of the problem immediately. When the item is very big, it may obstruct the airway and create the "café coronary" (discussed on pp. 194–95). Even when the air passages remain open, something stuck in the esophagus requires immediate attention.

What should be done?   In an older child or adult who's aware that something is stuck in the food pipe, the item may be washed down with water or a soft food such as bread. In a small child, when the symptoms of gagging, distress or coughing suggest that something is caught in the esophagus, no attempt should be made to dislodge it unless the child is having trouble breathing. Instead, call the Emergency Medical Service or take the child to the nearest emergency room. There's no need for alarm as long as the child is breathing all right, but the foreign body must be removed by a physician using an endoscope. An adult may require the same service if the object remains in the esophagus after a few attempts to wash it down.

Can a caustic substance damage the esophagus?   Yes, ingestion of substances such as lye, Chlorox, Drano or acid may burn the esophagus and cause it to narrow from scar formation. The condition, esophageal stricture, may appear years after the injury as a cause of difficulty in swallowing.

What's the treatment for caustic burn of the esophagus?   First, prevention is important: keep potentially harmful things away from the youngster (see Chapter 7). When a harmful ingestion does occur, do not attempt to induce vomiting. Call the Emergency Medical Service or take the child to a hospital emergency room. Examination with an esophagoscope is necessary to assess the extent of the damage, and treatment with prednisone may help to prevent esophageal stricture. The child should be admitted to the hospital for observation and treatment.

What if an esophageal stricture develops?   The narrowing may be enlarged by use of a bougie, a candle-shaped object that can be swallowed and withdrawn to dilate the esophagus. Small and large bougies are available, and the dilations have to be done periodically. Surgery is another possibility: the narrowed esophagus can be replaced with a section of intestine.

What about heartburn?   This symptom is due to irritation of the lower esophagus by stomach acid. The pain is dull and resembles a steady pressure beneath the breastbone; in some instances it is severe enough to mimic a heart attack—it may even radiate to the shoulder and arm. Other symptoms are sour belching and watering of the mouth. The person with severe esophagitis may experience nausea and vomiting following meals.

What causes heartburn and esophagitis?   A small muscle normally protects the lower esophagus from stomach acid. A weakness in this muscle or an increase in pressure inside the abdomen may overcome the muscle and propel acid upward. Obesity and wearing a tight belt or corset are two causes. Lying down right after a meal is another, because it's easier for fluid

401

to run sideways than in the uphill direction it has to take if you're sitting or standing. Sitting down after a meal may also favor heartburn by compressing the abdominal contents. Hiatus hernia is often the cause of persistent heartburn.

What is hiatus hernia?　In this condition, a small part of the stomach slides into the chest alongside the esophagus. Stomach acid easily reaches the lower esophagus, and the hernia itself may be pinched between the muscles of the diaphragm to cause additional problems.

What is the treatment for hiatus hernia?　The person should avoid heavy meals in favor of frequent, smaller feedings. Spicy foods are out, and so is lying down or sitting down after eating. Weight loss is helpful if obesity is present. Elevating the head of the bed on eight-inch blocks may help to prevent symptoms during the night. Antacids can be used to relieve the heartburn. It is possible to repair hiatus hernia surgically, but the results of the operation are often disappointing and the person would be better off by relying on medical treatment.

What are the characteristics of cancer of the esophagus?　Progressive difficulty in swallowing is the main symptom of this form of cancer, which also causes dull pain beneath the breastbone. Eventually the person, usually a middle-aged or older man, cannot swallow even liquids. Caught early, esophageal cancer may be successfully treated by surgery, so an upper GI series should be done when even the least difficulty in swallowing develops.

What is gastritis?　An irritation of the stomach causing heartburn and a sensation of pressure low in the chest. Other symptoms include loss of appetite, nausea and vomiting, sometimes of blood-tinged material. The most common cause of gastritis is excessive use of alcohol or aspirin. Treatment includes taking antacids and avoiding materials that may harm the stomach: alcohol, coffee, cigarettes, aspirin and spicy or sharp-edged foods.

What is an ulcer?　It is a wearing away of the surface of a body lining. A peptic ulcer of the stomach or duodenum (the first part of the small intestine) is caused by a relative excess of stomach acid. A circular defect, usually less than half an inch in diameter, the ulcer crater is usually situated in the duodenum.

How common is peptic ulcer?　One out of every ten persons can expect to develop one at some time during life.

Who is most susceptible?　Men are four times as susceptible as women, and factors that increase the risk are stress, unhealthy eating habits, cigarette smoking, excessive use of alcohol or coffee and lack of adequate rest. Ingestion of aspirin, Butazolidin, Indocin, Clinoril, prednisone, cortisone and other antiarthritic drugs favors ulcer development. Some persons are naturally more susceptible than others, and a tendency to develop ulcers may run in families.

What are the symptoms of a peptic ulcer?   Discomfort, described as pain or a hunger sensation, occurs in the upper abdomen in a predictable manner: it is worse when the stomach is empty and is relieved by eating or ingesting antacid. The pain is not usually present the first thing in the morning and is intensified in the afternoon and evening. Symptoms tend to appear an hour or two after a meal. The person may be able to localize the discomfort to one tender area the size of a silver dollar located two or three inches above the navel.

What are the complications of a peptic ulcer?   An ulcer may bleed, obstruct the flow of food from the stomach or perforate through the lining of the stomach or duodenum. A perforated ulcer is a medical crisis requiring immediate therapy. The person develops severe abdominal pain and the belly muscles undergo a boardlike spasm as acid, enzymes and other stomach contents spill into the abdominal cavity. Vomiting is the main symptom of obstruction, but weight loss accompanies the inability to eat solid foods for fear of throwing them up. Bleeding is a more frequent complication than obstruction or perforation, and the person may vomit the blood or pass it in the stools. Vomited blood may have a coffee-grounds appearance from being broken down by stomach acid. Blood in the stools has a tarry black appearance which, once you've seen it, is hard to mistake for anything but digested blood.

What is the treatment for a peptic ulcer?   Treatment is aimed at relieving the person's symptoms and preventing complications. At one time bland diets and milk and cream were used to treat ulcer. Now it is known that milk, which does give some relief of symptoms, may actually stimulate acid production and that most ulcer victims will get well if they are simply placed in the hospital and given a nutritious diet. Causative factors such as smoking and aspirin ingestion must be curtailed. Antacids are used one hour after eating and again every hour or two between meals to neutralize excess acid. Liquid antacid tends to be more potent, but less portable, than tablets. Cimetidine is a drug whose purpose is to inhibit the secretion of stomach acid. It has been helpful in treating many persons, but the side effects include diarrhea, dizziness, muscular pain, rash and a depression of the white blood cell count. The most important measure in treatment is simply to let the person rest for two or three weeks.

When is surgery indicated to treat an ulcer?   When a complication occurs. A perforation has to be sealed, and a bleeding or obstructing ulcer may have to be removed along with a portion of the stomach. When an ulcer causes severe pain and does not respond to medical treatment, surgery may be considered, but in such cases a second opinion should be sought.

How often is surgery necessary?   Five or 10 percent of ulcer victims may eventually require surgery.

Can an ulcer return following treatment?   Yes, it may recur following medical treatment or appear in a different place even after surgical removal of part of the stomach. The ulcer-prone individual has to avoid injurious habits that might favor a recurrence.

How common is cancer of the stomach?   It is much less common in the United States than it was before World War II. The incidence is greater in blacks and persons of Oriental extraction than in other groups. Worldwide, the highest incidence of stomach cancer occurs in Japan.

What are the symptoms of cancer of the stomach?   Weight loss and abdominal discomfort are the main symptoms. Sometimes abdominal pain similar to that of an ulcer is noted, and the pain may be relieved by ingesting food or antacid. Vomiting, loss of appetite, a change in bowel habits and the sensation of being filled too quickly at the table are additional symptoms. Anemia may develop and lead to breathlessness on exertion and easy fatigability.

What causes stomach cancer?   The cause is unknown, but an interesting observation is that it is more likely to occur in a person who has previously had surgery for duodenal ulcer. Thus, a person who develops a recurrence of ulcer symptoms following surgery should be investigated for malignancy. Persons with blood group A are at slightly greater risk of developing stomach cancer, and persons with pernicious anemia (see p. 362) are thought to have a one-in-ten chance of eventually developing stomach cancer.

What is the treatment for cancer of the stomach?   If possible, the cancer should be removed surgically. Chemotherapy and radiation therapy are sometimes used along with surgery or instead of it for an inoperable cancer.

What is the prognosis for cancer of the stomach?   The overall five-year survival rate is 10 percent, but early diagnosis and surgery will greatly increase the likelihood of a cure.

THE INTESTINES

How do the intestines work?   Food, water and nutrients are absorbed from the intestines as the ingested material is squeezed along through twenty feet of absorptive surface. In the large intestine, or colon, bacteria break large particles into small ones and muscular contractions compress the material into the firm substance that is eliminated as feces.

What are the symptoms of intestinal disease?   The common ones are loss of appetite, nausea, vomiting, abdominal pain and diarrhea. Constipation may occur as a symptom of intestinal disease or may exist in its own right. Belching and gassiness are troublesome symptoms that don't necessarily reflect disease. Weight loss is an uncommon but serious symptom of intestinal disease.

What causes loss of appetite?   A common cause is "intestinal flu," a viral infection. Nausea, vomiting, abdominal pain and diarrhea may accompany the infection. Pneumonia, kidney infection, liver disease or any serious illness may interfere with appetite, as may worry or tension.

What conditions most frequently cause weight loss?   Mild weight loss may accompany intestinal flu or any other illness. Weight loss occurring in spite of an increased appetite suggests diabetes or hyperthyroidism. Cancer of one of the body's organs usually results in weight loss. Two infrequent but serious causes are malabsorption and anorexia nervosa.

What is anorexia nervosa?   It is a poorly understood condition occurring usually in teenage girls and is characterized by an almost total loss of appetite and an actual aversion to food.

How common is anorexia nervosa?   The severe form is not uncommon among schoolgirls who are in their middle teens and, usually, from a middle-class or upper-socioeconomic background. The disease is almost twenty times more common in young women than in young men.

What are the symptoms of anorexia nervosa?   A previously healthy teenager begins to lose weight. The person may claim to be eating a lot when it's clear she's not. She may claim to be dieting to improve her figure, but it soon becomes obvious that there's more to it than that. Some young women even induce vomiting. A loss of forty pounds or more within several months is not unusual, and the nutritional lack may be compounded by the use of laxatives so that a bowel movement will occur every day. Menstrual periods become sparse or stop, and the person shows a tendency to withdraw from contact with others.

405

What causes anorexia nervosa?   It is thought to be a psychiatric condition resulting from conflicts that occur during the turbulent period of adjustment following puberty. Some doctors have theorized that the abnormality may be in the hypothalamic region of the brain.

What's the treatment for anorexia nervosa?   The purpose of medical treatment is to keep the person from starving to death, which may occur in a severe instance of anorexia nervosa. Hospitalization is advisable, and a nurse who can gain the person's trust is best suited to guide her into healthy eating habits. Psychotherapy may prove useful in resolving the problem.

What's the long-term outlook for someone with anorexia nervosa?   Weight loss may recur after an initial period of treatment, but most persons with this condition recover after two or three years of difficulty, apparently "outgrowing" it. Certain patients with anorexia nervosa may, however, continue to have severe adjustment problems.

What are the symptoms of malabsorption?   It causes weight loss and bulky, foul-smelling stools. The feces have a greasy consistency, are often light yellow in color, and float on the surface of the toilet water. It's not unusual for feces to have this appearance following a bout of intestinal flu, but in this instance the stools quickly return to normal. Bulky stools—reflecting poor absorption of fats—may persist for months or years in someone with malabsorption. Other symptoms of this condition include abdominal pain, loss of appetite and gassiness.

What causes malabsorption?   An intestinal allergy to wheat and other grains, known as celiac disease or nontropical sprue, is the most common cause of chronic malabsorption in the United States. Sometimes an inherited lack of intestinal enzymes, such as lactase deficiency, is responsible for the malabsorption; sometimes it is caused by pancreatitis (see p. 416).

What's the treatment for malabsorption?   Though this is not always necessary, the person may be hospitalized under the care of a gastroenterologist, given a thorough workup and placed on an appropriate diet. In some instances an antibiotic such as tetracycline is useful in the treatment. In the case of lactase deficiency, where the person cannot tolerate milk because of a lack of this digestive enzyme, long-term avoidance of the offending foods may be necessary.

Is malabsorption like a food allergy?   Some forms of it are, but most food allergies are much less severe and are more likely to cause mild diarrhea, stomach upset or headache after the offending food is ingested. Many children develop diarrhea from milk allergy, and still other persons are allergic to eggs, corn, fruit, peas, other vegetables, chocolate, food additives or food coloring. The allergy may also cause rash (hives), stuffy nose, runny nose, wheezing, cough or excessive mucus production from the throat. Food allergy may be responsible for some instances of hyperactive behavior in children.

How are food allergies diagnosed?   The most helpful tool is a closely kept record of the symptoms produced by eating a given food. An allergist can make the diagnosis by testing for specific substances or by putting the person on an elimination diet. The diet lists all the foods in a particular group, and the idea is to eliminate those that may be causing problems. If symptoms improve during two weeks of avoiding the food, the chances are good that food allergy is responsible.

Are all food reactions allergies?   No. This is an area in which a great deal of work remains to be done. It seems clear, however, that some people cannot tolerate certain foods because of enzyme deficiencies or other variances in their digestive or metabolic processes.

What's the treatment for food allergies?   The causative food or foods must be eliminated from the diet. In the case of a mild allergy to eggs or milk, one may be able to eat one or two portions of the food each week without having difficulties, and in some instances foods can be reintroduced after a period of time with no apparent problems.

What may cause abdominal pain?   A list of causes is given in the accompanying chart. Many of these conditions have already been discussed, and some will be discussed later in this chapter.

CAUSES OF ABDOMINAL PAIN

Common
  Menses
  Irritable colon
  Constipation
  Heartburn
  Peptic ulcer
  Intestinal flu
  Appendicitis
  Gall bladder attack

Less common
  Endometriosis

Pancreatitis
Hepatitis
Kidney infection
Sickle cell anemia
Twisted ovary or ovarian cyst
Diabetic nerve damage
Lead poisoning
Diverticulitis

Uncommon
   Tubal pregnancy
   Intestinal obstruction
   Porphyria
   Ulcerative colitis
   Regional enteritis
   Peritonitis from any cause
   Cancer of an abdominal organ

What is irritable colon?   Also known as spastic colitis and nervous stomach, this condition affects an estimated 10 or 20 million Americans. The onset is usually in early adulthood, and the symptoms include attacks of cramping abdominal pain and diarrhea triggered by the ingestion of rich or spicy foods or a stressful life situation. A college student may develop diarrhea and stomach cramps before an examination; a job applicant may note symptoms before an interview. Long periods of freedom from symptoms are typical of irritable colon, and in many instances constipation occurs in between attacks of diarrhea.

What's the treatment for irritable colon?   The person should be examined by an internist or gastroenterologist. Simply knowing the cause of the condition and how common it is may prove therapeutic. Some people have found relief from a diet which includes an adequate quantity of fiber supplied by roughage or bran cereal. Large meals should be avoided, as should spices, peppers and garlic. Since they may aggravate the problem, laxatives should not be taken. Symptomatic relief may be obtained by the use of an antispasmodic drug.

What is colitis?   It is an inflammation of the colon. Ulcerative colitis is a much more severe condition than irritable colon. It causes diarrhea and, often, the passage of blood in the stools. The diagnosis must be made by colon studies, and treatment is with sulfasalazine by mouth or steroid hormones, which are often given by retention enema.

What is regional enteritis, or ileitis?   An illness related to ulcerative colitis which tends to occur in children and young adults, though it may also occur in older people. The diagnosis must be made by a pediatrician, internist or gastroenterologist, and treatment may consist of steroids, but surgery may be necessary if complications occur.

What is diverticulitis?　Small pockets or outpouchings known as diverticula may develop in the large intestine. These occur in a fourth of persons over the age of forty and in half of those over the age of sixty. The diverticula are most often found in the left lower colon. It has never been determined why they develop, but dietary lack of roughage is suspected to be the main contributor. Diverticulitis occurs when material from the colon gets trapped in the outpouching to cause an infection.

What are the symptoms of diverticulitis?　A mild attack causes pain in the lower left side of the abdomen, and constipation and mild fever may occur. In a more severe attack, the pain is steady, may be associated with soreness to the touch, and tends to worsen during walking or any other movement.

What is the treatment for diverticulitis?　Antibiotics, such as ampicillin, may relieve the attack. Enemas should be avoided. Some persons get symptomatic relief by placing a hot water bottle over the lower abdomen. In a severe attack, surgical removal of the inflamed diverticulum may be necessary.

Do other symptoms ever develop from a diverticulum?　Yes, severe hemorrhage may occur from a diverticulum, causing wine-colored stools or bright red bleeding from the bowels. Surgery is often necessary to stop the hemorrhage.

What is porphyria?　It's a rare, inherited defect in the synthesis of materials that make up red blood cells. Acute intermittent porphyria begins in the teenage years or twenties and causes attacks of severe abdominal pain, sometimes following the ingestion of a barbiturate. The person with porphyria should wear a Medic-Alert bracelet (see p. 343) and avoid barbiturate-containing drugs, such as Donnatal and sleeping pills.

What may cause vomiting?　Dietary indiscretion and drinking too much may cause this problem, but a more common cause is intestinal flu (see p. 175). Vomiting may accompany pneumonia, appendicitis (see p. 158), hepatitis, peptic ulcer, pancreatitis, uncontrolled diabetes, kidney disease, food poisoning and intolerance to certain pain-relieving drugs. Bleeding into the stomach or upper intestine may cause vomiting from the irritative effects of the blood. Persistent vomiting suggests an intestinal obstruction.

What is intestinal obstruction?   The condition occurring when the passageway through the bowels is blocked. Among the causes are peptic ulcer, inguinal hernia, postoperative adhesions, volvulus (twisting of the bowel), intussusception (telescoping of the bowel) and cancer. Sometimes, in a condition called reflex ileus, the bowel loses its capacity to propel nutrients forward and a similar result occurs. This condition, also known as paralytic ileus, is most apt to accompany peritonitis (see below).

Who is most susceptible to developing this condition?   It is most likely to occur in someone who has had abdominal surgery. Bands of scar tissue known as adhesions may form in response to talc or cornstarch from the surgeon's gloves, cellulose fibers from the surgical drapes or sponges, or the rough surfaces the bowel may be exposed to after the abdominal architecture has been disrupted. After ten or twenty years, an adhesion may form into a tight band that traps and pinches off the passageway through the bowel. Peritonitis may also produce adhesions.

Children are most susceptible to deformities of the bowel, and certain illnesses may cause intestinal obstruction during infancy (see p. 159). In a man, an inguinal hernia (see p. 411) may obstruct the intestine. Benign or malignant tumors may also cause obstruction.

What are the symptoms of intestinal obstruction?   Vomiting, cramping abdominal pain and constipation occur. The abdomen becomes distended. Large quantities of body fluids pour into the dilated loops of bowel, causing dehydration, and fluid loss is accentuated by the persistent vomiting.

How is intestinal obstruction diagnosed?   In some instances the person's bowel sounds are so loud that they may be heard without a stethoscope, or rhythmic squeezing motions may be seen coursing across the abdomen. X-rays will show that the loops of intestine are widely dilated and indicate whether the problem is in the small or the large intestine.

What's the treatment for intestinal obstruction?   Immediate hospitalization under the care of a pediatrician, internist or gastroenterologist is indicated, and a general surgeon should be called in for consultation. Passage of a suction tube into the stomach may lessen the amount of distention, but surgery is usually necessary to relieve the obstruction.

What is peritonitis?   An infection of the peritoneum, the clear, glistening lining of the bowel, liver, pancreas and inner surface of the abdomen.

What may cause peritonitis?   Wounds due to a gunshot or stabbing are the most common cause: the missile or knife blade punctures the bowel or another organ, spilling its contents into the abdominal cavity. Natural causes of peritonitis include ruptured appendix (see p. 158), ruptured gall bladder, intestinal perforation from unrelieved obstruction, ruptured diverticulum and pelvic inflammatory disease.

What are the symptoms of peritonitis?   The abdomen is painful and tender to the touch. Movement increases the pain. The person has no appetite and may vomit even in the absence of eating. Swelling of the abdomen reflects the generalized distention of the intestine which accompanies peritonitis and which is caused by the infection.

What's the treatment for peritonitis?   The treatment consists of diagnosing the cause of the condition and, if possible, correcting it. Surgery may be necessary to seal off a perforated ulcer or appendix or to close off a hole in the intestine resulting from a wound. The general measures include antibiotics, fluid therapy and the avoidance of food or liquid by mouth until the peritoneal inflammation has subsided.

What is an inguinal hernia?   It is a muscular defect in the abdominal wall just above the groin, and its incidence is ten times as frequent in men as in women. The site for the hernia in a man is where the testicles were drawn into the scrotum during fetal life; the opening may gradually enlarge enough for a loop of small bowel to slip into the scrotum.

How is the hernia diagnosed?   Often it is apparent by the appearance of a bulge in the groin or scrotum. Smaller hernias can be felt by a physician during physical examination. Pain may be experienced in the area. Slippage of intestine through the inguinal opening may cause the scrotum to enlarge to the size of a softball. In most instances the hernia can be reduced by having the person lie down and then pushing the intestine back into the abdomen.

What is the treatment for hernia?   Surgery is indicated to correct the muscular defect if the hernia is causing pain. Wearing a truss to seal off the opening and prevent the intestine from passing into the scrotum is sometimes advised, but the truss has a tendency to slip and may pinch off a loop of bowel, causing a potentially dangerous situation.

Can hernia occur in women?   Yes, but the cause and location are usually different from those in men. The hernia is most likely to occur in the mid-groin through the opening where the main artery (femoral artery) passes from the abdomen to the thigh. Obesity and multiple pregnancies predispose to femoral hernia in a woman, and surgery is curative.

411

What's the main complication of a hernia?   The person whose hernia contains a loop of intestine is subject to intestinal obstruction if the loop becomes pinched off ("strangulated") and trapped inside the hernia. The problem is heralded by the sudden onset of pain and swelling in the hernia followed by the symptoms of bowel obstruction.

What is the treatment for strangulated hernia?   Surgery must be done to relieve the obstruction and repair the hernial defect.

What is constipation?   The term is used to describe the discomfort from fewer than normal bowel movements and/or feces of a hard consistency. However, it may be perfectly healthy to skip a day without a bowel movement, and there are no rigid rules about frequency or "regularity."

What causes constipation?   The causes are thought to be lack of exercise, lack of enough fluid and lack of adequate roughage in the diet. There seem to be people who are "normally constipated," and the condition, whether for psychological or dietary reasons, may sometimes run in families.

What is the treatment for constipation?   The importance of exercise can be shown by the fact that children, constantly in motion, are rarely constipated. Adults who jog, play tennis or walk regularly are unlikely to be constipated. But exercise alone is not enough, because sufficient fluid has to be taken in to keep the feces moist and to lubricate its passage. This may require two quarts of fluid a day. By holding moisture in the colon and increasing the intestinal bulk, roughage, such as fruits and vegetables or unprocessed bran, will promote normal bowel action.

Is fiber important?   Yes, a high intake of roughage or fiber may prevent constipation, hemorrhoids, diverticulosis and appendicitis, ameliorate the symptoms of irritable colon and reduce the incidence of cancer of the colon. One can eat bran cereal as is or added to other foods or enough fruits and vegetables to get a high fiber intake. The quantity of roughage one needs must be determined individually. Too much fiber in the diet could cause diarrhea.

Should laxatives be taken regularly?   Many over-the-counter products contain intestinal irritants. Because these interrupt the body's normal reflexes for bowel emptying, they tend to be habit-forming. Laxatives may also interfere with intestinal absorption.

How do you quit laxatives?   Decrease the dose gradually over two or three weeks while adding roughage to the diet, drinking more fluids and exercising. If constipation occurs, take an enema for relief.

412

Should enemas be used to relieve constipation?   The use of an enema is preferable to the use of laxatives, but as mentioned before, adequate amounts of exercise, fluid and high-fiber foods are the preferred way to manage this problem.

What if exercise isn't possible because of physical disability?   The person who requires a purgative should use milk of magnesia. Prescription stool softeners may prove adequate. Or a powdery preparation known as Metamucil can be mixed with liquid and taken two or three times a day to give bulk to the stool and allow normal bowel action. An enema or a suppository is preferable to using an irritative laxative.

What are hemorrhoids?   They are enlarged veins surrounding or just inside the anus. They may occur during pregnancy or with liver disease, but the usual cause is straining at stool.

What are the symptoms of hemorrhoids?   They may bleed or be painful after heavy straining at stool, which causes them to protrude. They may itch, and their presence may make it difficult to clean properly after a bowel movement. Pain is especially severe if a clot forms in one of them. Bleeding is the most serious effect of hemorrhoids, and bright red blood is noted on the toilet tissue or the surface of the feces.

What's the treatment for hemorrhoids?   Relief of constipation will prevent hemorrhoids from forming or cause them to shrink in size. A hemorrhoid that protrudes painfully should be pushed back in. Warm baths twice a day will give relief if a clot forms in a hemorrhoid; usually the clot will dissolve on its own in several days, or a physician can remove it through a small cut. When rawness or pain is present, certain over-the-counter creams and ointments, as well as a prescription suppository preparation, may provide relief. Some forms of this preparation come with an anti-inflammatory steroid added. Surgery may become necessary when bleeding persists or when hemorrhoids continue to cause discomfort despite relief of constipation. Hemorrhoids occurring during pregnancy usually leave after the baby is born.

What's the treatment for itching of the anus?   Among the reasons for itching in this region are untidy wiping habits, allergy to toilet tissue, soap or a garment, the wearing of tight pantyhose or undergarments that trap moisture in the area, and "nervous itching" (neurodermatitis). The treatment of the first cause is better cleanliness. Plain white soap is less likely to cause an allergy than colored or perfumed bars. One is also less likely to be allergic to plain white toilet tissue than to colored, perfumed or specially treated paper. The woman troubled with itch should choose cotton undergarments and avoid girdles, especially in the premenstrual days when itching is very common. Jeans or similar pants that hold the buttocks tightly together may have to be discarded in favor of looser-fitting clothing. Cotton pads coated with glycerin and a 50 percent solution of witch hazel are available without a prescription. They can be used after wiping and two or three other times during the day to provide symptomatic relief from itching and to keep the anus dry. The use of baby powder between the buttocks after a bath will also promote dryness. In the case of neurodermatitis, an anti-inflammatory cream may be prescribed to interrupt the itch-scratch cycle.

What is an anal fissure?   A small tear or slit in the anus caused, usually, by passage of a very firm stool. The fissure is painful and may bleed. Spontaneous healing is the rule, but a neglected fissure could develop into a deep ulcer requiring surgery. The treatment is to keep the area clean, take hot tub soaks for relief of pain, and to use the measures mentioned above to avoid constipation.

What causes pain in the anal region?   An injury to the tailbone may cause dull pain in the anal area, especially after long periods of sitting. The pain worsens during a bowel movement. Treatment consists of avoiding consti-pation, sitting on a firm surface while driving, and massage and stretching of the anal muscles by a physician. Surgical removal of the coccyx (tailbone) may be necessary when all other forms of treatment fail.

Proctalgia fugax is a distressing pain in the lower rectum and anus occurring usually in men in their twenties or thirties. The cause is unknown. Typically, the man is awakened by the pain in the middle of the night. He feels the urge to pass gas or have a bowel movement, neither or which may be possible. The pain tends to subside in thirty minutes or an hour. A hot bath or upward pressure on the anus may give relief. Though the attacks of fleeting rectal pain may recur for months or years, the condition eventu-ally leaves as mysteriously as it appeared.

What causes diarrhea?   Most often it's due to intestinal flu or to an irritable colon. A bacterial infection of the intestine such as shigellosis causes diarrhea (see p. 178), and so may malabsorption, food allergy, disease of the pancreas or immune deficiency disease. The person with severe diabetes may experience attacks of diarrhea due to nerve damage caused by the diabetes.

What's the treatment for diarrhea?   The treatment is to correct the cause, but symptomatic relief can be obtained by using anti-diarrheal preparations, commonly available or prescribed by a physician, which increase the bulk in the intestine and absorb the water. Anti-spasmodics are also used. Spicy foods should be avoided, and the emphasis placed on getting enough liquids and, as tolerated, eating bland foods, such as mashed potatoes, rice, and bread. Persistent diarrhea requires medical attention.

What causes belching?   It may result from overeating, swallowing air or indigestion, as from gall bladder disease, a rich diet, carbonated beverages or beer. Esophagitis is a cause of belching (see p. 401).

What's the treatment for belching?   Eating slowly and avoiding tension at mealtime may reduce air swallowing. Smaller meals consisting of bland foods may help. Medical evaluation is indicated for persistent belching, and antacids may provide relief.

What causes gassiness?   The most frequent causes are constipation, eating very fast, stress, gall bladder disease, intolerance of foods such as milk and milk products, and the ingestion of gas-producing foods. Among the foods that cause gassiness are milk, beans, apples, peas, broccoli, cauliflower, eggplant, celery, bell peppers, pork and rich or greasy foods. Drugs that promote gassiness are aspirin, calcium, vitamin C and iron tablets.

What's the treatment for gassiness?   Avoiding the cause is usually effective. Some persons get relief from using Gelusil or Mylanta. Medical evaluation is indicated for persistent gassiness to rule out any serious problem, but little is known about treating gassiness itself.

What are the symptoms of cancer of the colon?   Abdominal discomfort, weight loss and a change in bowel habits are the most frequent symptoms. Constipation alternating with diarrhea may occur when the tumor is in the left portion of the colon. Cancer in the right side of the colon is more likely to bleed and produce anemia, so that weakness and fatigue are early symptoms.

How common is cancer of the colon?   It kills 50,000 Americans each year, and is the second leading cause of cancer death in women and men, behind cancers of the breast and lung, respectively.

Who is most susceptible to this cancer?   The incidence is the same in both sexes and the peak age of onset is sixty to seventy. Persons with a family history of colon cancer are twice as susceptible to the disease. An inherited condition causing growth of polyps in the colon also greatly increases the risk. Cancer of the colon is thought to be more common in those with a diet

415

low in fiber content who have been exposed to food additives and other possible carcinogens for many years.

What is the treatment for colon cancer?   The best treatment is surgery to remove the tumor. An operation known as a colostomy can be done when a tumor that cannot be completely removed has caused intestinal obstruction. In this procedure, part of the colon is brought out through an opening in the abdominal wall so that the person's fecal material can be routed around the obstruction and collected in colostomy bags. Sometimes a temporary colostomy is done to allow healing even when the colon cancer has been completely removed.

What is the prognosis of colon cancer?   The five-year survival rate is 50 percent, but the figure goes up to 85 percent if the cancer is caught early. An examination of the stool which detects microscopic traces of blood is an important tool for early detection of colon cancer.

THE PANCREAS

Where is the pancreas located?   This fish-shaped gland lies in a fold between the stomach and the duodenum, the first part of the small intestine. Its tail nearly touches the spleen in the left upper abdomen, while its head fits snugly into a loop of duodenum near the place where bile empties into the intestine.

What does the pancreas do?   It produces insulin as well as enzymes that help in the digestion of carbohydrates, fats and proteins.

What may go wrong with the pancreas?   The gland may become inflamed (pancreatitis), lose its ability to make digestive enzymes (pancreatic insufficiency) or become malignant (pancreatic cancer).

What are the symptoms of pancreatitis?   Following alcohol consumption or a heavy meal, the person develops severe upper abdominal pain. Worse than the distress of an ulcer, the pain occurs two or three inches above the navel and radiates through to the back. Lying down makes the pain worse and sitting up may give some relief. Vomiting and distention of the abdomen occur as the attack progresses.

What causes pancreatitis?   The usual cause is excessive drinking for a period exceeding six years, but gallstones also may be at fault and sometimes the cause remains obscure. The attack itself may follow an alcoholic binge.

What is the treatment for pancreatitis?   Hospitalization is indicated and the person has to be fed intravenously for several days to a week. The management should be by a gastroenterologist. A fluid-filled mass known as a pseudocyst may form in the pancreas and require surgical removal.

What's the outlook after an attack of pancreatitis?   The great majority of persons survive the initial attack, but continued drinking may lead to other attacks. Relapsing pancreatitis rarely occurs except in an alcoholic, and such persons may have abdominal pain every few days. Each attack further insults the pancreas and sets the stage for the development of pancreatic insufficiency.

What are the symptoms of pancreatic insufficiency?   Weight loss and malabsorption of food may result from an inadequate supply of digestive enzymes. Diabetes may also occur.

What is the treatment for pancreatic insufficiency?   Symptomatic relief can usually be obtained by taking the pancreatic enzymes in tablet form several times a day. Insulin therapy may be needed for diabetes.

What are the symptoms of cancer of the pancreas?   The early symptoms are weight loss and vague abdominal pain. Jaundice, a yellowish discoloration of the skin and mucous membranes, may occur when the cancer is in the head of the pancreas obstructing bile flow into the intestine. Back pain is an early symptom in a fourth of persons with pancreatic cancer. Occasionally, malabsorption from pancreatic insufficiency is a symptom of cancer of the pancreas.

How common is cancer of the pancreas?   It is the fourth leading cause of cancer death, and 25,000 new cases are diagnosed each year. The frequency of pancreatic cancer is increasing.

Who is most likely to develop cancer of the pancreas?   It's twice as common in men and is more frequent among heavy drinkers, diabetics and those who smoke. The average age at onset is fifty-five, but the chance of having pancreatic cancer seems to rise with advancing age.

What's the treatment for pancreatic cancer?   Removal of the tumor is the only effective treatment, but by the time the diagnosis is made the cancer has often spread beyond the pancreas.

What's the survival rate for pancreatic cancer?   The five-year survival rate is less than 5 percent.

417

THE LIVER AND GALL BLADDER

Where is the liver located? It is nestled high in the right side of the abdomen, protected by the rib cage, back and chest. In normal persons the tip of the liver may be felt beneath the rib cage during deep inspiration.

How big is the liver? It weighs three or four pounds: the largest organ in the body.

What does it do? It has dozens of functions based on its role as a processing plant for the nutrients that are absorbed from the intestine. It uses these raw materials to make body chemicals, blood-clotting factors and the proteins that circulate in the blood. The liver also breaks down drugs and other chemicals that are ingested.

One of the liver's main functions is to make and excrete bile. This green substance is stored in the gall bladder and released after meals to help in the digestion of fats. Heme pigment that is left over from broken-down red blood cells is excreted into the bile. Liver disease, liver damage or an obstruction of the bile duct causes these pigments to accumulate in the bloodstream and stain the skin and mucous membranes the yellow color of jaundice.

What are the symptoms of jaundice? The whites of the eyes are the first to show the yellowish tint, and the jaundice is more readily visible under natural light. Since bile is responsible for the normal brown color of the stools, its lack may cause the feces to turn a light gray or cream color. Intense itching may accompany severe jaundice, and the urine may turn dark yellow or brown.

What are the causes of jaundice? The most common cause is hepatitis (see p. 178). Cirrhosis of the liver is another cause, and jaundice may accompany an anemia caused by rapid breakdown of red blood cells. Obstruction of the bile ducts may result from gall stones or cancer of the liver or pancreas.

Can drugs cause jaundice? Yes, and two that may damage the liver are isoniazid (INH) and pyrazinamide (PZA), drugs used to treat tuberculosis. The latter is used infrequently, but INH is often given to someone whose TB skin test has become positive. The older the person, the greater the likelihood of liver damage from INH, and liver tests should be done each month while one is taking this drug. Chlorpromazine (Thorazine) is a tranquilizer that may cause jaundice and liver damage. The problem is most apt to arise in one receiving the drug at high doses during institutional care. Ilosone, a form of erythromycin, may cause liver damage and is less safe than other forms of this antibiotic. Male sex hormones (androgens) given by mouth or injection may damage the liver. Birth-control pills may cause jaundice or liver damage, as well as the growth of a benign tumor of the liver (see p. 7). Other drugs that may damage the liver are Indocin, Motrin, Clinoril, Butazolidin, Tandearil and acetaminophen if it is taken in a high dosage.

What is cirrhosis of the liver?   It is a progressive scarring of the liver that disrupts its normal architecture, causes it to shrink and harden, and eventually leads to liver failure.

How common is cirrhosis of the liver?   The seventh leading cause of death in the United States, it accounts for an estimated 30,000 deaths a year. Cirrhosis is twice as common in men as in women.

What causes cirrhosis?   Alcoholism is responsible for three out of four instances of cirrhosis. The other causes are postnecrotic cirrhosis that follows some instances of viral hepatitis, hemochromatosis from excessive iron absorption (see p. 361) and biliary cirrhosis, an uncommon form of the disease occurring mainly in women and not associated with alcohol intake.

How likely is an alcoholic to develop cirrhosis?   Cirrhosis is present in three-fourths of persons who drink a pint of whiskey a day for fifteen years or longer, and the disease may be noted after only five or six years of very heavy drinking.

What are the symptoms of cirrhosis?   Jaundice may appear after a bout of heavy drinking, and other symptoms include weakness, abdominal discomfort, nausea and loss of appetite. Vomiting of blood may reflect esophageal varices (enlarged veins in the lower esophagus due to the cirrhosis). Distention of the abdomen reflects an outpouring of water into the abdominal cavity; it is caused by an elevated pressure in the portal vein, the main vessel between the intestines and the liver. Fluid may also accumulate in the legs and feet to cause swelling.

What is the treatment for cirrhosis?   A nutritious diet and the avoidance of alcohol are the only successful measures for alcoholic cirrhosis. Steroid hormone therapy, surgery to widen the bile ducts and measures to remove iron from the body may prove helpful for cirrhosis due to viral hepatitis, biliary cirrhosis or hemochromatosis, respectively. Various medical and surgical procedures are used to control severe hemorrhage from esophageal varices.

What is liver failure?   This condition occurs when the organ has lost over 90 percent of its functioning capacity. Confusion, disorientation and coma

419

are the symptoms. Because nitrogen-containing foods add to the problem, a person with incipient liver failure may note confusion or grogginess for several hours after eating a piece of meat. Cases are on record of a severe cirrhotic losing consciousness after eating a hamburger. The treatment is to reduce the intake of protein, correct the associated medical problems and provide vitamins, fluids and other nutrients as tolerated.

What is the long-term outlook for the person with cirrhosis?   Two-thirds of cirrhotics are dead within five years of the onset of symptoms such as jaundice, but the prognosis is better when symptoms are mild and complications haven't yet occurred. Those who stop drinking show a much better survival rate.

How common is cancer of the liver?   It causes 8,000 deaths a year in the United States.

What causes the cancer to develop?   It seldom occurs except in someone with cirrhosis of the liver, and one in five cirrhotics will eventually develop liver cancer.

A type of liver cancer known as angiosarcoma has developed in persons exposed to the chemical vinyl chloride. The role of aflatoxin in causing liver cancer also is under study. A by-product of a mold, aflatoxin is found in many grains and in peanut meal. Tumor of the liver has resulted from the use of birth-control pills (see p. 7), but the great majority of such tumors are not cancerous.

What is the treatment for cancer of the liver?   To date, no effective treatment has been found. Survival for more than a few years is unusual.

What is the gall bladder?   It is the storage sac for bile that is found just below the liver and attached to the main bile duct.

What causes gallstones?   The cause is not known, but the stones show a tendency to develop in those with a family history for them and may result from an excessive content of cholesterol in the bile. Pregnancy, obesity and a diet rich in fat predispose to gallstones.

How common are gallstones?   Fifteen million Americans have them, and 300,000 gall bladder removals are done each year for gallstones. Women have three or four times the risk of men, and American Indians are especially susceptible. Gallstones seldom develop under the age of thirty-five, but may occur in American Indian women in their teens or twenties.

How many gallstones may occur in one gall bladder? Anywhere from one to a hundred, and the severity of symptoms is not usually related to the number of stones that are present.

What are the symptoms of gallstones? Indigestion characterized by abdominal discomfort, gassiness and belching occurs an hour or two after eating, especially after a large meal of rich foods. In a severe attack, the person has distressing abdominal pain and may vomit several times. Chills and fever may occur. Jaundice appears in several days if a gallstone passes into and obstructs the bile duct.

What is the treatment for gallstones? Anyone with a gallstone attack should be hospitalized. When the diagnosis is obvious and general health is good, early surgery is indicated. When the diagnosis is uncertain or the patient's health won't permit surgery, medical treatment consists of antibiotics, fluid therapy and medicine for the relief of pain. Elective removal of the gall bladder can be done several months later, and the bile duct must be explored to make sure that all the stones have been removed from it.

What happens after the gall bladder is removed? In most instances the body adjusts quite well to the absence of the gall bladder. The upper part of the bile duct enlarges and acts as a storage area for bile. Some persons do have difficulty following gall bladder surgery, but usually the problem is a gallstone that is still in the bile duct. Occasionally, repeat surgery is necessary.

What if the person with gallstones has only mild symptoms and has never had an attack? Though gall bladder removal in this instance is an elective procedure, some physicians believe the operation is indicated to prevent more severe attacks and to protect the person from developing gall bladder cancer. Other physicians favor cautious observation of the patient. It is best to get a second opinion before having surgery for asymptomatic gallstones.

Under what circumstances does gall bladder cancer develop? It rarely develops except in someone with a long-standing history of gallstones, and is a relatively uncommon cancer.

What's the treatment for gall bladder cancer? The gall bladder and any part of the liver that is cancerous must be removed.

What's the prognosis for gall bladder cancer? Only 5 percent of the victims of this malignancy are alive five years later. In those in whom a cure is achieved, the cancer is usually found incidentally during routine surgery for gallstones.

THE SPLEEN

What is the spleen?   It is a filter for the blood that removes old or damaged red blood cells, bacteria or foreign particles that get into the blood. It also makes antibodies and releases lymphocytes that aid in body defenses.

Where is the spleen located?   High in the left side of the abdomen, protected by the ribs, chest and back.

How big is the spleen?   This disc-shaped purple organ weighs only a fourth of a pound and is not normally large enough to be felt during an examination. A spleen that can be felt by the examiner is considered enlarged and abnormal.

What may cause the spleen to enlarge?   Some causes are:
· Infections, such as infectious mononucleosis, malaria and infected heart valve.
· Malignancy of the blood or lymph nodes, such as leukemia, lymphoma, Hodgkin's disease or primary polycythemia.
· Anemia due to rapid breakdown of red blood cells.
· Juvenile rheumatoid arthritis or lupus erythematosus.
· Cirrhosis of the liver with elevated pressure in the portal vein.
· Hereditary diseases of metabolism, such as Tay-Sachs disease or Gaucher's disease.

What's the main risk from an enlarged spleen?   It is more susceptible to injury or rupture. Splenic rupture has occurred in persons with infectious mononucleosis just from overzealous palpation of the organ by a physician. The person with an enlarged spleen who plays a contact sport is at greater risk of splenic rupture, which is heralded by collapse due to shock from hemorrhaging into the abdomen. Surgical removal of the spleen is the only way to stop the bleeding and save the person's life.

What's the treatment for splenic enlargement?   The treatment is aimed at the underlying disease, and regression in the size of the spleen is a sign of improvement. Splenic removal may be indicated to treat certain kinds of anemia, lymphoma or bleeding complications from cirrhosis of the liver or a deficiency of blood platelets (see p. 370).

Can one do without the spleen?   Yes, but because the spleen is an important source of antibodies, a child under five whose spleen is removed is more likely to have a severe or fatal infection of the bloodstream. Adults tolerate splenic removal better than children do, but even so, problems may occur. People who have had a splenectomy are particularly susceptible to pneumococcal infections, and fatalities have resulted from an overwhelming infection. This underscores the need for such individuals to be immunized by the vaccine that has been developed against most strains of pneumococcal bacteria (see p. 170). Persons who've previously lost their spleen should contact their doctor and ask about receiving this important vaccine.

THE KIDNEYS

What are the kidneys?   These two organs, weighing a third of a pound each, are situated high in the back of the abdomen where they're protected by the lower ribs and a thick mound of fat. They filter chemical wastes out of the blood and at the same time control the body's fluid content. They do this by forming urine.

How is urine made?   The kidneys are richly supplied with blood, and as it passes through the kidneys its liquid part is removed and squeezed through a million small tubules in each kidney. Only the water and minerals needed by the body are resorbed from the tubules; the rest, unwanted material, is allowed to continue through the tubules and be excreted as urine.

How much urine is formed each day?   Of the 180 quarts of fluid that filter through the kidneys each day, a quart or a quart and a half is converted to urine. The volume of urine depends on the amount of perspiration as well as that of fluid intake. It's because of the kidneys that you can drink as much water as you want without having to worry about whether the body needs the extra fluid, and the reason that you can tolerate periods of low fluid intake is that the kidneys have the ability to conserve water by reducing urine output.

What causes kidney disease?   Conditions that may harm the kidneys are infections (p. 180), blockage of the urinary tract as the result of an enlarged prostate (p. 80), high blood pressure (p. 392), and diseases such as diabetes and Bright's disease, which affect the substance of the kidneys.

How common is kidney disease?   About 13 million Americans suffer from it, and kidney failure is a major source of disablement among adults. Three million Americans are bothered by kidney stones.

What are the symptoms of kidney disease?   The person with kidney infection may have back pain or abdominal pain, nausea, vomiting, chills and fever. A burning sensation when urinating is a sign of bladder or kidney infection, as is urine with a cloudy color or a strong odor. Blood in the urine also signals a bladder or kidney problem.

What may cause bloody urine?　The most frequent causes are a bladder infection, a kidney stone or bleeding from the prostate. Conditions that are sometimes responsible include Bright's disease, a tumor of the bladder or kidney, or trauma to the back. The urine may be bright red, dark red or tinged with pink, though microscopic amounts of blood may not change the color of the urine.

Does red or pink urine always indicate the presence of blood?　No. A woman may lose some menstrual blood at the time of urination, and if this is an unusual occurrence, mistakenly suspect that her urine is bloody. Foods that can impart a red or pinkish tinge to the urine include beets, rhubarb and candy or jellies containing aniline dyes. Danthron, an ingredient in certain laxatives, can turn the urine pink, and pyridium, a bladder sedative that may be prescribed for an infection, will turn the urine a psychedelic brown or orange color. A slight amount of pink staining of the urine is normal during the first few days of a baby's life.

What causes kidney stones?　The recognized causes include gout, hyperparathyroidism, kidney infection and excessive intake of milk, antacids or vitamin D. Kidney stones are more common in those who work outdoors. This has led to speculation that work requiring strenuous exertion and accompanied by marked sweating favors stone formation during the temporary periods of reduced urine output.

What are the symptoms of a kidney stone?　Agonizing pain begins in one side of the back and radiates to the abdomen and groin. The pain comes in spells that makes the person double over. Nausea and vomiting occur, and the urine contains blood, though not always a grossly visible amount.

What's the treatment for a kidney stone?　The person should be hospitalized under the care of a urologist. Most stones will pass spontaneously within one to three days. Medicine is given to relieve pain, control infection and promote a high urine output. Surgical removal of the stone becomes necessary when it doesn't pass on its own. Measures to prevent stone formation include a high fluid intake and eradication of kidney infection. Continuous therapy with orthophosphates or thiazide diuretics has been effective in preventing a recurrence of kidney stones. In people with uric-acid stones, medication is given to lower the body's uric-acid content. Alkalinization of the urine may cause such stones to dissolve.

What is Bright's disease?   Also known as glomerulonephritis, it is an inflammation of the kidneys resulting from the body's overreaction to a strep throat or a streptococcal infection of the skin. The immune reaction isn't primarily directed against the kidneys, but these organs suffer the most damage.

What are the symptoms of Bright's disease?   Bloody urine and swelling of the feet and face occur, and the person may complain of headache, loss of appetite and weakness. The illness may run a short course and disappear in a few weeks, or hang on for years to eventually cause kidney failure.

Who is most susceptible to Bright's disease?   Children are more susceptible than adults, and persons with allergic problems such as asthma show an increased susceptibility. Frequent bouts of strep throat also increase the risk. Certain forms of the illness run in families.

What's the treatment for Bright's disease?   Treatment should be given by a nephrologist, and consists of steroid hormones and immunosuppressive drugs. The patient should be checked by a physician once or twice a year so that recurrence can be detected and treated.

What's the long-term outlook for someone with Bright's disease?   The outlook for most persons with this disease is good. Perhaps one in ten such individuals develops a chronic form of the illness which may cause kidney failure ten to twenty years later.

What is dropsy?   In medical parlance, dropsy refers to a condition of generalized edema or swelling of the body. It may be caused by heart failure (see p. 384) or kidney disease, and in the latter instance doctors speak of it as nephrosis. Kidney conditions that may produce swelling in the hands, feet, legs and face include Bright's disease, diabetes, lupus erythematosus (see p. 239), lead poisoning or a reaction to the anticonvulsant drug Tridione.

What is the treatment for dropsy?   Treatment is directed at the underlying cause. When a kidney condition is responsible, steroid hormones and diuretics may be chosen in the treatment.

What other conditions may harm the kidneys?   Diabetes may cause kidney failure after fifteen or twenty years of the disease, and kidney cysts and chronic kidney infection are other causes of kidney damage.

What causes chronic kidney infection?   Due to the proximity of the urethra to the other pelvic openings, women show an increased susceptibility to bladder and kidney infections. Infrequent urination may promote the susceptibility to infection. For poorly understood reasons, the kidney infection may not respond completely to antibiotics and may persist as a low-grade inflammation that flares up from time to time and eventually causes kidney failure. An obstruction to the flow of urine at any point between the kidneys and the outside favors an infection, as in a man with an enlarged prostate.

How common are kidney cysts?　　Cystic disease of the kidneys is an inherited disease affecting one in every 500 persons. The extent and distribution of the cysts, fluid pockets that replace part of the kidney, vary greatly. Death from kidney failure may occur during childhood, or the cysts may be found incidentally during autopsy of an elderly individual.

What's the best way to avoid drug or chemical damage to the kidneys?
　　Don't use the drug phenacetin, which is in headache remedies containing the traditional APC ingredients: aspirin, phenacetin and caffeine. Overuse of aspirin may also damage the kidneys. The best way to avoid taking a harmful prescription antibiotic is to choose a physician who understands the toxicities as well as the benefits of drugs. Even then, check into the drug's side effects before you take it. Many of the injectable antibiotics that might be used in a hospital setting are potentially harmful to the kidneys. Among these are streptomycin, kanamycin, polymyxin-B and amphotericin-B. Sometimes it is necessary to accept a trade-off between a drug's benefits and toxicity, but never when a safer drug would work as well. The key is, of course, to choose a physician whose judgment you trust.

　　People whose work brings them into contact with mercury, carbon tetrachloride, ethylene glycol or any potentially harmful chemical should ask for reassignment, find other work or take great precautions to avoid exposure on the job. The danger of these agents is twofold: they're capable of being absorbed through the skin to damage the kidneys, and the damage gets worse the longer the exposure continues.

What is kidney failure?　　It is a condition resulting from a loss of the functioning capacity of the kidneys. An acute form may occur in shock. Other causes of acute failure are exposure to kidney-damaging drugs or chemicals, or a severe bout of Bright's disease or lupus erythematosus. Chronic kidney failure is a condition that begins slowly and may show gradual progression to complete loss of kidney function.

What are the symptoms of kidney failure?　　Loss of appetite, nausea and vomiting may occur, as may weakness and fatigue from anemia. Headache and visual problems may reflect the high blood pressure which accompanies

426

kidney failure. The volume of urine slowly diminishes, and the person may note swelling of the legs, wrists and feet.

What is the treatment for chronic kidney failure?   A diet low in meat may help, and salt and fluid intake have to be balanced against the person's needs and ability to process them. Associated hypertension must be controlled. Blood transfusions may be necessary from time to time. The person whose kidney failure continues to progress may eventually need therapy with dialysis or a kidney transplant.

What is dialysis?   This is a process for the removal of waste products from the blood. Through a special connection the arterial blood is shunted into a kidney machine. Inside the machine the blood flows through many coils lined with cellophane and surrounded by a solution of sugar, water and certain minerals. Waste products from the blood pass through the cellophane and into the fluid by the process of diffusion. Purified blood is continually returned to the veins just as unpurified blood continues to flow into the machine. Several hours are needed for one treatment, and most persons require three treatments a week.

How many people are currently on dialysis?   About 45,000 Americans are being treated by dialysis at an annual cost of over $1 billion. The federal government, through Medicare, provides funds for dialysis for anyone who needs it.

How long is survival possible on dialysis?   One can survive indefinitely on dialysis, and many persons in this country are alive after fifteen or sixteen years of maintenance dialysis.

Are there any alternatives to dialysis?   Two: kidney transplantation and a new form of dialysis known as continuous ambulatory peritoneal dialysis (CAPD). In the latter procedure the person's abdominal cavity becomes the site of dialysis. Several times a day the person lets dialysis fluid run into the abdomen through an indwelling tubing put in for this purpose. Waste products diffuse out of the small blood vessels lining the peritoneum and pass into the fluid, which is drained out of the abdomen by gravity after five hours. The main benefit is that the person isn't tied down to a kidney machine and can go about his or her ordinary activities while the dialysis is taking place. Still another benefit is the cost: about a third of that for dialysis with a kidney machine.

What is the main risk from CAPD?   There is a greater risk of developing peritonitis if germs accidentally get into the abdomen along with the fluid, but most instances of infection can be quickly controlled with antibiotics.

Since this type of dialysis is a relatively new procedure, its long-term safety and usefulness remain to be assessed.

How many people are using the new form of dialysis?   Hundreds of persons with kidney failure have switched to CAPD, and many more are expected to take up this form of dialysis in the next few years. Information about it can be obtained by writing the National Kidney Foundation, 116 East 27th Street, New York, N.Y. 10016.

How common is a kidney transplant?   Kidney transplantation is now a recognized form of therapy, and more than 7,000 transplants have been done in this country. But for lack of enough donors, more would have been done.

Where are donor kidneys obtained?   From a living relative if the person has one who is a good tissue match and is willing to donate a kidney. (The donor can live normally with only one kidney.) An identical twin serves as the best possible match, and a brother or sister usually as the next best. Most transplanted kidneys are obtained from persons who die accidentally or from a disease not involving the kidneys.

What are the chances for a successful transplant?   Half of transplanted kidneys remain viable after two years, and the success rate is greater when the donor is a living relative. More than a third of transplanted kidneys are still functioning five years after the transplant, and continued function for more than ten years after the transplant is not unusual.

When rejection occurs it usually does so within the first three months, and the person can always return to dialysis therapy.

How common is cancer of the kidney?   It is one of the leading causes of cancer, and 15,000 Americans develop it each year.

What are the symptoms of cancer of the kidney?   Fever and blood in the urine are the main symptoms, and some persons develop back and abdominal pain similar to that of a kidney infection. Weight loss and awareness of an enlargement in the abdomen are other symptoms.

Who is most susceptible to this cancer?   Kidney cancer occurring in children, known as Wilm's tumor, almost always strikes a child under five. In an adult, cancer of the kidney tends to occur between the ages of twenty and fifty. Persons with a family history of kidney cancer are more susceptible to this malignancy.

What's the treatment for cancer of the kidney?   The kidney containing the tumor is removed, and the person is treated with X-irradiation before or after surgery to kill tumor cells that can't be removed. Drugs such as actinomycin-D and vincristine are given to treat Wilm's tumor.

What's the prognosis for cancer of the kidney?   A third of adults are alive five years after treatment, but the prognosis for children with Wilm's tumor is much better. The two-year survival rate is 80 to 90 percent, and many of these children remain free of disease long enough so that they are considered cured.

Bibliography

Alk, Madelin (ed.). *The Expectant Mother.* New York: Trident Press, 1967.

American Cancer Society. *1979 Cancer Facts & Figures.* New York: American Cancer Society, 1978.

American National Red Cross. *Advanced First Aid & Emergency Care.* New York: Doubleday, 1973.

American National Red Cross. *Standard First Aid & Personal Safety.* New York: Doubleday, 1973.

Annon, Jack S. *Behavioral Treatment of Sexual Problems: Brief Therapy.* New York: Harper & Row, 1976.

Arnett, Frank C., Jr. "The Implications of HL-A W27," *Annals of Internal Medicine,* 84: 94, 1976.

Austen, W. Gerald. "Heart Transplantation after Ten Years," *New England Journal of Medicine,* 298: 682, 1978.

Bailar, John C. III. "Mammography: A Contrary View," *Annals of Internal Medicine,* 84: 77, 1976.

Barnes, Barbara E. "Dermatomyositis and Malignancy. A Review of the Literature," *Annals of Internal Medicine,* 84: 68, 1976.

Barnes, Robert W. "Diagnosing Vascular Disease with Noninvasive Tests," *Consultant* (December 1978), p. 56.

Baxter, C.R. "Present Concepts in the Management of Major Electrical Injury," *Surgical Clinics of North America,* 50: 1401, 1970.

Beeson, Paul B., and Walsh McDermott. *Textbook of Medicine.* 14th ed. Philadelphia: W.B. Saunders, 1975.

Berard, Costan W., et al. "Current Concepts of Leukemia and Lymphoma: Etiology, Pathogenesis, and Therapy," *Annals of Internal Medicine,* 85: 351, 1976.

Biermann, June, and Barbara Toohey. *The Diabetic's Sports and Exercise Book: How to Play Your Way to Better Health.* Philadelphia: Lippincott, 1977.

Billups, Norman F. *American Drug Index.* Philadelphia: Lippincott, 1977.

Bing, Elisabeth. *Six Practical Lessons for an Easier Childbirth.* New York: Bantam, 1969.

Bonner, James R. "Stinging Insect Allergy—What to Do for the Patient," *Consultant* (September 1978), p. 49.

Boston Women's Health Book Collective. *Our Bodies, Ourselves.* New York, Simon and Schuster, 1971.

Braney, Marie Louise. "The Child with Hydrocephalus," *American Journal of Nursing,* (May 1973), p. 828.

Brewer, Gail Sforza, with Tom Brewer. *What Every Pregnant Woman Should Know: The Truth about Diets and Drugs in Pregnancy.* New York: Random House, 1977.

Brody, Jane E. "Personal Health," *The New York Times,* December 15, 1976, C10.

———. "Personal Health (Epilepsy)," *The New York Times,* April 19, 1978, C13.

———. "Personal Health: There Are Improved Techniques for Breast Reconstruction," *The New York Times,* June 14, 1978, C17.

Burkitt, Denis P. "If your diet lacks fiber . . ." *Life and Health* (July 1977), p. 21.

Cates, Willard Jr., et al. "The Intrauterine Device and Deaths from Spontaneous Abortion," *New England Journal of Medicine,* 295: 1155, 1976.

Charney, Evan, et al. "Childhood Antecedents of Adult Obesity: Do Chubby Infants Become Obese Adults?" *New England Journal of Medicine,* 295: 6, 1976.

Cline, Martin J., et al. "Bone Marrow Transplantation in Man," *Annals of Internal Medicine,* 83: 691, 1975.

Cohen, Ruth. "A new look at breast feeding," *Consultant* (September 1978), p. 173.

Cole, Warren H., et al. "Cardiopulmonary Resuscitation," *Journal of the American Medical Association,* 198: October 24, 1966.

Committee on Cutaneous Health and Cosmetics. *The Hair You Can Do Without.* Chicago: American Medical Association, 1972.

Conn, Howard F. *Current Therapy, 1978.* Philadelphia: W. B. Saunders, 1978.

Consumer's Union. "Estrogen: Doctors' Complete Update on Dangers, Needs," *Vogue* (April 1977), p. 86.

Coronary Risk Handbook, American Heart Association, Dallas, Tex.

Crile, George Jr. *What Women Should Know about the Breast Cancer Controversy.* New York: Macmillan, 1973.

Dalessio, Donald J. "Medical Maxims on Headache," *Consultant* (February 1976), p. 52.

Davis, Adelle. *Let's Eat Right to Keep Fit.* New York: Harcourt Brace Jovanovich, 1970.

Deaton, John. "Just What the Doctor Ordered," *Texas Monthly* (February 1977), p. 120.

———. *Below the Belt: A Book About the Pelvic Organs.* Palisade, N. J.: Franklin Publishing Co., 1978.

———. *Love and Sex in Marriage: A Medical Doctor's Guide to the Sensual Union.* Englewood Cliffs, N. J.: Parker Publishing Co., 1978.

Dee, Ronald. "New interest in sclerotherapy for varicose veins," *Consultant* (June 1977), p. 123.

Diamond, Seymour, and William Barry Furlong. *More than Two Aspirin; Hope for Your Headache Problem.* Chicago: Follett, 1976.

Dick-Read, Grantly. *Childbirth Without Fear: The Original Approach to Natural Childbirth.* New York: Harper & Row, 1972.

Dolger, Henry, and Bernard Seeman. *How to Live with Diabetes.* 4th ed. New York: Norton, 1977.

Donaldson, James A. "How to Recognize and Manage Middle Ear Fluid." *Consultant* (August 1976), p. 99.

Douglas, R. Gordon, Jr. "Flu Shots: Are They Indicated This Year?" *Consultant* (October 1978), p. 23.

Eden, John. *The Eye Book.* New York: Viking, 1978.

Engleman, E.G., et al. "Letter to the Editor," *New England Journal of Medicine,* 285: 1489, 1971.

Fink, Max. "Electroshock Therapy: Myths and Realities." *Hospital Practice* (November 1978), p. 77.

Finnerty, Frank A., Jr. "Hypertension: Current Management," *Consultant* (February 1978), p. 127.

Fisch, Irwin R., and Jess Frank. "Oral Contraceptives and Blood Pressure," *Journal of the American Medical Association,* 237: 2501, 1977.

Fixx, James F. *The Complete Book of Running.* New York: Random House, 1977.

Flood, Thomas M. "Diet and Diabetes Mellitus," *Hospital Practice,* 14: 61, February 1979.

Fraser, David W., et al., "Legionnaires' Disease: Description of an Epidemic," *New England Journal of Medicine,* 297: 1189, 1977.

Friedman, H. Harold, and Solomon Papper. *Problem-Oriented Medical Diagnosis.* Boston: Little, Brown, 1975.

Friedman, Meyer, and Ray H. Rosenman. *Type A Behavior and Your Heart.* New York: Knopf, 1974.

Glass, Thomas G., Jr. *Management of Poisonous Snakebite.* San Antonio, Tex.: Thomas G. Glass, 1976.

Goldschlager, Nora, et al. "Treadmill Stress Tests as Indicators of Presence and Severity of Coronary Artery Disease," *Annals of Internal Medicine,* 85: 277, 1976.

Gregory, Ian, and Donald J. Smeltzer. *Psychiatry, Essentials of Clinical Practice.* Boston: Little, Brown, 1977.

Gucker, Thomas. "The Child with a Limp," *Consultant* (May 1976), p. 91.

Guyton, Arthur C. *Textbook of Medical Physiology.* 4th ed. Philadelphia: W.B. Saunders, 1971.

Haberman, Helen, and Allene Talmey. "New Cures for Headaches," *Woman's Day* (May 1977), p. 40.

Haggerty, Robert J. "Sore Throats and Tonsillectomy," *New England Journal of Medicine,* 298: 453, 1978.

Harrison, Len C. "Current Concepts: Insulin Resistance in Obese Diabetic Patients," *Consultant* (February 1979), p. 64.

Hatcher, Robert A., Gary K. Stewart, et al. 8th ed. *Contraceptive Technology, 1976–1977.* New York: John Wiley, 1976.

———. 1978–1979. 9th ed. New York: John Wiley, 1978.

Hellman, Louis M., and Jack A. Pritchard. *Williams Obstetrics. 14th ed.* New York: Appleton-Century-Crofts, 1971.

Hemenway, William G., and Marion P. Downs. "Deafness in Children: Early Detection is the Key to Therapy," *Consultant* (July 1974), p. 105.

Henderson, John. *Emergency Medical Guide.* 4th ed. New York: McGraw-Hill, 1978.

Hennekens, Charles H., and Brian MacMahon. "Oral Contraceptives and Myocardial Infarction," *New England Journal of Medicine,* 296: 1166, 1977.

Hirsch, Jules. "The Adipose-Cell Hypothesis," *New England Journal Medicine,* 295: 389, 1976.

Hunt, Morton. *Sexual Behavior in the 1970s.* Chicago: Playboy Press, 1974.

Imbus, Harold R. "Hearing loss: the key to successful therapy." *Consultant* (November 1975), p. 75.

Jacobson, Howard N. "Diet in Pregnancy." *New England Journal of Medicine,* 297: 1951, 1977.

Jayson, Malcolm I.V., and Allan St. J. Dixon. *Understanding Arthritis and Rheumatism.* New York: Pantheon, 1974.

Jelliffe, Derrick B., and E.F. Patrice Jelliffe. " 'Breast is Best': Modern Meanings," *New England Journal of Medicine,* 297: 912, 1977.

Jones, Howard W., Jr., and John H. Rock. "On the Reanastomosis of Fallopian Tubes after Surgical Sterilization," *Fertility and Sterility,* 29: 702, 1978.

Kannel, William B. "Hypertension is Never Benign!" *Consultant* (March 1977), p. 31.

Kaufman, Sherwin A. *From a Gynecologist's Notebook, Questions Women Ask.* New York: Stein & Day, 1974.

Kavanagh, Terence. *Heart Attack? Counterattack!* New York: Van Nostrand Reinhold, 1976.

Kempe, C. Henry, et al., *Current Pediatric Diagnosis & Treatment.* 5th ed. Los Altos, Cal.: Lange Medical Publications, 1978.

Koch, Richard, and Kathryn Jean Koch. *Understanding the Mentally Retarded Child: A New Approach.* New York: Random House, 1974.

Krupp, Marcus A., and Milton J. Chatton. *Current Medical Diagnosis and Treatment.* Los Altos, Cal.: Lange Medical Publications, 1974.

Lanson, Lucienne. *From Woman to Woman.* New York: Knopf, 1975.

Leboyer, Frederick. *Birth Without Violence.* New York: Knopf, 1975.

Leyden, James J. "Getting to the root of the dandruff problem," *Consultant* (November 1976), p. 32.

Luce, John M. "Chiropractic—Its History and Challenge to Medicine," *The Pharos* (April 1978), p. 12.

Mahoney, Maurice J. "Prenatal Diagnosis of Duchenne's Muscular Dystrophy," *New England Journal of Medicine,* 297: 968, 1977.

Malt, Ronald A., and Frederick G. Guggenheim. "Surgery for Obesity," *New England Journal of Medicine,* 295: 43, 1976.

Markovits, Andrew S. "What to Tell Your Patients about Intraocular Lenses." *Consultant* (December 1978), p. 87.

Masters, William H., and Virginia E. Johnson. *Human Sexual Response.* Boston: Little, Brown, 1966.

———. *Human Sexual Inadequacy.* Boston: Little, Brown, 1970.

May, Lawrence A. *Getting the Most Out of Your Doctor.* New York: Basic Books, 1977.

McCauley, Carole Spearin. *Pregnancy After 35.* New York: Dutton, 1976.

McDade, Joseph E. "Legionnaires' Disease: Isolation of a Bacterium and Demonstration of Its Role in Other Respiratory Disease," *New England Journal of Medicine,* 297: 1189, 1977.

McMillan, Julia A., Frank A. Oski, et al. "Iron Absorption from Human Milk, Simulated Human Milk, and Proprietary Formulas," *Pediatrics,* 60: 896, 1977.

McNamara, Joan, and Bernard McNamara. *The Special Child Handbook.* New York: Hawthorn Books, 1977.

Mennuti, Michael T. "Prenatal genetic diagnosis: Current status." *New England Journal of Medicine,* 297: 1004, 1977.

Meyers, Frederick H., et al. *Review of Medical Pharmacology.* 3rd ed. Los Altos, Cal.: Lange Medical Publications, 1972.

Miller, Benjamin F., and Lawrence Galton. *The Family Book of Preventive Medicine.* New York: Simon and Schuster, 1971.

435

Miller, Robert H., and James R. Cantrell. *Textbook of Basic Emergency Medicine.* St. Louis: C.V. Mosby, 1975.

Miller, Sigmund Stephen. *Symptoms: The Complete Home Medical Encyclopedia.* New York: Thomas Y. Crowell, 1976.

Milunsky, Aubrey. "Prenatal diagnosis of genetic disorders." *New England Journal of Medicine,* 295: 377, 1976.

——. *Know Your Genes.* Boston: Houghton Mifflin, 1977.

Moody, Paul Amos. *Genetics of Man.* New York: Norton, 1967.

Moore, Mary E., and Stephen N. Berk. "Acupuncture for Chronic Shoulder Pain," *Annals of Internal Medicine,* 84: 381, 1976.

Murdock, R., and Eva Joyce. "Home Accidents to Children under 15 Years —Survey of 910." *British Medical Journal* 3, July 13, 1974, p. 103.

Murphy, George E. "Suicide and Attempted Suicide," *Hospital Practice* (November 1977), p. 73.

Nathan, David G., and Frank A. Oski. *Hematology of Infancy and Childhood.* Philadelphia: W.B. Saunders, 1974.

911, The Emergency Telephone Number. Publication no. 2205–0003 (May 1973). Washington, D.C.: U.S. Government Printing Office.

Nirschl, Robert P. "Tennis (Elbow), Anyone?" *Consultant* (February 1974), p. 89.

Nolen, William A. "What We Now Know about Breast Cancer." *McCall's* (July 1978), p. 32.

Nyhan, William L., with Edward Edelson. *The Heredity Factor.* New York: Grosset & Dunlap, 1976.

Ong, Beale H. *Doctor's Call Hour.* New York: Wyden, 1977.

Orkin, Milton, and Howard I. Maibach. "Current Concepts in Parasitology: This Scabies Pandemic," *New England Journal of Medicine,* 298: 496, 1978.

Orlando, Joan, et al. "Effect of Ethanol on Angina Pectoris," *Annals of Internal Medicine,* 84: 652, 1976.

Pantell, Robert H., et al. *Taking Care of Your Child: A Parents' Guide to Medical Care.* Reading, Mass.: Addison-Wesley, 1977.

Paradise, Jack L., et al. "Limitation of Sore-Throat History as an Indication for Tonsillectomy," *New England Journal of Medicine,* 298: 409, 1978.

Philipp, Elliot. *Overcoming Childlessness, Its Causes and What to Do about Them.* New York: Taplinger, 1975.

Physicians' Desk Reference, 1978. 32nd ed. Oradell, N. J.: Medical Economics, 1978.

Pool, J. Lawrence. *Your Brain and Nerves.* New York: Scribner's Sons, 1973.

Public Health Service, "Breast Self-Examination." Publication no. (NIH) 76–649. Washington, D.C.: U.S. Department of Health, Education, and Welfare.

Reuben, David. *The Save Your Life Diet.* New York: Random House, 1975.

Riley, Harris D., Jr. " 'Rocky Mountain' Spotted Fever," *Hospital Practice* (April 1977), p. 51.

Rockwood, Charles A., et al. "History of Emergency Medical Services in the United States," *Journal of Trauma,* 16: 299, 1976.

Roe, Robert L. "Some Guidelines to the New Drugs for Rheumatic Diseases," *Consultant* (July 1977), p. 21.

Romney, Seymour L., et al. *Gynecology and Obstetrics: The Health Care of Women.* New York: McGraw-Hill Co., 1975.

Root, Leon, and Thomas Kiernan. *The Doctor's Guide to Tennis Elbow, Trick Knee, and Other Miseries of the Weekend Athlete.* New York: David McKay, 1974.

Rose, Louisa. *The Menopause Book.* New York: Hawthorn Books, 1977.

Rosenblatt, Ruth. "Mammography and other Procedures in Breast Cancer Diagnosis," *Consultant* (January 1978), p. 121.

Rosenfield, Allan G. "Injectable Long-acting Progestogen Contraception: A Neglected Modality," *American Journal of Obstetrics and Gynecology,* 120: 537, 1974.

Roth, Oscar, and Lawrence Galton. *Heart Attack!* Philadelphia: Lippincott, 1978.

Saarinen, Ulla M. "Need for Iron Supplementation in Infants on Prolonged Breast Feeding," *Journal of Pediatrics,* 93: 177, 1978.

Sack, David A., et al. "Prophylactic Doxycycline for Travelers' Diarrhea," *New England Journal of Medicine,* 298: 758, 1978.

Sauer, Gordon C. *Manual of Skin Diseases.* 3rd ed. Philadelphia: Lippincott, 1973.

Schein, Clarence J. *A Surgeon Answers.* New York: G.P. Putnam's Sons, 1973.

Seaman, Barbara, and Gideon Seaman. *Women and the Crisis in Sex Hormones.* New York: Rawson Associates Publishers, 1977.

Shafer, Nathaniel. "The Meaning of Tremors," *Consultant* (August 1976), p. 68.

Shapiro, Howard I. *The Birth Control Book.* New York: St. Martin's Press, 1977.

Shaw, Charles R., and A. Clark Griffin. *When You Need Help with Cancer.* New York: William Morrow, 1973.

Silber, Sherman. "Microscopic Vasectomy Reversal," *Fertility and Sterility,* 28: 1191, 1977.

Silverio, John, and Anna M. Sesso. "Accidental Childhood Poisoning in Pennsylvania," *Journal of School Health,* 44: 514, 1974.

Smith, David W. *Recognizable Patterns of Human Malformation.* Philadelphia: W.B. Saunders, 1970.

Smith, David W., and Ann Asper Wilson. *The Child with Down's Syndrome (Mongolism).* Philadelphia: W.B. Saunders, 1973.

Smith, Donald R. *General Urology.* Los Altos, Cal.: Lange Medical Publications, 1975.

Snyder, Solomon H. *The Troubled Mind: A Guide to Release from Distress.* New York: McGraw-Hill, 1976.

Speroff, Leon. "Which Birth Control Pill Should Be Prescribed?" *Fertility and Sterility,* 27: 997, 1976.

Stedman's Medical Dictionary. 23rd ed. Baltimore: Williams & Wilkins, 1976.

Sweet, Richard D., and Fletcher H. McDowell. "Five years' Treatment of Parkinson's Disease with Levodopa," *Annals of Internal Medicine,* 83: 456, 1975.

Tatum, Howard J. "Clinical Aspects of Intrauterine Contraception: Circumspection 1976," *Fertility and Sterility,* 28: 3, 1977.

Taussig, Helen B. " 'Death' from Lightning—and the Possibility of Living Again," *Annals of Internal Medicine,* 68: 1345, 1968.

Testa, N. Noel. "Surgery for Arthritis: What Can—and Cannot—Be Done," *Consultant* (November 1978), p. 142.

The Canadian Cooperative Study Group. "A Randomized Trial of Aspirin and Sulfinpyrazone in Threatened Stroke," *New England Journal of Medicine,* 299: 53, 1978.

Thomson, David L., and Boy Frame. "Involutional Osteopenia: Current Concepts," *Annals of Internal Medicine,* 85: 789, 1976.

Toft, Anthony D., "Thyroid Function after Surgical Treatment of Thyrotoxicosis," *New England Journal of Medicine,* 298: 643, 1978.

Wertz, Richard W., and Dorothy C. Wertz. *Lying-In: A History of Childbirth in America.* New York: Free Press, 1977.

Whelan, Elizabeth. *Preventing Cancer: What You Can Do to Cut Your Risks by Up to 50 Percent.* New York: Norton, 1977.

Williams, Robert H. (ed.). 3rd ed. *Textbook of Endocrinology.* Philadelphia: W.B. Saunders, 1962.

Zinn, Walter J., and Herbert Solomon. *The Complete Guide to Eye Care, Eyeglasses and Contact Lenses.* New York: Frederick Fell, 1977.

Zizmor, Jonathan, and John Foreman. "The Fine Art of Looking Years Younger." *Woman's Day* (April 1976), p.22.

———. "An End to Needless Fears," *Woman's Day* (July 1976), p.22.

Index